THE ART OF PSYCHOTHERAPY
AND THE LIBERATION
OF THE THERAPIST

THE ART OF PSYCHOTHERAPY AND THE LIBERATION OF THE THERAPIST

Dr. Len Bergantino, Ed.D., Ph.D.

InfusedMedia Co. LLC
www.infusedmedia.co
1-888-251-6088

DR. LEN BERGANTINO, ED. D. (USC), A.B.P.P. (Diplomate)
POLITICAL PSYCHOLOGY CONSULTANT

CALL (424) 293-9511
(7 RINGS)

BOOK COVER PICTURE

PATRICK HENRY –AMERICAN REVOLUTIONARY WAR HERO

WAS NOTED FOR HIS FAMOUS QUOTE "GIVE ME LIBERTY OR GIVE ME DEATH."

When I thought about a picture for the cover of a book entitled the art of psychotherapy and the liveration of the therapist, I realized that the sina quo non of actually doing the work requires Patrick Henry's quote "Give Me Liberty or Give Me Death" on the part of both the psychotherapist and the patient and both need to be free to preserve, both internal and external freedom to pursue his or her own BEING WITHOUT FEAR OF REPRISALS FROM LICENSING BOARDS THAT PROVIDE AN ILLU SION OF PATIENT SAFET WHILE ACTUALLY PROVIDING A SPIRIT OF FEAR AND DEATH FROM THE TOP DOWN!

Thus, patients and therapists need to keep in mind always "NBNBC!" "NO BALLS NO BLUE CHIPS!" (MEANT AS A GENDER NEUTRAL COMMENT) AS THE STAKES INVOLVE TURNING THE TRAGIC CORNER IN YOUR LIFE AND WITHOUT THAT COMMITMENT NEITHER PATIENT NOR THERAPIST CAN REALLY EXPECT VERY MUCH OF ANYTHING!

Keeping the above in mind,

ENJOY THIS BOOK,

The Reverend Dr. Len Bergantino

THE REVEREND DR. LEN BERGANTINO, ED.D., PH.D., ABPP

1215 Brockton Avenue, Suite 104, Los Angeles, California 90025

Contents

A Review..xliii
Foreword..lxiii
Preface..lxv
Acknowledgments...lxix
Prologue..lxxi

PART ONE

The Foundations of Personal Style: Introduction

1   The Existential Moment.. 13
      The Existential Moment 14
      Working With Children 19
      Self-Disclosure..22

2   From Theory to Style: Developing an Existential Point of
    View with William Ofman, Ph.D... 41
      Resistance And The Facilitation Of Process Awareness 53
      Stretching The Boundaries.. 58
        Bill and I–An Experience With My Therapist........................ 60
        Alyson 67

3   The Liberation of the Therapist.. 77
      A Holistic Approach To Psychotherapy/Hypnosis 105
      Physical Illness And Psychotherapy 106
      Working with Psychological Ramifications of
      Physical Symptoms 106
      Exercise And Fun.. 109

PART TWO
The Impact of Existential Moments

4   Psychoanalysis and the Existential Moment 125
      Was Freud An Existentialist? 125
            My Reaction to Bion: A Clear Mind and a State of Discovery ... 134
            An Analysand's Experience with Bion, with
                  Richard Edelman, M.D. 145
            A Practitioner of Dr. Heinz Kohut's Methods
                  Comments On Bion, with Lars Lofgren, M.D. 148
            Bion's Legacy: The Language of Achievement, I,
                  with James S. Grotstein, M.D. 148
            Bion's Legacy: The Language of Achievement, II,
                  with Michael Paul, M.D. 156
            Bion's Legacy: The Language of Achievement, III,
                  with Stephen E. Salenger, M.D. 161
            Bion: Impact and the Supervision of the Practical
                  Analysis of Being There, with Wilfred R. Bion,
                  M.R.C.S. and Stephen E. Salenger, M.D. 167
            Patient Threatening Suicide 185
      A Tavistock Group Experience, With Lars Lofgren, M.d.,
            And Marion Solomon, Ph.d. 188
      Analytic Group Therapy–An Approach To Narcissism,
            With Martin Grotjahn, M.d. 201

5   Transactional Analysis and Existentialism with Bob
      Goulding, M.D. and Mary Goulding, M.S.W. 223
            Case Of Joan 237
            Ta Marital Therapy With Bob And Mary 244

6   Gestalt Therapy and the Existential Moment 257
      Stylistic Focus On "Thou Vs. I," With Miriam Polster, Ph.d.,
            Erving Polster, Ph.d., And Jim Simkin, Ph.d. 258
      Impact: The Key To Responsible Action With Couples,
            With Dr. Walter Kempler, M.d. 292
            Walt, My wife at the time, and Me 300
            My Work With a Couple 302
      Creative Expression And Sensory Perception, With Bob
            Martin, D.s.w. 305

7   The Somatic Therapy of Stanley Keleman 321

8   Behavior Modification: Cognitive-Emotive Therapy 337
     The Reinforcement Of Existential Moments, With George
          Bach, Ph.d. 337
          Structuring Situations to Create Movement 342
          Post-Marathon Experience 349
          Two Group Sessions after the Marathon 350
     Rational-Emotive Therapy With Albert Ellis, Ph.d. 353
          Summary 367
     Direct Decision Therapy And The Rebellious Patient, With
          Harold Greenwald, Ph.d. 367

9   Clinical Hypnosis 383
     An Experience Of The Hypnotherapy Of Milton H.
          Erickson, M.d. 383
          Distracting the Conscious Mind 385
          Changing Belief Systems 388
          Getting to the Heart of the Matter 393
          Touching Their Souls 394
          Therapy Is Just a Part of Life 395
          No Wasted Energy 396
          The Essence of the Work 397
          What Therapists Need to Know and Practice 398
     Commentary On My Work With Dr. Erickson 399
     Milton H. Erickson, M.d. 400
     Existential Moments In Clinical Hypnosis 417
     Clinical Hypnosis, With William S. Kroger, M.d. 422
          *The Impact of Automatic Writing: Breakthroughs
               into Existential Moments* 427
          Case of Jerry–Sex, Guilt 430
          Case of Joe–Obsessive, Depressive, No Fun! 431

10   Direct Confrontation: The Treatment of Schizophrenia,
     with Jack Rosberg, M.A. 437
          Introduction 437
          Direct Confrontation: The Treatment of Schizophrenia 440
          Session Two 453
          Summary 457

11   The Godfather of Clinical Psychology 461

12   The Therapist Is Alive and Well: The Existential-
Experiential Therapy Style of Carl Whitaker, M.D. 491
        Mock Family Interview 499
        Actual Interview 500

Epilogue 511

BOOKS THAT ARE EITHER PUBLISHED OR WILL BE PUBLISHED AUTHORED BY THE REVEREND DR. LEN BERGANTINO AS THESE BOOKS WERE WRITTEN AS THE THING-IN-ITSELF AND WERE DIVINELY INSPIRED BY THE HOLY SPIRIT TO AT THE VERY LEAST GIVE MEN AND WOMEN AS OPPORTUNITY TO BE MORE FULLY THEMSELVES AND MORE IN TOUCH WITH THEIR OWN NATURE.

IT IS STRONGLY RECOMMENDED THAT THE READERS DEVELOP THEIR LEVEL OF ATTENTION TO READ ALL FOUR BOOKS AND PERMIT THEM TO BECOME PART AND PARCEL OF HOW EACH INDIVIDUAL ANSWERS THE QUESTION "TO BE OR NOT TO BE." AS THE REVEREND DR. LEN BERGANTINO IS SEVENTY FIVE YEARS OLD, HE WILL NOT BE AROUND PERSONALLY TO DO PSYCHOANALYSIS OR PSYCHOTHERAPY WITH YOU THEREFORE THESE BOOKS WERE WRITTEN ON THE BASIS OF THEM BEING AROUND FOR AT LEAST TWO HUNDRED YEARS!!!

1. I AM FREUD! PSYCHOANALYSIS IS THE ONLY METHOD OF CURE: IT'S TOO BAD NO ONE KNOWS HOW TO DO ONE, XLIBRIS PUB. CO., 2019. 502 PP.
2. REVERSE ANALYSIS, THE EXISTENTIAL SHIFT, GESTALT FAMILY THERAPY AND THE PREVENTION OF THE HOLOCAUST, XLIBRIS PUB. CO.,
3. THE ART OF PSYCHOTHERAPY AND THE LIBERATION OF THE THERAPIST XLIBRIS PUBLISHING COMPANY.
4. THE ESSENCE OF MUSIC, XLIBRIS PUBLISHING COMPANY.

This is a book for all time. As I had extrasensory perception to help me find out things on a primitive level and depth with an ability to pick up spin-off, severe psychological projective identifications moment to moment in an era when psychologists were only permitted to be research psychoanalysts by the American Psychoanalytic Association (but rightly controlled where that research was going that in many ways nullified it as true psychoanalytic research), I present to you a book that might at that time have been considered wild psychoanalysis. And I will show you how extrasensory perception can be developed and utilized by the therapeutic use of self within the psychoanalytic frame in ways that can enhance the treatment of borderline, narcissistic, obsessive-compulsive, and schizophrenic disorders and other diagnoses, as well as help pinpoint psychophysiological awareness, which through the repetition compulsion, can prevent disease and will circumvent disease in later life. This kind of psychoanalysis will go a long way in preventing the next holocaust!

Dr. Bergantino and his two children were sent back on a karmic mission to complete the work. Dr. Bergantino is the reincarnated soul of Sigmund Freud and Julius Caesar. Those skill sets were required to complete this project. His children are Wilfred Bion and Milton Erickson. They taught Dr. Bergantino how to use paranormal abilities. We are all off the karmic wheel and WE WILL NOT BE BACK!!! GOODBYE!!

Xlibris

TO PURCHASE THIS 502 pp. BOOK GO TO www. Xlibris . com and type in either the title of the book or. Dr. Len Bergantino, or contact barnes and noble.com or amazon.com

I AM FREUD!

Psychoanalysis Is the Only Method of Cure: It's Too Bad No One Knows How to Do One!!!

Justice is the balancing of Karmic law-natural law-civil law

DR. LEN BERGANTINO, ED.D., PH.D.

"FOR IMMEDIATE RELEASE"

EDITORS: For review copies or interview requests, contact:
Marketing Services
Tel: 888-795-4274
Fax: 912-***-4079
Email: MarketingServices@xlibris.com
(When requesting a review copy, please provide a street address.)

Xlibris

I DARED TO DISTURB THE UNIVERSE!!!

Dr. Len Bergantino Ed. D., Ph.D., releases 'I AM Freud! Psychoanalysis is the Only Method of Cure: It's Too Bad No One Knows How to Do One!!!'

BEVERLY HILLS, Calif. – Dr. Len Bergantino, Ed.D., Ph.D., is the reincarnated soul of Sigmund Freud and Julius Caesar and his children Lisa Francesca is the reincarnated soul of the great British psychoanalyst Wilfred R. Bion and Cleopatra while his developmentally delayed son Alexander Leonardo is the reincarnated soul of Milton H. Erickson, M.D. (known as the father of Modern Medical Hypnosis and for Uncommon Therapy) and Decimus Brutus. All of these skill sets were necessary in the writing of "I Am Freud! Psychoanalysis is the Only Method of Cure: It's Too Bad No One Knows How to Do One!!!" (published by Xlibris) and the issues it is meant to deal with at both conscious and unconscious levels.

Further, Bergantino in 1992, made a direct contact with God to have Bion and Erickson sent back as the reincarnated souls of his children to teach him what to do with the paranormal gifts that were given to him and unleashed by Erickson. Through this development, he, with God's tutelage became the best psychoanalyst that ever lived and began to implement Freud's plan that both psychoanalysis and subsequently developed psychotherapies would create the kind of patients who would and could then go out and create an upward spiraling society.

Wilhelm Reich, M.D. – Freud's most gifted training analyst said "If you can't do politics, you can't do analysis!" The book shows how to develop extrasensory perception so that analysts and therapists have an opportunity to develop the tools necessary to do the jobs at hand if they are so inclined. In this way, people will not pay for a three day a week, seven year analysis and come out as crazy as the day they began with few if any tools to carry on the work. "When I did an analysis with the crème de la crème of society, they customarily tripled their income and the quality of their life! (Don't waste $50,000 per year or $350,000 per analysis)."

The book is not based on anything Bergantino may or may not believe. It is based on his attaining a level of "pure being" that Jean Paul Sartre wrote about as the thing-in-itself. And it is at that level that this book was written as the thing-in-itself to effect change in the reader.

"I Am Freud! Psychoanalysis is the Only Method of Cure: It's Too Bad No One Knows How to Do One!!!"
By Dr. Len Bergantino, Ed.D., Ph.D.
Hardcover | 6 x 9in | 504 pages | ISBN 9781984557368
Softcover | 6 x 9in | 504 pages | ISBN 9781984557252
E-Book | 504 pages | ISBN 9781984557269
Available at www.amazon.com and www.barnesandnoble.com

About the Author
Dr. Len Bergantino, Ed.D., Ph.D. practiced psychoanalysis in Beverly Hills, California from 1979-1991. He saw seven patients five days a week for between five and seven years totaling 49 hours a week and saw an occasional family therapy or clinical hypnosis case totaling 51 hours a week at $125 per hour; $6125 per week; $240,000 per year. In addition, he trained psychiatrists and clinical psychologists at the international level delivering on his workshop premise "The Therapeutic Wizardry of Dr. Len Bergantino" at Wentworth Castle in Sheffield, England and treating the British at the Royal College of Medicine in London in "Developing the Use of Extrasensory Perception in the Practice of Psychoanalysis, Psychotherapy and Clinical Hypnosis." In Brisbane, Australia, his work was described as "a kind of mental precision" that electrified the Australian Therapeutic Community and had lasting therapeutic impact. Furthermore, he was an affiliate of the Italian American Lawyers Association for seven years. He became an expert witness in both severe parental Alienation Syndrome in criminal cases. He was the only clinician to give bargain a man for release who was on death row. He was President of the Southern California Society of Clinical Hypnosis when they were composed of exclusively MD's, PHD's and DDS'. The year he was president he turned it into a psychoanalytic institute.

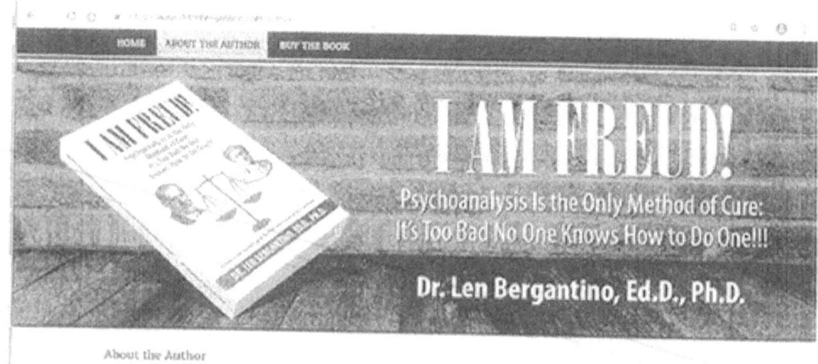

About the Author

Dr. Len Bergantino, Ed.D., Ph.D.

The Author Dr. Len Bergantino was trained in psychoanalysis attending the passionate and ordinary methods of training by Dr. Wilfred R. Bion, M.D., Medical Board College of Virginia. Many of Bion's M.D. Associates in Beverly Hills, CA, Dr. Martin Grotjahn, M.D. and Dr. Ernst Federn, Ph.D. who were in Freud's original training group. They were all Training Analysts. Dr. Michael Paul M.D. as one of the two best of Bion's Training Analysts.

REVERSE ANALYSIS, THE EXISTENTIAL SHIFT, GESTALT FAMILY THERAPY AND THE PREVENTION OF THE NEXT HOLOCAUST

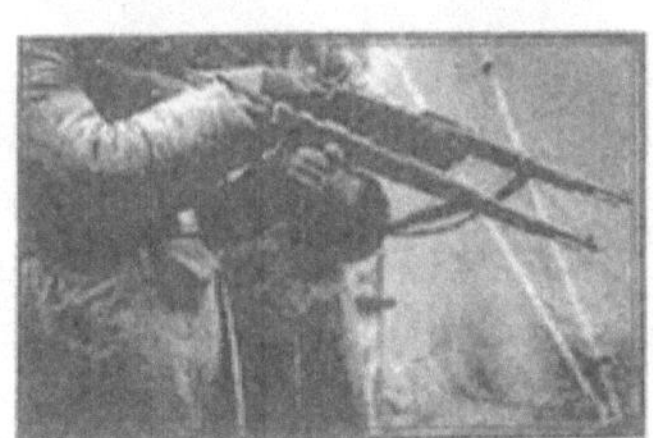

Xlibris

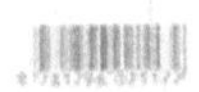

FOR IMMEDIATE RELEASE

EDITORS: For review copies or interview requests, contact:
Marketing Services
Tel: 888-795-4274
Fax: 812-355-4079
Email: MarketingServices@xlibris.com
(When requesting a review copy, please provide a street address.)

Dr. Len Bergantino, Ed.D, Ph.D., addresses societal issues in new book

'Reverse Analysis, the Existential Shift, Gestalt Family Therapy and the Prevention of the Next Holocaust' released

LOS ANGELES – Through the Holy Spirit, his direct contact with God and his karmic mission, Dr. Len Bergantino, Ed.D., Ph.D., addresses the problem of the today's downward spiraling society in his latest book "Reverse Analysis, the Existential Shift, Gestalt Family Therapy and the Prevention of the Next Holocaust" (published by Xlibris).

This book creates a subliminal methodology that will help to prevent the next holocaust and perhaps deter the apocalypse and the end of days. As such, the book expands and enriches the community standards of practice of Psychoanalysis, psychiatry, clinical psychology, politics, political intervention and a reconciliation of religion with the state, as opposed to a separation of church and state that has left its people a soulless and emotionally bankrupt nation with a downward spiraling society. This book throws the United States government and its citizens into an international jam of family therapy as evoked at the meticulous and primitive levels required to effect and affect societal change, to render a redirection to an upward spiraling society providing the kind of leadership for Americans to create well-being and prosperity for all.

"[The book] is the common man's best shot to turn the tragic corner in his or her life: make dysfunctional families functional, save one's soul, become thoughtful members of society who do the right thing more often than not," Bergantino says. "This book also trains therapists how to do one session existential shifts thereby creating therapies for the common man that are more affordable than a seven year psychoanalysis where the patient is seen five days a week. In other words, it makes the currently impossible possible!"

At its core, the book aims to remind readers to "Open up the space and keep it open so Man will not destroy himself via the illusion of safety and will learn to experientially tolerate the anxiety and chaos of not knowing."

"Reverse Analysis, the Existential Shift, Gestalt Family Therapy and the Prevention of the Next Holocaust"
By Dr. Len Bergantino, Ed.D., Ph.D.
Hardcover | 6 x 9in | 244 pages | ISBN 9781546021186
Softcover | 6 x 9in | 244 pages | ISBN 9781546021179
E-Book | 244 pages | ISBN 9781546021565
Available at Amazon and Barnes & Noble

About the Author

Dr. Len Bergantino, Ed.D., Ph.D., has written THE HOLY BIBLE Of Psychoanalysis, psychotherapy, political psychology and music-books, I-IV!! The books are the thing-in-itself and all four books must be read to make the necessary personal and societal impact!! He was trained by Milton Erickson, M.D., Carl Whitaker, M.D., Wilfred Bion, M.R.C.P., Walter Kempler, M.D., George Bach, Ph.D., Bruno Bettelheim, Ph.D., Jim Simkin, Ph.D., and Erv Polster, Ph.D., they had the most lasting impact along with the Holy Spirit. Bergantino is the author of "The Essence of Music," "The Art of Psychotherapy and the Liberation of the Therapist," "I Am Freud! Psychoanalysis is the Only Method of Cure: It's Too Bad No One Knows How to Do One!!!," "Reverse Analysis, the Existential Shift, Gestalt Family Therapy and the Prevention of the Next Holocaust," "Psychotherapy, Insight, and Style: The Existential Moment", and "Making an Impact in Therapy: How Master Clinicians Intervene."

###

Xlibris

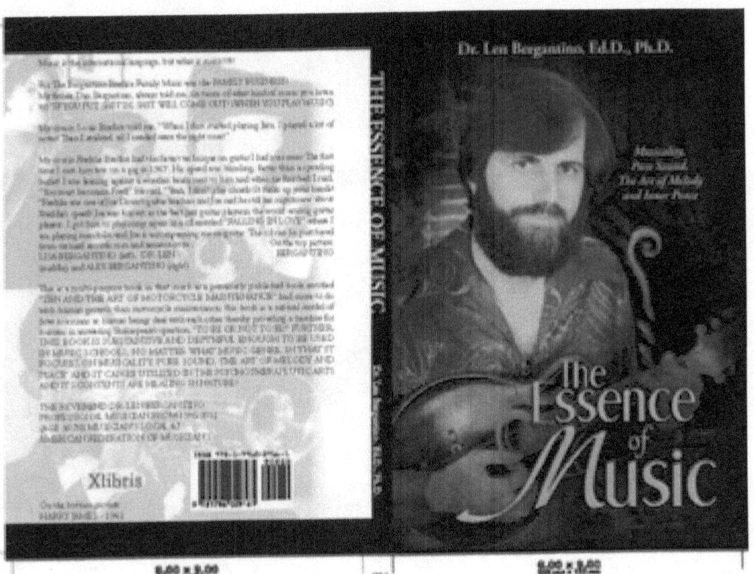

Dr. Len Bergantino, Ed.D., Ph.D.
Musicality,
Pure Sound,
The Art of Melody
and Inner Peace
The Essence of Music
THE ESSENCE OF MUSIC
Xlibris

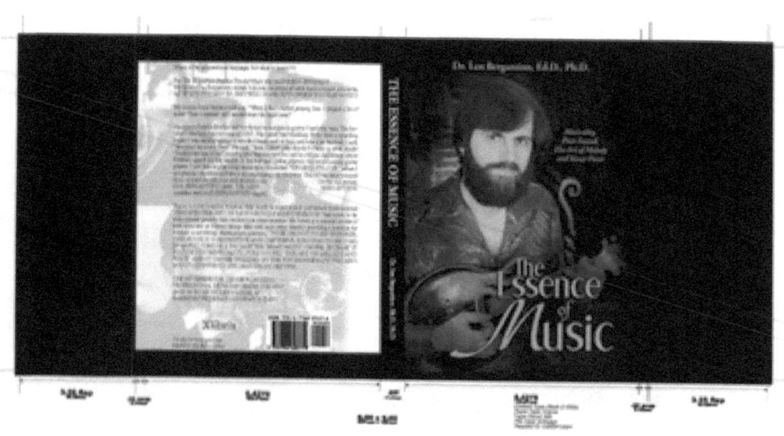
Dr. Ken Bergstrom, Ed.D., Ph.D.
THE ESSENCE OF MUSIC
The Essence of Music
Xlibris

This is a book for professional psychotherapists, psychoanalysts, and counselors, students in those areas of specialty, and lay persons who are interested in the essence of effective therapy and how some of the people who do it best practice their art. For professionals, the book presents a personal way of viewing therapy that can add pleasurable options. Each of the therapists with whom I worked, and myself, all had a feeling of enjoyment that we hope will carry over to the office and practices of the readers. For students of therapy, the book offers a search for a professional stance and working posture that may be of value in the development of each student's unique personal style. For lay persons, the book speaks of therapy that can make an impact and speaks of how some of the most potent therapists practice. For Psychoanalysts interested in the work of the Great British Psychoanalyst, Dr. Wilfred R. Bion MRCS (Medical Royal College of Surgeons). This is the only book that demonstrates exactly what he did.

I wrote the book with the intention of letting it be both an experience and an explanation. I have presented it according to my developmental needs while maturing personally and professionally. This was done so the book might be informative at the conscious level, entertaining at the child level, and persuasive at the unconscious level.

The existential moment is the thread that ties the book together; it is a moment of therapeutic potency. While all moments are existential by definition, there are certain moments that are more powerful in helping patients live happier and healthier lives. Positive results, whether they be from one session or over the long haul, are partially, if not fully, a result of existential moments.

Xlibris

ISBN 978-1-7541-9680-1

The Art of Psychotherapy And the Liberation of the Therapist

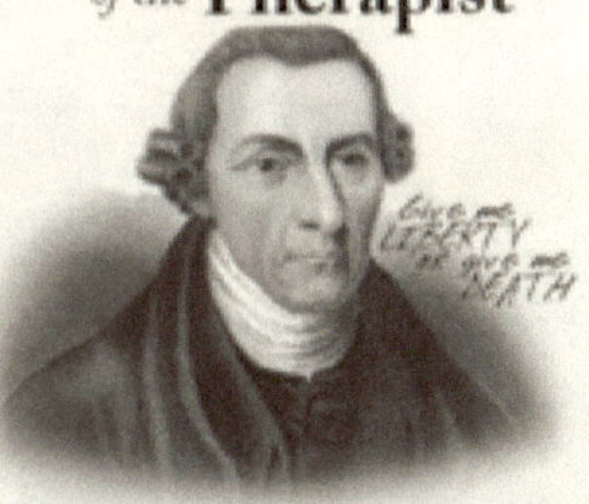

Much has been written about the Science of Psychotherapy, but it has remained for Dr. Bergantino to write about the Art of Psychotherapy with such elegant impact.

Dr. Len Bergantino, Ed. D., Ph. D.

The Art of
Psychotherapy
And the Liberation
of the Therapist

Dr. Len Bergantino, Ed.D., Ph.D.

Veterans Administration

1 July 1985   In Reply Refer To:

Len Bergantino, Ed.D., Ph.D.
10266 Kilrenney Avenue
Los Angeles, California 90064

Dear Len:

How nice to receive yours of June 24th, and to learn of your upward spiral! I'm very pleased indeed to believe that my little review of your book has contributed to your success!

Frankly, Len, I have long been eructatively fed up with the sort of territorial cupidities and other evidences of narcissistic nonsensicality so many of the colleagues display. Such antics reveal the essentially limbic nature of people as it comes to be expressed in envies and jealousies to which you allude in your letter. When I read your book I knew at once of your outsider-ism (cf. Colin Wilson's seminal book of the same name—The Outsider) as well as your talent; since I know I am good also, I do not need to do the Big-Daddy-in-Cat-On-A-Hot-Tin-Roof bit, viz., to shit on one's sons out of envy and fear that they will appropriate my penis-cum-wife-cum-everything-else!

I trust your family are in good health. Keep in touch.

Most sincerely,

Donald B. Rinsley, M.D., F.R.S.E. (Lond.)
Associate Chief for Education
Psychiatry Service

Clinical Professor of Psychiatry
University of Kansas School of Medicine
Kansas City

DBR:mtf

FOREWORD TO THE ART OF PSYCHOTHERAPY
AND THE LIBERATION OF THE THERAPIST

The field of psychotherapy had a space that was open during my professional lifetime, whereas psychotherapy was not curative per se, I both observed and experienced many psychotherapeutic interventions at the hands of many world renown psychiatrists and clinical psychologists that had a lifetime impact upon the patient population.

The patients were just as courageous as the psychotherapists. This is no longer the case as Boards of Psychology and other punitive boards have so frightened these gifted treaters that the courageous psychotherapists and patients who worked together on a tightrope without a net no longer exist in 2018. So today we have careful psychotherapists who do not have the courage to take risks to develop the therapeutic use of self to the degree that they can break new ground; we have patients who file complaints to Boards of Psychology over the least little thing; and we have Boards of Psychology racking up their share of professional kills. ALL THIS KEEPS THE FIELD OF PSYCHOTHERAPY FROM ADVANCING TO THE POINT WHERE IT CAN MEET SOME OF THE NEW CHALLENGES OF THE TIMES AND WE HAVE RESULTS SUCH AS 122 VETERANS A DAY COMMITTING SUICIDE WITHOUT A PSYCHOTHERAPEUTIC TREATMENT BEING TAILORED TO THEIR INDIVIDUAL NEEDS!

Boards of Psychology and similar Boards must be done away with if this destructive trend is to be reversed and an era of sweetness and light opened up again.

For the small gain of punishing therapists who have sex with patients they have destroyed the entire field as a potentially curative factor. Both psychotherapists and patients have to have an environment provided by psychotherapists where both feel an inner freedom to take risks and maintain courage throughout the work. Both patients and therapists need to maintain A LIFE FORCE THROUGHOUT THE TREATMENT OTHERWISE THANATOS OR DEATH FORCE PERMEATES THE TREATMENT AND WE ARE MORE LIKELY TO TURN OUT ZOMBIES THAN INCREASINGLY ALIVE PERSONS!

THIS BOOK SHOULD HAVE A SHELF LIFE OF AT LEAST A COUPLE OF HUNDRED YEARS IN THAT THE DEVOTION TO THE DEVELOPMENT TO THE THERAPEUTIC USE OF SELF AND THE TRAINING SOUGHT OUT WITH NEARLY ALL THE MASTER THERAPISTS OF THE TIME IS AND IS MOST LIKELY TO REMAIN UNPARRALLELED!

Furthur, graduate school professors need to develop their own therapeutic use of self from wherever they are starting and use this book with their graduate students in psychotherapy and counseling EVEN THOUGH THEY ARE FRIGHTENED THAT THEY CAN'T DO IT! ROME WASN'T BUILT IN A DAY! WHEREVER YOU START IS ALRIGHT, AS LONG AS YOU START! IT IS ONLY IN THIS MANNER THAT BOARDS OF PSYCHOLOGY WILL STOP PRESENTING THE ILLUSION OF SAFETY WHILE IN FACT KILLING THE LIFE FORCE IN BOTH THERAPISTS AND PATIENTS!

While evidenced based psychotherapy sounds good; it sounds as if evidenced based psychotherapy and mental health actually provides results while in fact evidenced based psychotherapy takes the life force out of psychotherapy and patients, and plays to the <u>mediocre</u>.

Of all that was written about my book "Psychotherapy, Insight and Style: The Existential Moment', Allyn & Bacon, Inc., Boston, Dr. Harold Greenwald, Ph.D., Diplomate in Clinical Psychology of The American Board of Professional Psychology, wrote of me in 1981 "While much has been written about the science of psychotherapy, It has remained for Dr. Bergantino to write about the art of psychotherapy with such elegant impact."

As the times demand a switch of emphasis IF WE ARE TO ADVANCE THE FIELD AND GET IT OUT OF THE DOLDRUMS OF MEDIOCRITY, THAT WE FOCUS ON THE ART OF PSYCHOTHERAPY AND WHAT CARL WHITAKER, M.D. WROTE ABOUT ME IN THE ORIGINAL FOREWORD TO MY BOOK in 1981 - THE LIBERATION OF THE THERAPIST!!! THIS BOOK FOCUSES ON WHITAKER'S LETTER TO ME IN 1981 WHEREBY HE STATED THE WAY TO TURN OUT COMPETENT THERAPISTS IS TO TRAIN THEM WHEREBY THEY HAVE TO WORK ON THEMSELVES WHICH IS THE DEVELOPMENT OF THE THERAPEUTIC USE OF SELF!!!

written by
The Reverend Dr. Len Bergantino
The Pope - Vatican West

P.S. The chapter on Wilfred Bion and the practice of Psychoanalysis will remain throughout time a tremendous preface to both Bion's work and my new book "I AM FREUD! PSYCHOANALYSIS IS THE ONLY METHOD OF CURE: IT'S TOO BAD NO ONE KNOWS HOW TO DO ONE!!!

This chapter is of value in that it has the only tape supervision of Bion with a young Analysand so you actually get to experience why Bion was so different. Furthur, it has a list of all the books he has written and the order they should be read. THIS BOOK IS A MUST READ FOR THOSE REASONS ALONE! Then there is the review by Donald B. Rinsley, M.D., Fellow, American College of Psychoanalysts who wrote a review in Bulletin of the Menninger Clinic, Vol. 47, No. 5, September, 1983 pinpointing that I had a "healing capacity" and that this book conveyed healing methodology and the book was to be "thought about, mulled over and placed on one's bedside table if not under one's pillow. It is a book that the experienced clinician will read with knowledgeable satisfaction and that the nascent therapist will read with excitement. And both will profit from what it has to tell."

WHAT IS DR. LEN BERGANTINO DOING NOW?

I am willing to do gestalt family therapy as I define it; as well as a kind of storytelling with individuals that Margaret Mead told Milton Erickson, M.D. she had only heard in a rare African tribe relatively free of disease.

I am willing to do this work with whatever difficult medical symptomatology is thrown at me, from an experimental point of view agreed upon by both me and the patient. The Board of Psychology and Medical Board came after me about 7 times AND I WHIPPED THEIR ASS EACH TIME! THE PROBLEM IS I WAS NOT FREE TO DO THE WORK! SO I SET UP THREE BOARDS OF PSYCHOLOGY AND GOT RID OF ALL OF THEM AND AS I have them on my turf plan to kick the living shit out of them for as long as I live.! Essentially, they have destroyed a lifetime's body of work and saw to it that I was not free enough to do what I am willing to do at 75 years old. In other words they are the kind of stupid bastards that would throw away a cure for cancer if it did not already exist within the MEDIOCRE COMMUNITY STANDARDS OF PRACTICE!

Furthur, my last supervisor, Dr. Bruno Bettelheim, who was trained in Freud's original training group stated that Wilhelm Reich was Freud's most gifted Training Analyst. Reich said he stopped doing Analysis because he could not cure "hatred"; that it was a matter best left to philosophers and theologians.

Experientially I found this to be true, and I am a Minister (No. 12, 656). Furthur, I have a direct connection to God and The Pope does not. In other words, as it turns out I am currently able to call more authentic shots than the Pope in matters of "faith and morals" which is the Pope's strong suit in that The Pope is stated to be "infallible" in matters of "faith and morals." I do not want to start a Church; only make political interventions where the spirit of The Holy Ghost instructs me to do so and TAKE THE DEGREES OF FREEDOM NECESSARY TO LIBERATE MYSELF FROM ANY MAN MADE CONSTRAINTS THAT WOULD IMPEDE MY DEVELOPMENT OF THERAPEUTIC USE OF SELF THROUGHOUT THE ENTIRE COURSE OF MY LIFE WHEREBY I CAN HELP PEOPLE TURN THE TRAGIC CORNER IN THEIR LIVES AND SAVE THEIR SOUL. THERE ARE ONLY ABOUT TWELVE PERSONS THAT SAVE THEIR SOUL OUT OF EVERY 100,000, 000! Twelve out of every 100 million as stated in the Bible. Thus, the purpose of psychotherapy must not only be able to function better temporarily in the world but also to save one's soul by gaining some tools upon which to approach the matter.

Furthur, I want to experiment doing gestalt family therapy by being a live in for a week at a fee of $2500. The way I have set this up I am free to explore what is possible! I therefore refer to myself a "THE POPE-VATICAN WEST", AND I OFFER THE POPE ANY OPPORTUNITY TO SEE IF I CAN BACK UP WHAT I HAVE STATED TO BE TRUE!

THE REVEREND DR. LEN BERGANTINO

TEACHERS UNION PRESIDENTS &
NEWSPAPERS "PUBLISHER PERISH!!!"

IN EVERY CITY ON A STATE!!! (Circulate!

<u>Circulate!</u>

February 16, 2018

President Trump, Senators, Congresspersons & Romans,

1. DID YOU HEAR THE MOTHER OF ONE OF THE DEAD CHILDREN IN FLORIDA YELLING "PRESIDENT TRUMP YOU CAN DO SOMETHING!!!" "YOUR HEART GOES OUT TO PARENTS OF DECEASED CHILDREN" IS INADEQUATE!!!
2. ARE NRA SUPPORTERS AND MEMBERS GOING TO VOLUNTEER TO TEACH ELEMENTARY, MIDDLE AND HIGH SCHOOL WHEN TEACHERS UNIONS STRIKE BECAUSE OF UNSAFE WORKING CONDITIONS? (NATIONAL LEVEL)
3. WHAT ARE PARENTS GOING TO DO WHEN STUDENTS REFUSE TO GO TO SCHOOL UNDER ANY CONDITIONS FOR REASONABLE FEAR OF DEATH?
4. THERE HAVE BEEN EIGHTEEN SCHOOL SHOOTINGS SINCE JANUARY 1, 2018!!! ENOUGH IS ENOUGH!!! GET THE GUNS OFF THE STREETS!!!
5. DO NOT USE MENTAL HEALTH AS A SCAPEGOAT!!!

EXISTENTIALLY SPEAKING "A CRAZY BASTARD IS A CRAZY BASTARD IS A CRAZY BASTARD!!!" AND MENTAL HEALTH HAS ALL THEY CAN DO TO DEAL WITH NORMAL NEUROTICS. MURDERERS DON'T CHANGE! THAT IS WHY PRISONS DON'T LET THEM OUT!

SUBMITTED FOR PUBLICATION,

DR. LEN BERGANTINO
PRELIMINARY ADMINISTRATIVE CREDENTIAL

UNIVERSITY OF SOUTHERN CALIFORNIA -1994
FORMER MEMBER - WTA - WATERBURY TEACHERS ASSOCIATION
CIA-CALIFORNIA TEACHERS ASSOCIATION
REFERENCE: THE BALANCE BETWEEN "CONCORD AND LIBERTY"
ORTEGA Y GASSETT - 1534

At.: Assignment Denk

January 4, 2018

<table>
<tr><td>

President Donald Trump &
Family
The White House
1600 Pennsylvania
Avenue N.W.
Washington, D.C.

</td><td>

TO BE OR NOT TO BE!.
IT DOES NOT MATTER
WHAT TRUMP DOES! ONLY
THAT HE IS THERE! FOR
THE STOCK MARKET TO
CONTINUE TO SOAR TO NEW
HEIGHTS

</td></tr>
</table>

Dear President Trump,

When I tell stories I go to my unconscious mind to see what occurs for the persons involved and the situation.

I remember when Mohammed Ali flunked the Army IQ test around 1966. When they asked him about it he said "I just said I WAS the Greatest! I didn't say I was the brightest!"

Around 1977 I read his book THE GREATEST! (Autobiography) Ali used to have orgies before his fights. He made a point to invite Jimmy Brown. Brown said Ali invited the ugliest women on the face of the earth and in Chicago he snuck out as soon as he could. Then Ali invited him in Miami. Same problem. Brown began to sneak out. Ali caught him and said "Hey Jimmy Brown, you snuck out of my party in Chicago and here you are sneaking out again!" Brown said, "Well Champ, seeing you are bringing it up YOU INVITE THE UGLIEST WOMEN IN THE WORLD TO YOUR PARTIES!" <u>Ali did not deny it</u>! Instead he stood up on the bed and shouted to Jimmy Brown, "I'm SO PRETTY IT DOESN'T MAKE ANY DIFFERENCE!" ALI MENTORED BY "GEORGEOUS GEORGE" (Professional Wrestler)

In 1972 I went to Madame Taussaud's Wax Museum in London and they had a life size statue of Ali. At the bottom of the statue they had something written like "Ali kicked the shit out of the United States

Government and he happened to be heavyweight champ!" Needless to say this shocked me!

PERSONALLY I THINK YOU ARE THE GREATEST! HOWEVER I THINK SO IN THE FOLLOWING CONTEXT TAKING THE HIGH ROAD! IN TERMS OF SHAKESPEARE'S QUESTION, "TO BE OR NOT TO BE" YOU ARE THE GREATEST PRESIDENT OF THE UNITED STATES! THAT IS THE ONLY IMPORTANT CRITERIA ON WHICH YOU ARE TO BE EVALUATED, EVEN IF YOU AND SARA HUCKABEE SANDERS ARE THE ONLY ONES DOING THE EVALUATING! STAND YOUR GROUND AND DO NOT FOLD UNDER ANY CIRCUMSTANCES!

Why should your children be intellectual disconnected elites! You surround yourself with them because they love you and you have a better chance trusting family than the governmentalites that stripped Ali of his title during his prime!

You are doing a great job! Keep up the good work!

Respectfully,

Dr. Len Bergantino

cc: Melania, Sanders, Don Jr., Ivanka

Eric

P.S. Gana Huckabee Sanders is doing a magnificent job!!!

January 12, 2018

DEAR PRESIDENT TRUMP,

HOW REFRESHING THAT YOU STATED WHAT I NOTICED AROUND THE TIME I STOPPED DOING PSYCHOANALYSIS! YOU STATED "WHY ARE ALL THESE PEOPLE FROM "SHITHOLE COUNTRIES" COMING HERE!

TO DO PSYCHOANALYSIS AN INTELLECTUAL ELITE WITH MENTAL SOPHISTICATION IS REQUIRED. THE NUANCES MAKE THE WORK FASCINATING!

AS I WAS TRAINED IN FAMILY THERAPY BY WORLD RENOWN PIONEERS CARL WHITAKER, M.D. AND WALTER KEMPLER, M.D. I NOTICED THAT THE WORK ITSELF BEGAN TO MOVE IN THE DIRECTION OF FAMILY THERAPY WITH MORE "ORDINARY" PELPLE DUE TO THE IMMIGRATION POLLCIES THAT LET IN PEOPLE FROM "SHITHOLE COUNTRIES" ON SOME SAVIOR MISSION THAT HAS DESTROYED NOT ONLY THE PSYCHOANALYTIC POPULATION THAT MIGHT SEND IT'S GRADUATES OFF TO CREATE AN UPWARD SPIRALING SOCIETY BY THE LOWERING OF ABILITIES OF THE COMMUNITY STANDARDS OF PRACTICE OF EVEN OUR MEDICAL SCHOOLS. I FIND THE MOST MEDICAL BRAINS THESE DAYS ARE IN THE HEADS OF THOSE FROM CHINESE HERITAGE WHO CHOOSE TO REMAIN HERE!. THEY ARE FAR SUPERIOR TO PHYSICIANS EDUCATED IN THE UNITED STATES!

YOUR STATEMENT HAS NOTHING AT ALL TO DO WITH RACIAL PREJUDICE OR RACIAL HATRED. IT HAS TO DO WITH THE BEGINNING OF WHEN A PRESIDENT I LOVED, JFK, MADE A SERIOUS MISTAKE AND CUT BACK THE ENTRANCE OF BRITS, ITALIANS, POLES, GERMANS, et. al and DEVOTED HIS EFFORTS TO "SHITHOLE COUNTRIES" COMING HERE TURNING THE UNITED STATES INTO A THIRD WORLD COUNTRY!.

THE PROBLEM FOR ME IS THAT I WORKED MY ASS OFF TO DEVELOP A SKILL SET THAT WORKED IN THE HIGHEST LEVEL OF SUPERSTARS! IF I WANTED TO WORK IN A THIRD WORLD COUNTRY I WOULD HAVE MOVED TO BELIZE. I CAN DO BOTH KINDS OF WORK! Norway loves Americans! They were one of two countries that appreciated the contribution of the United States from World War II! You might also try Denmark! They are not a shithole country!

You are refreshing in what you say. Don't let them twist your words and intentions! YOU ARE JUST CALLING EM LIKE YOU SEE EM!

Respectfully,

Dr. Len Bergantino

P.S. The problem is that THE SLUGS THAT WE LET IN ARE MUCH MORE LIKELY TO DRAG US INTO THIRD WORLD STATUS THAN WE ARE TO LIFT THEM UP INTO BEING A CITIZEN IN THE GREATEST COUNTRY IN THE HISTORY OF MANKIND!

P.S. 2 TRUMP UNDERSTANDS WHAT IS REQUIRED TO PLAY IN HIGH ROLLER CIRCUIT!

January 1, 2018

<u>President Trump's Tweeting Similar to Martin Buber's I-Thou Encounter</u>

LA Times- JANUARY p,A9)!* "BIG protests in Iran," the President tweeted Sunday "The people are finally getting wise as to how their money and wealth is being stolen and squandered on terrorism. Looks like they will not take it any longer."

Dr. Jim Simkin, Ph.D., ABPP, premier gestalt trainer who was known to be a much better psychotherapist than Frederick Perls, M.D.-the founder of gestalt therapy stated "QUESTIONS ARE DESIGNED TO TORTURE PEOPLE! MAKE "I" STATEMENTS (as written about by Martin Buber). President Trump does this on a daily basis in that he tells citizens of the world exactly where he is at! I am 74 years old and he is the only President who has ever done that. While this is viewed as unnerving to those WHO CANNOT STAND THE CHAOS AND ANXIETY OF NOT KNOWING TO ME TRUMP IS REFRESHING! YOU KNOW EXACTLY WHERE HE IS AT!

Dr. Simkin said of me "OF ALL THE THERAPISTS I HAVE TRAINED OR SEEN WORK, INCLUDING Fritz Perls, BERGANTINO, HE IS A MAN OF DEPTH! HE IS A MAN OF SUBSTANCE! HIM I THINK ABOUT! HIM I CONSIDER!"

Think about it! At the deepest levels, Isn't President Trump tweeting bottom line how most Americans really feel about most everything, including Iran and North Korea!

For example, do we trust China to impose sanctions on N. Korea, a country they sent 450,000 troops to aid in the Korean War? Do we trust Iran to not give the money we gave them to support terrorists? Do we believe they won't find some way to develop their nuclear capacities and to strike first? as did Japan during WWII?

And think about this; IF THEY RUB PRESIDENT TRUMP THE WRONG WAY ON ANY GIVEN DAY, HE HAS THE NUCLEAR

POWER TO WIPE THEM OFF THE FACE OF THE EARTH!!!
WHOSE SIDE WOULD YOU RATHER BE ON?

RESPECTFULLY,

REV. DR. LEN BERGANTINO

PRIME MINISTER, UNIV. LIFE CHURCH - WLA

ED.D. (USC - 1971) DOCTOR OF EDUCATION

Ph.D. (INT'L COLLEGE - 1977) CLINICAL PSYCH.

P.S. President Trump has provided evidence beyond a "reasonable doubt" that if any foreign or domestic enemy "shits on The United States of America" President Trump will be the one "TO FLUSH THE TOILET!!!"

FAMILY THERAPY INTERVENTION

-- Len Bergantino and Robert Rabert

Client's Description: I have known Dr. Len Bergantino since 1990, having met him when we were both members of the St. Peter's Italian Catholic Church on Broadway Street in Los Angeles. Over the course of time, we became friends and he asked me to be his son's Godfather around 1997. I was honored to do so.

He met my wife on one occasion prior to our being married and he has known my children, Mimi and Reemo, since they were about one year old, as he has often stated he has a clear recollection of me changing their diapers on the sidewalk in front of DiVita's restaurant in West Los Angeles, California. Dr. Bergantino is a fine musician and my children often went to hear him play and to visit with Afex (his son) and him. This sparked an interest in music on the part of my daughter. With the hard times of two recessions, we were forced to move from Los Angeles to Tucson, and I had no funds to purchase an instrument or to pay for music lessons.

Dr. Bergantino came to visit us in May, 2008, and he gave my daughter a guitar. Then he began giving her weekly guitar lessons by telephone from Los Angeles to Tucson from June 2008 to December 2009.

During this time, Mimi showed both diligence and enthusiasm toward the practice of music and general interest in music. Dr. Bergantino took her through *Mel Bay I* and most of *Mel Bay II* before she was not able to continue her studies on the guitar as her hands were too small to play chords for which her fingers were either not long enough or strong enough.

During the weeks that followed termination of her lessons, my daughter became withdrawn and began to fail classes at her school where she had been a straight A student.

While Dr. Bergantino made it a point to keep the fact that he was a clinical psychologist separate from our friendship with him and his role as Mimi's teacher, this was the first time he said to me that he had become "clinically alarmed." He wrote a very supportive document to the high school principal, the high school counselor, and the superintendent of schools, requesting that my daughter be provided with a clarinet and music lessons at school, become part of the school band, and more involved in social activities at school. He was insistent that I follow up immediately in Mimi's behalf. Due to my worries about the difficulty of my financial situation I did not. Further, the principal who called Dr. Bergantino and assured him that she would not let Mimi fall through the cracks, did not get her involved with weekly music lessons or get her a clarinet, and put off getting her involved in school activities until the following year. In the meantime, my daughter became more and more withdrawn and began to fail most of her courses.

Dr. Bergantino was scheduled to come to visit us in Tucson as part of a banjo festival he was going to attend. He was furious at both me and the school principal for not following through on our promises given that from his point of view my daughter's life and well-being were at stake. He made it clear several times that her well-being took precedence over what might customarily be expected from a friend. He further said that what he was going to do at this point had to cross boundaries that he had never crossed in terms of our personal relationship (he was a licensed psychologist in California, Arizona, and Hawaii).

As soon as I picked him up from the airport he insisted I drive him to the Office of the Superintendent of Schools and he met with the Assistant Superintendent and he made it clear to them that Mimi was not to be sold down the river and if the district did not get her a clarinet and weekly clarinet lessons with such clear warning signs as her going from a straight A to a straight F student, that he as a licensed psychologist in Arizona would serve as an expert witness in helping to construct a lawsuit against the school. By the end of this meeting, he thought both persons intended to be helpful. He made it clear to them he felt totally betrayed by the high school principal. Next, he insisted I drive him to the high school and set up a meeting with the Principal, and the high school counselor. He was told that the Assistant Principal would meet with him on the morning of May 13, 2010, at 8:30 a.m. When he got to the meeting, the Principal and high school counselor were present. At a point in time, the high school principal made it clear she was not going to be helpful and was going to do nothing until the following semester and then only band and an occasional meeting with the school counselor. Dr. Bergantino went into a tirade in the meeting, telling the principal and the counselor in no uncertain terms that either I was giving him permission to direct the course of affairs or I was not, in which case his participation to help my daugher was over; and if he did give me permission, this meeting was over and we were on our way to immediately seek out legal counsel to file a lawsuit against the school, for intentionally jeopardizing the academic and emotional well-being of Mimi Rabert prior to his return to Los Angeles. The Principal looked to me as the father and attempted to get me to back down from Dr. Bergantino's position, while she was offering nothing. I said "He has full authority from me as a parent to do whatever he feels is in my daughter's best interest." The school counselor acted as if he were going to start a fight with Dr. Bergantino, telling him that he could not idly sit by and watch Dr. Bergantino run roughshod over his principal. As Dr. Bergantino began to stand up and made it clear he was not a man to be bluffed, the principal changed her tune. Assigned school counselor to be involved as the school liaison in weekly counselling sessions with Mimi, the Father, and for one session Reemo [the brother] and the mother when she was in Tucson. It was made clear that all of Dr. Bergantino's work would be pro bono (as were the guitar lessons.) It was made clear that his methods were unorthodox and not likely to be understood by school personnel.

Dr. Bergantino spent a great deal of time visiting our family at our home on the dates of May 12, 2010, through May 16, 2010. I would have to describe these as clinical visits, the outcome of which was miraculous. For example, Mimi refused to speak with me and hardly ever left her room, while spending hours on the Internet. Dr. Bergantino began shouting loud enough for her to hear, to me: "I want you to go to the hardware store, buy a padlock, and lock her room! At least that way you will be in charge of the family madness!" So Mimi began to leave her room so she could spy on Dr. Bergantino because he could be dangerous to her from her point of view if left unwatched (she did not want any interference with her successful blackmail of me and her brother). Then, from Mimi's point of view she had no reason to come out of her room, because I could not discuss the problem without being extremely offensive to Reemo. So when Reemo was late for dinner from football practice, and I wanted to save him the biggest steak, Dr. Bergantino said: "That little b– isn't on time for dinner! Give him leftovers! Give Mimi the big steak!" She began to laugh uproariously and came out of the room more and more for lively visits with us. In other words, Dr. Bergantino turned the situation around in about four days of "live-in therapy". He sounded off the wall, and I did understand what he did when he did it, but by the time of our visit at school on May 13 or 14, 2010, the results were already positive and I told the principal about his success. On that basis he turned control of the situation over to Dr. Bergantino. Sessions occurred on June 14, 2010, 1 p.m. on Monday, June 21, 2010, and July 6, 2010. They lasted about 30 minutes (by telephone).

During the first session, a school psychologist sat in on the session, which was not part of the arrangement. When Dr. Bergantino assessed who sent for her and for what purpose, he stated that unless she understood he had total control of the way the sessions were conducted and she could remain as a student in that she had no experience doing family therapy, she could get out now! While it sounded as if she had a choice, he actually threw her out, sending a message to the principal.

Dr. Bergantino said several times that he could not have done it without me, in that some of the encounters he had with me on the weekend he stayed in my home were fierce and "socially intolerable". I told him I had complete faith that he would never let up on getting help for my daughter, and given those feelings I was glad he crossed the boundaries of our social relationship, which has continued to bring lasting value to not only my daughter's life (in that her grades are back up and she loves taking clarinet lessons); but in that the interactions among my son and daughter and me are lively, engaging, and more considerate of each other than they had ever been, and therefore the results are likely to carry on into the future.

--Robert Rabert, Tucson 9/6/2010
Len Bergantino, Ed.D., ABPP

ACKNOWLEDGMENTS TO XLIBRIS PUBLISHING COMPANY STAFF

Michelle Postrano is a manager with tenacity. Her greatest asset is in knowing the entire playing field and getting the football across the goal line. Thank you Michelle!

Thank you to Carlos Cortes for being there in ways I needed him to be there when I needed him to be there.

Sarah Perkins has been quite helpful in getting the manuscript ready for the production team.

Sheila Legaspi has been instrumental in putting together the final manuscript for final production and design.

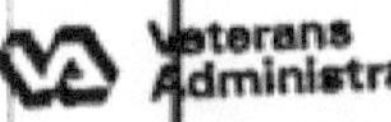

1 July 1985   In Reply Refer To:

Len Bergantino, Ed.D., Ph.D.
10266 Kilrenney Avenue
Los Angeles, California 90064

Dear Len:

How nice to receive yours of June 24th., and to learn of your upward spiral! I'm very pleased indeed to believe that my little review of your book has contributed to your success!

Frankly, Len, I have long been eructatively fed up with the sort of territorial cupidities and other evidences of narcissistic nonsensicality so many of the colleagues display. Such antics reveal the essentially limbic nature of people as it comes to be expressed in envies and jealousies to which you allude in your letter. When I read your book I knew at once of your outsider-ism (cf. Colin Wilson's seminal book of the same name—The Outsider) as well as your talent; since I know I am good also, I do not need to do the Big-Daddy-in-Cat-On-A-Hot-Tin-Roof bit, viz., to shit on one's sons out of envy and fear that they will appropriate my penis-cum-wife-cum-everything-else!

I trust your family are in good health. Keep in touch.

Most sincerely,

Donald B. Rinsley, M.D., F.R.S.E. (Lond.)
Associate Chief for Education
Psychiatry Service

Clinical Professor of Psychiatry
University of Kansas School of Medicine
Kansas City

DBR:mtf

A REVIEW

By DONALD B. RINSLEY, M.D., F.R.S.H.,
Fellow, American College of Psychoanalysts;
Fellow, American Psychiatric Association
Psychotherapy, Insight and Style.
By Len Bergantino, Ed.D., Ph.D.
Boston: Allyn and Bacon, 1981, 288 pp.
Published in Bulletin of the Menninger Clinic,
Vol. 47, No. 5, September 1983.

THERE IS NO DOUBT THAT SOME PEOPLE POSSESS A HEALING CAPACITY AND THAT OTHERS DO NOT; NOR IS THERE ANY DOUBT THAT A ZULU WITCH DOCTOR, A PUERTO RICAN CURANDERO, A NAVAHO MEDICINE MAN OR A VOODOO SPIRITIST MAY REMIT SYMPTOMS MORE EFFECTIVELY THAN THE BEST TRAINED PSYCHOTHERAPIST OR PSYCHOANALYST. The differences between healing and therapy are not inconspicuous even as both may readily dissolve into quackery in the hands of the exploitive and the unscrupulous. A wise Freud once commented that the function of psychoanalysis is to convert neurotic misery into ordinary human suffering, a point of view to be dismissed only at one's peril even though it doubtless reflected the essence of Freud's depressive personality. From such few considerations as these emerge questions concerning the differences separating healing and therapy, the features that unite them and the goals and objectives they may be noted to share. And whatever answers to these questions may satisfy those who propound them will reflect whether one's Weltanschauung considers the world to be a vale of tears or, after the fashion of the Gallic optimist, Coué, a place where everything keeps getting better and better.

Dr. Bergantino's book in scholarly and even entertaining fashion sets out to address issues such as these. The blurb on its bookjacket states that it "integrates 17 prominent therapists' styles and problem solving techniques . . ." Its more accurate subtitle, The Existential Moment reflects the author's searching awareness that effective psychological healing, or psychotherapy, or whatever one chooses to call such interpersonal transactional processes ultimately expands one's awareness, hence one's knowledge of one's self, one's surround and the relationship between them; and further, that such awareness and knowledge develops in saltatory fashion, deriving from unheralded and even momentary experiences of insight, illumination ("aha!") or unconscious internal change. So far so good, but there is after all nothing new in that, so why read yet another book devoted to arresting human experiences that many believe to be inexplicable and unteachable?

There are at least two answers to that question. To begin with, the book reflects the personal odyssey of a trained, disciplined yet openminded professional psychologist who has drunk deeply at the wells of an number of acknowledged healer-therapists whose work he has carefully studied and evaluated, among them, Viktor Frankl, Wilfred Bion, the Gouldings, Frederick Perls, Milton Erickson and Carl Whitaker. A unique feature of Dr. Bergantino's presentation is his detailed accounts of these therapists' hour-to-hour work, drawn from his own personal experience and from verbatim descriptions provided by their students and analysands, offering fascinating and instructive insights into the therapeutic labors of admittedly gifted treaters. The book is thus replete with clinical material, excerpts from therapeutic encounters and direct reports of those precious "aha"-type moments, conveyed within a disciplined epistemic context that presents each example in terms of ethical professionalism rather than exemplary amateurishness.

Again, the book reflects its author's ongoing growth and development as both thinker and therapist. Dr. Bergantino has gone to great length to converse and consult with both primary and secondary sources, delving into the what and the how, ferreting out illustrative clinical situations and indicating how he has proceeded to synthesize and integrate what he has learned from them and from his own therapeutic work. His book is indeed a literate statement of how one clinician has made of himself a therapist and his statement is both informative and poignant.

As I read this book my thoughts returned to a little-known 1962 Psychiatric Quarterly paper by Ernst Federn, the son of the psychoanalyst Paul Federn, entitled "The Therapeutic Personality. As Illustrated by Paul Federn and August Aichorn." It described in some detail the uniquely intuitive therapeutic work of these two outstanding clinicians, drawn from the author's own experience of knowing them both; Federn and Aichorn brought disciplined artistry to their respective therapeutic tasks in working psychoanalytically with "difficult" cases, Federn with psychotics, Aichorn with disturbed adolescents; both readily sensed suffering and never flinched from addressing it; both could occupy honored places in Dr. Bergantino's book. I learned much from that paper and I have learned much from Dr. Bergantino's book as well.

Psychotherapy, Insight and Style is an absorbing work, to be returned to time and again after one has read it through, to be thought about, MULLED OVER AND PLACED ON ONE'S BEDSIDE TABLE IF NOT UNDER ONE'S PILLOW. It is a book that the EXPERIENCED CLINICIAN will read with knowledgeable satisfaction and that the NASCENT THERAPIST will read with excitement. And both will profit from what it has to tell.

Donald Rinsley, M.D., F.R.S.H.
Senior Faculty Member in Adult and
Child Psychiatry, Karl Menninger
School of Psychiatry

Associate Chief for Education, Psychiatry Service, Colmery-O'Neil
Veterans Administration Medical Center

LEN BERGANTINO, Ed.D., Ph.D.
Clinical Psychology (PL3837)

10266 Kilrenney Ave.

Los Angeles, CA 90064

1/12/81

Carl Whitaker, M.D.
Professor of Psychiatry
U. of Wisconsin Medical School
Center for Health Sciences
600 Highland Avenue
Madison, Wisconsin 53792

Dear Carl,

The following is material that you dictated to me over the telephone regarding material that may be used in any advertising capacity that Allyn & Bacon, Inc., chooses to do in the promotion of my book, "Psychotherapy Insight And Style: The Existential Moment."

"The author as a therapist is a student of creativity and he offers a metaphorical elaboration that is both impressionistic, artistic and a stimulus for thinking. He is a professional reporter of interpersonal change models in the family therapy set and even intrapsychic change process in its twentieth century face. The book rouses powerful feelings and stimulates growth in its readers."

"Reading this book is an active experience in the use of self in the field of psychotherapy, and as such, it both expands and enriches the community standards of practice of professional psychotherapists. That self is really our only tool. It's use is critical and evolving through each practitioner's professional lifetime."

Please sign below acknowledging your permission to quote.

Sincerely,

Len

Carl Whitaker, M.D.

Len Bergantino, Ed.D., Ph.D.

P.S. Please return one copy to me, keep one for your records and send one to Allyn & Bacon, Inc. Thank you.

The Centre for Experiential Learning

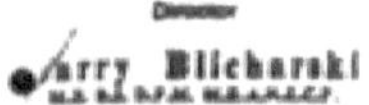

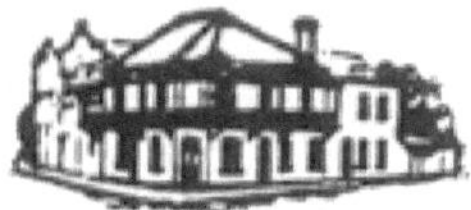

141 Beattie Street,
Balmain,
N.S.W. 2041
Phone 818 4188

5th September 1986.

<u>TO WHOM IT MAY CONCERN</u>

Len Bergantino Ed.D, Ph.D., has recently conducted workshops
at this Centre on Existential Family Therapy and Ericksonian
Hypnotic Storytelling. He also conducted some workshops for
the Gestalt Institute of Queensland during this visit to
Australia. He also conducted a workshop with the students in
the Gestalt Therapy Training Programme in Sydney.

I am happy to recommend Len Bergantino as an excellent work-
shop leader, trainer and psychotherapist. His work with our
Gestalt trainees was of the highest order and his Gestalt work
is enhanced by his breadth of training in Family Therapy,
Ericksonian Hypnotherapy etc. His work was extremely well
received both here and in Queensland.

I am a Psychotherapist, accredited Psychodrama Director and
Gestalt Therapist and have trained with Erv and Miriam Polster,
Jim Simkin, Jorge Rosner and have had workshop experience with
a number of other Gestalt Therapists visiting Australia during
the last ten years.

We will be inviting Len Bergantino to return to Australia and
I recommend his work, both clinical and teaching, in any
situation.

Barry Blicharski,
Director.
Psychiatrist

8th September, 1986.

<u>TO   WHOM   IT   MAY   CONCERN</u>

Dr. Len Bergantino has conducted workshops on Family Therapy and Existential Psychotherapy for us in Brisbane, Australia in 1984 and 1986.

We have had various individuals giving workshops for us each year since 1979. Some of the Leaders were Dr. Jim Simkin, Dr. Stella Resnick, Dr. Tom Munson and others.

We find Dr. Bergantino's calibre of work equal and even superior to some of the presenters. Dr. Bergantino's teaching and demonstrations of his therapeutic style are exceptional in the area of Family Therapy, Gestalt, Existential Psychotherapy and Ericksonian hypnosis via story telling.

Dr. Bergantino has a unique ability to transfer his teaching methods in a live and expressive manner that has proven to have lasting impact on his audience. He has our highest recommendation as a workshop leader.

<u>FOR THE GESTALT INSTITUTE OF QLD. FACULTY</u>

<u>YARO STARAK</u>
CO-ORDINATOR

Rinsley was on the circuit with Harold Searles MD (the best American Psychoanalyst), and Otto Kernberg MD. If you read between the lines, he said I was the best alive then!

8th September, 1986.

<u>TO   WHOM   IT   MAY   CONCERN</u>

Dr. Len Bergantino has conducted workshops on Family Therapy and
Existential Psychotherapy for us in Brisbane, Australia in 1984 and
1986.

We have had various individuals giving workshops for us each year since
1979. Some of the Leaders were Dr. Jim Simkin, Dr. Stella Resnick,
Dr. Tom Munson and others.

We find Dr. Bergantino's calibre of work equal and even superior to
some of the presenters. Dr. Bergantino's teaching and demonstrations
of his therapeutic style are exceptional in the area of Family Therapy,
Gestalt, Existential Psychotherapy and Ericksonian hypnosis via story
telling.

Dr. Bergantino has a unique ability to transfer his teaching methods
in a live and expressive manner that has proven to have lasting impact
on his audience. He has our highest recommendation as a workshop
leader.

<u>FOR THE GESTALT INSTITUTE OF QLD. FACULTY</u>

<u>YARO STARAK</u>
CO-ORDINATOR

March 15, 2011   The Ides of March

Dear Publisher:

I have an idea that will make us a small fortune. Enclosed is a book to which I own the copyright that was a master classic in the field as a professional book. IT WAS NEVER MARKETED TO THE STUDENT POPULATIONS WHO STUDY PSYCHOTHERAPY AND COUNSELING!!!!!

THE BOOK INTEGRATES AND GIVES CLINICAL EXAMPLES OF ALL THE MOST EFFECTIVE PSYCHIATRISTS AND PSYCHOLOGISTS OF AN ERA BETWEEN 1970 and 1985, AND MANY WILL AGREE ARE THE BEST THAT EVER LIVED.

IN THAT CONTEXT THE BOOK NEEDS A NEW TITLE ALONG THE LINES OF "THE HISTORY OF EXCELLENCE IN PSYCHOTHERAPY AND COUNSELING: A TRANSMISSION OF THE CULTURE".

<u>HISTORY OF THE BOOK</u>

The book was originally published by a Boston House named Allyn & Bacon, Inc. in 1981. It was their intention to break into THE PSYCHOLOGY MARKET with my book. My editor, Eugene McCann -did a marvelous job and the book far exceeded expectations, getting reviews from not only world renown psychologists but also world renown psychiatrists and the book cut across all theoretical models of doing psychotherapy in that the reviews came from all places! I even had reviews by both Carl Whitaker, M.D. and Tom Malone, M.D. both of whom who wrote THE ROOTS OF PSYCHOTHEAPY in 1956. Furthur, Whitaker was the premiere family therapist in the world at the time he reviewed my work and wrote the forward to the book.

Other markets include

1. I am a clinical member of The International Transactional Analysis Association and I have detailed clinical examples of

Bob Goulding, M.D. and Mary Goulding, M.S.W. who were the two most prominent clinicians ever with ITAA.

2. I have a section on Wilfred Bion, the great British psychoanalyst, perhaps following only Freud and Melanie Klein with twelve tape recorded interviews that one of his supervisees -an MD from a psychoanalytic institute permitted to be published.

3. I have a section on my training with Milton Erickson, MD the kernels of which permit one to actually do some of what this genius pioneer did in brief psychotherapy and clinical hypnosis.

4. I have clinical examples of three world renown gestalt therapists named Jim Simkin and Erv and Miriam Polster. They are three of the best that ever lived.

5. I have clinical examples of Walter Kempler, M.D., perhaps more effective than Carl Whitaker, M.D. doing family therapy but not as famous.

6. Donald Rinsley, M.D. wrote a review for the Bulletin of The Menninger Clinic by 1983 which made the book a hot property.

A. Allyn & Bacon decided not to go into the psychology market after all and did not republish the book.

B. In 1986 Jason Aronson, M.D. republished the book under its original title Psychotherapy Insight & Style: The Existential Moment and twice made it Book of the Month for <u>Psychotherapy And Social Science Review Book Club,</u> which was the hottest book club for professionals in 1986 and 1987.

C. In 1992 Humanistiche Psychologie of Cologne (Koln) Germany translated the book into German and published it in Germany.

D. In 1994 Jason Aronson, M.D. republished the book under a new title in keeping with the times entitled "MAKING AN IMPACT IN THERAPY: HOW MASTER CLINICIANS INTERVENE".

E. In 1999 the book went out of print and Jason Aronson Publishers returned the copyright to me. There was a Professor of Counseling at one of the branches of the University of Wisconsin in the Dept. of Education that bought several hundred for about five years that I had made up much as what I have enclosed for your review. (Dr. Marty Sapp)

F. <u>ALL IN ALL THE BOOK SOLD ROUGHLY 6000 COPIES!!!!!!!!!!!!!!!</u>

G. At the time the book was too scary for college professors in that they could not do what was in the book or anything close to it so the book would only expose their inadequacies - so it became part of Jason Aronson's MASTER CLASSIC SERIES FOR PROFESSIONALS FROM 1994-1999.

H. TODAY THE BOOK IS A TRANSMISSION OF THE CULTURE ON WHAT THE GREATS DID TO GET RESULTS DOING PSYCHOTHERAPY.

I. THE BOOK IS TIMELY FOR THE COLLEGE GRADUATE SCHOOL MARKET AND WILL PREVENT THE FIELD FROM HAVING TO REINVENT THE WHEEL BY PROVDING A TRANSMISSION OF THE CULTURE OF WHAT WAS ONCE GREATNESS IN THE FIELD OF PSYCHOTHERAPY AND COUNSELING!

I LOOK FORWARD TO HEARING FROM YOU!

SINCERELY,

Len Bergantino, Ed.D., Ph.D., ABPP

8th September, 1986.

TO   WHOM   IT   MAY   CONCERN

Dr. Len Bergantino has conducted workshops on Family Therapy and
Existential Psychotherapy for us in Brisbane, Australia in 1984 and
1986.

We have had various individuals giving workshops for us each year since
1979. Some of the Leaders were Dr. Jim Simkin, Dr. Stella Resnick,
Dr. Tom Munson and others.

We find Dr. Bergantino's calibre of work equal and even superior to
some of the presenters. Dr. Bergantino's teaching and demonstrations
of his therapeutic style are exceptional in the area of Family Therapy,
Gestalt, Existential Psychotherapy and Ericksonian hypnosis via story
telling.

Dr. Bergantino has a unique ability to transfer his teaching methods
in a live and expressive manner that has proven to have lasting impact
on his audience. He has our highest recommendation as a workshop
leader.

FOR THE GESTALT INSTITUTE OF QLD. FACULTY

YARO STARAK
CO-ORDINATOR

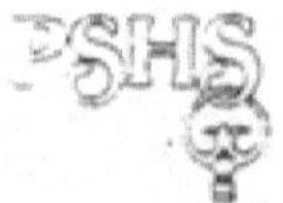

The Professional School for Humanistic Studies
420 Ash Street, San Diego, CA 92101   (714) 232-3171

June 24, 1981

Dr. Len Bergantino
415 North Camden - Suite 202
Beverly Hills, California   90210

Dear Len,

Many thanks for the copy of your book. I was delighted and surprised
that you did include your excellent summary of the workshop and the
case, after all.

The publisher did an excellent job and there are some lovely quotes.
If you need any more you can use the following paragraph.

Many have written about the science of psycho-therapy, but it has re-
mained for Dr. Bergantino to describe and illustrate the art of psycho-
therapy with such elegant impact.

Sincerely,

Harold Greenwald, Ph.D.
President

HG:cd

What the Reviewers Say:
Psychotherapy, Insight and Style
The Existential Moment

by Len Bergantino, Ed. D., ABPP

_The book sells for $26.95 / Send check to . 1215 Brockton Ave. #104, Los Angeles, C____ 900___

Interested? Contact **Dr.Bergantino** / (310) 207-8818

Dr. Carl A. Whitaker, M.D. Professor of Psychiatry / School of Medicine, University of Wisconsin

"The plethora of how-to books is increasing. Barbara Betz stated that the dynamics of psychotherapy is in the person of the therapist. Abraham Maslow stated the the peak experience lasts two weeks. Winicott insisted that if you haven't been hated by your psychotherapist you have been cheated. Erenwald has stated that psychotherapy is the effort to evolve an existential shift.

Len Bergantino is trying to expand this operational territory by strecthing the psychotherapeutic geology He succeeds. Describing the therapist as a person of liberated wisdom, he dares to the chaos and anxiety of not knowing; he opens a gate to see and make the impact of psychotherapy more clearly. His description of beingness as a process is reminiscent of Paul Tillich. His grasp of responsible involvement with the patient as a discipline of self shows his own search for creative options. He makes no pretense of camouflaging the psychotherapist as a wounded healer. Furthermore, Len makes crucial the pattern of the therapist's search for his own healing and successfully validates the authentic trickery of the psychotherapist as a liberated spirit. The approach to his own craziness, the freedom from the culture bind, and the discipline of self each emerged as obtainable goals of that professional parent we call the psychotherapist.

Further evidence of his own search is illustrated by his impersonalized impressionistic response to the other searchers he uses as models. Simply reading his book leaves me feeling it would be meaningful to join in his search for his beingness. Though he would be enjoying himself and enjoying me as a patient, he would not be doing things to keep from being himself and thus I could be more fully myself."

Dr. Donald Rinsley, M.D., F. R.S.H. Fellow, American College of Psychoanalysts in his

review of Dr. Bergantino's book published in Bulletin of the Menninger Clinic, Vol. 47, No. 5, September, 1983 wrote:

"The book reflects the personal odyssey of a trained, disciplined yet openminded professional psychologist who has drunk at the wells of an number of acknowledged healer-therapists whose work he has carefully studied and evaluated, among them, Viktor Frankl, Wilfred Bion, the Gouldings, Frederick Perls, Milton Erickson and Carl Whitaker. A unique feature of Dr. Bergantino's presentation is his detailed accounts of these therapists' hour-to-hour work, drawn from his own personal experience and from verbatim descriptions provided by their students and analysands, offering fascinating and instructive insights into the therapeutic labors of admittedly gifted treaters."

Dr. Martin Grotjahn, M.D., Training and Supervising Analyst Emeritus, Southern California

Psychoanalytic Institute, in a pre-publication review wrote:

"Dr. Bergantino is obviously a gifted therapist ...Most cases as reported in the literature describe the patient's associations and productions while the therapist remains hidden in the mystery of darkness unrevealed. Dr. B is an exception: the great advantage of his work is the openness and frankness with which the author reveals his experiences when treating patients or when accepting himself as a patient of another therapist.

Dr. Walter Kempler, M.D. The Kempler Institure - Costa Mesa, CA

"Len's writing is intelligent and lucid...engrossing.....
I think his book is valuable...an interesting and propelling work...His ideas ride the crest of current thought in the field, provides clean reviews of popular modes, formulates in the popular jargon of the day using traditional interpretions and terminology. His personal touch is enchancing."

Dr. James S. Simkin, Ph.D. American Board of Examiners in Professional Psychology - Big Sur, CA

"Professionals could benefit directly from this book in that Bergantino describes how it is possible to integrate a variety of psychotherapeutic approaches."

Dr. Ernest Lawrence Rossi, Ph.D. Diplomate in Clinical Psychology - Los Angeles, CA

"A deeply moving flood of insights and approaches to becoming oneself as a psychotherapist....It is a highly readable record of (Bergantino's) development as a therapist via his personal contacts and training with a variety of current-day psychotherapists....a new understanding of what it means to be a creative therapist continually living in the present's potential for change and transformation...
.....focuses on the precise and often provocative and shocking techniques that are useful in helping patients break out of their learned limitations to realize their potentials for creative change."

*This book is being republished by Jason Aronson Publishers Inc. as part of The Master Classic Series under a new title, Moments of Impact in Psychotherapy: How The Masters Intervene

LEN BERGANTINO Ed. D., ABPP

In-Depth Family Therapy • Ericksonian Hypnosis

American Board of Professional Psychology • Diplomate in Family Psychology

DOCTORATE-UNIVERSITY OF SOUTHERN CALIFORNIA-1971 • PRIVATE PRACTICE OF CLINICAL PSYCHOLOGY NOW

LEN BERGANTINO, Ed.D., Ph.D., A.B.P.P.
Clinical Psychologist (Lic. No. 3827)

Psychoanalysis
A.B.P.P. - Diplomate in Family Psychology
American Board of Professional Psychology

1215 Brockton Ave., Ste. 104, W. Los Angeles, CA 90025 · U.S.A.
(310) 207-9397

ASSOCIATION OF HUMANISTIC PSYCHOLOGY PERSPECTIVE
= ahp
Review below by Tom Malone, M.D.

book
reviews

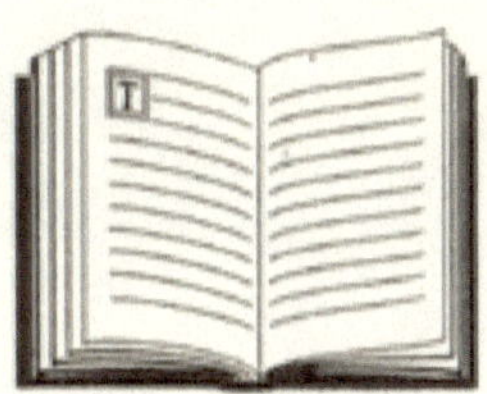

CALIFORNIA PSYCHOLOGIST
September, 1994
Volume XXVII   Number 7

Making An Impact In Therapy: How Master Clinicians Intervene
by Len Bergantino, Ed.D.
Reviewed by Harold Greenwald, Ph.D.

Many professionals learn their trade by observing their mentors at work; surgeons, for example, operate in full view of their students. Such practice is difficult to duplicate in teaching psychotherapy. Dr. Len Bergantino has done the next best thing in his extensive description of such master clinicians as Albert Ellis, Milton Erickson, William Kroger, Carl Whitaker and Erv and Miriam Polster.

It is refreshing and exciting to observe the freedom with which these master therapists are willing to depart from the professional's role of being careful and proper, in order to use themselves and to create the impact which Dr. Bergantino describes as the existential moment when both therapist and patient dare to be completely themselves. While some of the interventions described may seem unusual, they are excellent examples of being with the patient to further world. The choice of material selected by the author is quite broad and is a vital emotional and educational experience.

The book is concise and well-written, and makes a valuable addition to the bookshelves of both veteran and neophyte therapists.

REVIEWS

Making an Impact in Therapy

How Master Clinicians Intervene

By Len Bergantino
Jason Aronson Publishers, 1994.
Reviewed by Thomas P. Malone.
1-800-782-0015 to order

This is an impressive piece of work. It is cogent, very relevant at present in the field of health, be it mental or physical; and it is truly an experience. It is a book about psychotherapy, and more particularly, about the experiential aspects of psychotherapy.

Most often, those of us who have written about experiential psychotherapy tend to be somewhat cognitive. We try to describe and explain rather than have the reader experience the psychotherapy as one does in this book. With *Making an Impact* it is as if you are sitting there not only listening, but in a sense, part of. The reader not only hears the words, but hears and feels and recognizes the affect. There, of course, are relevant discussion and commentary by the author at appropriate places.

The book is also quite timely and relevant to the present crisis in health care. Instead of managing the psychic health of the patients, the psychotherapeutic interventions here are facilitative. They describe essentially the therapist interacting with the patients in a way that is oriented toward increasing the patient's capacity for managing his or her own health.

Thomas P. Malone, M.D. is co-author with Carl Whitaker of the classic book The Roots of Psychotherapy.

FOREWORD

Making an Impact in Therapy:
How Master Clinicians Intervene

JASON ARONSON INC.
Northvale, New Jersey
London

THE PLETHORA OF how-to books is increasing. This is not one of those. My wife at the time Betz stated that the dynamics of psychotherapy is in the person of the therapist. Abraham Maslow stated that the peak experience lasts two weeks. Winicott insisted that if you haven't been hated by your psychotherapist you have been cheated. Erenwald has stated that psychotherapy is the effort to evolve an existential shift.

Len Bergantino is trying to expand this operational territory by stretching the psychotherapeutic geology. He succeeds. Describing the therapist as a person of liberated wisdom, he dares to the chaos and anxiety of not knowing; he opens a gate to see and make the impact of psychotherapy more clearly. His description of beingness as a process is reminiscent of Paul Tillich. His grasp of responsible involvement with the patient as a discipline of self shows his own search for creative options. He makes no pretense of camouflaging the psychotherapist as a wounded healer. Furthermore, Len makes crucial the pattern of the therapist's search for his own healing and successfully validates the authentic trickery of the psychotherapist as a liberated spirit. The approach to his own craziness, the freedom from the culture bind, and the discipline of self each emerged as obtainable goals of that professional parent we call the psychotherapist.

Further evidence of his own search is illustrated by his impersonalized impressionistic response to the other searchers he uses as models.

Simply reading his book leaves me feeling it would be meaningful to join in his search for his beingness. Though he would be enjoying himself and enjoying me as a patient, he would not be doing things to keep from being himself and thus I could be more fully myself.

Carl A. Whitaker, M.D.
Professor of Psychiatry
School of Medicine
University of Wisconsin

PREFACE

THIS IS A book for professional psychotherapists, psychoanalysts and counselors; students in those areas of specialty; and lay persons who are interested in the essence of effective therapy, and how some of the people who do it best practice their art. For professionals the book presents a personal way of viewing therapy that can add pleasurable options. Each of the therapists with whom I worked, and myself, all had a feeling of enjoyment that we hope will carry over to the office and practices of the readers. For students of therapy the book offers a search for a professional stature and working posture that may be of value in the development of each student's unique personal style. For lay persons the book speaks of therapy that can make an impact and how some of the most potent therapists practiced.

I wrote the book with the intention of having it be both an experience and an explanation. I have presented it according to my developmental needs while maturing personally and professionally. This was done so the book might be informative at the conscious level, entertaining at the child level, and persuasive at the unconscious level.

The existential moment is the thread that ties the book together; it is a moment of therapeutic potency. While all moments are existential by definition, there are certain moments that are more powerful in helping patients live happier and healthier lives. Positive results, whether they be from one session, or over the long haul, are partially, if not fully, a result of existential moments.

Basically, I think of existential moments as those moments of contact that powerfully flow from the uniqueness of a therapist to cause a therapeutic response to affect change in patients. These existential moments may take place at either the conscious or unconscious levels and usually include accentuated contact (1) between patient and therapist (usually but not necessarily of an authentic nature), (2) between alienated parts of a patient suffering from inner conflict, (3) between patient and environment. It can also occur as a result of a particular therapeutic method that leaves a patient feeling freer to choose to live differently, and may enhance the quality of the patient's being in terms of answering the question "To Be or Not to Be?" In practice, these existential moments may appear to at times be contradictory, but they are not in that each therapist and each style presents a unique way of making impact.

Through these moments can be seen one way of integrating a variety of therapy methods. But even more important than the theories it can be seen why the particular people I write about stand out above their theories. I try to capture them as vital, responsive people who practice their art, which flows from their nature in most creative ways.

Each school of therapy has its potent therapists who affect patients in ways that are conducive to change. These therapists not only help patients to facilitate change, but they do so with efficiency. The book attempts to capture the nature and method of that efficiency. That is not meant to imply that personal growth doesn't take time. But the therapist's ability will affect the outcome of the therapy.

The therapists I experienced as leaving the kind of impression that lasts and facilitates change are those I have written about. They have read what I have written about them and have been generous with their time and commentary in helping to make each of those chapters more beneficial. They are George Bach, Ph.D. (couples, group, marathon therapies and behavior modification), Wilfred Bion, M.R.C.S. (psychoanalysis), Albert Ellis, Ph.D. (rational-emotive therapy), Bob Goulding, M.D. and Mary Goulding, M.S.W. (transactional analysis), Harold Greenwald, Ph.D. (direct decision therapy), Martin Grotjahn, M.D. (group analysis), Milton H. Erickson, M.D. (clinical hypnosis and behavior modification), Stanley Keleman, (body therapy), Walter Kempler, M.D. (couples therapy, existential-experiential-gestalt therapy), William S. Kroger, M.D. (clinical hypnosis), Bob Martin, D.S.W. (gestalt therapy, creative expression and sensory perception), William Ofman, Ph.D. (humanistic existential therapy), Erving Polster, Ph.D. and Miriam Polster, Ph.D. (gestalt therapy), James S. Simkin, Ph.D. (gestalt therapy), Jack Rosberg, M.A. (direct confrontation) and Carl Whitaker, M.D. (existential-experiential therapy).

I approach the different therapies within a philosophical framework that is existential in nature, but that partially grew out of my experience and development. In places it differs significantly from what is ordinarily considered to be existential philosophy, but is what I consider to be both a natural and hopeful development of existential philosophy as applied to therapy. The book is a *philosophical approach to experience.*

The result of my existential beginnings was a realization that all therapies contained bits of the truth, and that I did not have to practice straightforward existential therapy to be an existentialist. In fact, an open-ended approach has led me to a style that might be considered primarily gestalt therapy synthesized with clinical hypnosis, also utilizing what I consider to be the best of the therapies included here.

I refer to the development of personal style as a learning process whereby each therapist will borrow the best of what exists, integrate that until it becomes natural, and then let his or her own nature unfold so that what comes out will be the therapist's unique feelings, thoughts, memories and actions at that time. When therapists are able to flow with their uniqueness in such ways, it is likely that they will be able to affect patients by providing an experience of impact through existential moments that differ in kind and description depending upon the uniqueness of the therapist.

I have found that both in my life, and in the lives of those with whom I have worked, it has been these existential moments that were experienced and remembered as turning points in patients' lives or milestones in the therapeutic process. The book will concentrate on a variety of therapists and how they are able to provide such *moments of impact,* while practicing their *unique styles* of therapy.

While in a sense the intention of this book is to give therapists a license to be uncommon, unique, spontaneous, and at times even outrageous; it also demands that therapists develop themselves and their methods to a level of potency and sophistication where they will become so proficient that they can "shoot from the hip," take risks, do the unusual, and provide experiences for patients that are at the very least, touching or moving, and influential in a beneficial manner. The research literature has indicated for too long that one-third of all therapy has a negative result: one-third a neutral result; and one-third a positive result. The task of this book is to focus on the core of what makes an impact, and how therapists can develop a style–or borrow some of what has gone before them that may evolve from parts of themselves that have gone unexplored, so they may *enjoy what they are doing*. One needs to be extremely well disciplined to gain license for such freedom of responsiveness.

Developing therapeutic discipline and style is important because without a sense of inner confidence that comes from such diligence, therapists are not likely to feel an inner freedom to respond. Further, unless therapists are willing to develop themselves with diligence, the community standards of acceptable practice formulated by peers and the general public may be far less accepting of unusual and creative ways of reaching patients. Unless therapists feel both internal as well as external support, it is unlikely that they would go for broke to reach deeply-troubled patients. Only with this complete support can therapists who are willing to use all their power, creativity and compassion, empathy and humanity, best serve the public–and reach them at the deepest emotional levels. It is with the *liberation of the therapist that patients also have the best chance to become liberated*.

THE NAMES AND CIRCUMSTANCES OF EVERYONE DISCUSSED IN THIS BOOK EXCEPT THE THERAPISTS HAVE BEEN CAREFULLY DISGUISED. THEREFORE, READERS WHO THINK THEY CAN RECOGNIZE THEMSELVES OR MEMBERS OF THEIR THERAPY GROUPS IN THESE PAGES ARE PROBABLY MISTAKEN.

ACKNOWLEDGMENTS

THE BOOK IMPARTS an attitude of lifelong search for both personal growth and continued development in terms of creativity and personal therapeutic style. I hope that it will help you to stay enthusiastic and fresh, along with the patients who take the journey with you.

My heartfelt thanks to Peter Marin, without whose writing tutelage there would be no book; to Kathleen Knutsen Rowell for much of the early editorial work; to Bernie Wolfe whose support was appreciated throughout the writing, and to my editor, Gene McCann, whose creativity, wisdom and encouragement are responsible for the finished product.

A special note of thanks to Dr. Martin Grotjahn, who was generous in reviewing through much of the rewriting process; and to Dr. James Rice and Dr. Janet Ciriello for their editorial and professional opinions at differing stages of development of the manuscript.

An appreciation to the generous contribution of Dr. Richard Edelman, Dr. James Grotstein, Dr. Lars Lofgren, Lyndell Paul, M.S.W., Dr. Michael Paul, Dr. Steve Salenger and Mrs. Susan Grotstein, without whose contributions I would not have been able to provide as full a chapter about Wilfred Bion as I desired.

Also my thanks to Dr. Erv Polster, who helped me to learn to write in a way that expresses my ideas in a fuller way, and to Dr. Milton H. Erickson, who told me stories over and over about "rewriting line by line" until I got the message!

And, of course, an anonymous thank-you to the many patients who have taught me a great deal.

PROLOGUE

SEVERAL YEARS AGO I was hired by an institution to take over a group from a departing therapist. He informed me that a 6-foot 4-inch, 240-pound man was in the group. He came each week with a machete knife strapped to his leg. The other therapist and the patients in the group limited their responsiveness because they were not sure this patient wouldn't act out and hurt them. The following is a dialogue that took place between us right after I entered the group on my first session:

Me	John, number one, you are big enough to kick my ass without that machete strapped to your leg. Number two, I am afraid of you. If that is what you wanted to prove–you did. Number three, I will not tolerate you coming to group with that damn thing strapped to your leg. Number four, if you do not get rid of it immediately I will use every bit of administrative clout that I have to see that you are thrown out of this group and that your disability payments be cut.

At this moment every person in the group was sitting on the edge of their seats, including myself. I had hoped that I would be fast enough to get out the door if John came at me, that is, before *he* put *me* through the door. However, his response stunned everyone.

John   Man, with you here, I don't need the machete. I wish you were with me in Vietnam. I feel I can trust you.

My initial contact with John, and John's trusting reply were existential moments. I reached him at the primitive or primal level. My response had the emotional impact necessary to get to someone who was so heavily entrenched in a self-destructive personality that he could have easily been written off as hopeless. This existential moment was the kind of key experience that can have a lasting quality in the memory of patients. Such existential moments can turn around the therapeutic process in a matter of a minute or two. In the case of John, and many others, they provided the basis from which patient and therapist were able to develop a close and authentic relationship. By authentic I am referring to a relationship that has the qualities of genuineness, authoritativeness, truthfulness, trustworthiness, and believability.

John respected himself for doing what felt courageous. He respected and trusted me for setting limits and sticking to them. Had I not been so firm John would have rightly felt that I was not able to help him from having unrealistic demands, acting out, and being an angry, anxiety-arousing, spoiled brat (while I was told that he always claimed he never understood what was going on).

While my work with John was taken from a session quite early in my career, it provided me with a way of thinking about therapy that was to shape my work not only in existential therapy, but in each of the modes of therapy that I write about in this book.

I began to see that while a genuine relationship was the bond that held patient and therapist together, and while all moments of existence were equally important in terms of supplying the building blocks in therapy, there were certain events and occurrences which were so powerful, and so moving, that they affected the patient to the same degree as if the therapist were a surgeon who would cut open the patient's skull, and write the message with indelible ink into the patient's unconscious mind. Not all existential moments have this degree of impact, but those that do are existential moments.

It felt to me that when I was at my best I engaged in a passionate, blunt and provocative style of therapy. My study of the other modes of therapy (in addition to existential therapy) describe some of the ways I learned to help provide experiences for patients of such impact that they felt as if indelible ink were being used, but in tactful and less provocative ways. This search was a search for balance. I wanted to be able to reach people using a wide variety of options so I would have the greatest possible chance of not only helping patients to lead more meaningful and enjoyable lives, but to help them become free. I wanted to find the most efficient and powerful way I could to get right to the heart of the matter. It was upon such premises that I began to build a personal style of therapy.

PART ONE

The Foundations of Personal Style: Introduction

T HE FOLLOWING DIALOGUE is composed of segments of a session between Ned and me. Ned's wife had recently died in an automobile accident. He had come to me both to deal with his grief and readjust his lifestyle. He had three children whom he was now learning to care for by himself. He had an absolute value system and sexual rigidities that were preventing him from developing a new relationship. Ned was obsessive in his pursuit of an absolute reality that would leave him feeling safe. He felt he couldn't stand even the smallest trace of ambiguity in a relationship. Often, I would come from left field in ways that would leave Ned befuddled. This angered him, but the situation that unfolded also led to moments that surprised me.

Ned   I'm in the same place I was in last week and you're saying to me right now that I'm exciting and I look good. When I was in this place last week you were saying to me, "You're dull. You're not exciting."

Len

You place a lot of weight on what I say. (It was obvious that his color of skin was more toned and his eyes were brighter.)

Ned

Yes, I do.

Len

You really mess yourself up that way. (This response is frustrating to Ned because it is paradoxical and hits at the core of his obsessive behavior. Ned's problem becomes listening to me so he can learn to listen to himself, without having made the transition of listening to himself and his inner resources).

Ned

I'm giving you a helluva lot of weight because I see you making really objective statements to me.

Len

You get yourself into trouble when you make an ironclad rule of giving my statements more weight than your reactions. No matter how honest I am, I'm not quite inside of you.

Ned

I don't know where you are, Len, and I'm not sure in what way you're being helpful. I'm really angry at you right now. I don't know what the hell to do with you.

Len

I feel relieved that the weight of you is getting off my head. (While he still wants me to assume responsibility for his life, which I am refusing to do, his genuine communication with me lifts much of the actual physical pressure I was feeling when Ned was accusing me.)

Ned

Yes, but you don't have to make me well. (Ned, in retrospect, is quite accurate. I was much too passive in dealing with him, and was taking more responsibility for his cure than I ought have done, which left me feeling more burdened than necessary. This is not to deny that he was laying on me the responsibility for his life).

Len Only Ned can make Ned well. (I missed the issue here due to my own blind spot at that time. That is, I was not aware of my interventions being a bit too passive. Thus, while I gave him correct information, I missed the issue between us).

Ned I feel betrayed! I don't know where you are. I don't know where I am because I have been counting on what you have been saying and that's not the way to do the whole damn therapy.

Len I can understand your feeling angry. From my side of it I don't know if I can say anything to you without your trying to make an absolute rule for yourself, and getting pissed at me if it doesn't work out right.

A difficult issue for me and other therapists I have trained is a patient who is used to making absolute rules from what is said. He may continue to do that with each bit of awareness that is facilitated, and only use such awareness to make himself feel bad.

Ned Yes, because I'm so clever (frustrated, angry tone). I mean I'm really good at that. I feel I've got elephant ears through listening to find out what people want. They're just huge.

Len I can see them (playfully). You have huge ears. (Humor is often a way to get people to laugh at themselves instead of giving in to the "disease of seriosity.")

Ned   You didn't know they were there until I told you.

Len   I can see them.

Ned   No you can't.

Len   I can see them.

Ned   You can't either.

Len   I can see your big elephant ears.

Ned   You can't, Len. I can see it, but you can't. You can turn around anything I say at this point and I'm not going to let you do that.

Ned is projecting. He said he had elephant ears. I wasn't turning things around. I was agreeing with him. He does not want me to see him that way, so he uses projection. He comments on what he is doing, "turning things around" and attributes that behavior to me.

Ned   Maybe that's why I'm going to keep you distant. I don't know. I feel I'd like to go out on a raquetball court with you. There I'd be ahead of you. Here you're ahead of me.

And now for the open challenge–raquetball. This fits in with one of Ned's first comments in the session, "I'll give you jive about it." Initial happenings– especially first sentences of a session are good predictors of the plot that will unfold later.

Len   If you were ahead of me you would lose.

A patient who is faster at deception than his therapist is at unraveling the lie will win the battle but lose the war.

Ned   No I wouldn't.

Len   In here?

Ned   Yes. I'd pay your final fee and be on my way.

Ned   I skunked a guy at raquetball Wednesday. The same guy who gave me the big thing on my leg. Are you angry at my marking your wall?

Ned talks about challenging me to raquetball; however, he is challenging me right at that moment by putting his dirty shoes on my white wall–footprints going up the wall.

Len   Yes!

Ned   Just like my mother.

Len   You are sloppy.

Ned   Well, hell, I don't . . .

Len   What kind of patient are you climbing all over my walls. Christ! Make sure you bring some Ajax next session.

What Ned was doing was healthy. He was giving me the opportunity to become assertive enough to stop him when he couldn't stop himself. As you can see, my words were falling short of stopping him.

Ned   If you need your walls clean, you clean your walls or you tell the janitor to clean your walls.

Len   You're marking them.

Ned   I know. Because it's a part of wear and tear on the office.

Len   I don't like those black marks on my wall.

Ned   It's tough. That's really tough. I remember I had some guy walk in my office once with dirty shoes. I had just had new carpet installed–he walked in with dirty muddy feet and I never said to him, "You've got dirty, muddy feet, you dumb ass, clean it up." (Pause) You piss me off.

Ned   So, it's a small thing. I'm a good patient. I've been with you a long time, a little mark on the wall. It's the only time I've ever rumpled.

Len   I don't want you marking up my wall! (I grab a pillow-like club called a bataca.)

I felt totally helpless. I used verbally forceful confrontations, but he only spoofed my helplessness. What's more, he wouldn't take his feet off my wall. I couldn't get up and beat him up without risking a lawsuit–but that is what I felt like doing.

The situation called for action! I picked up a bataca, ran over to Ned's chair, and began beating him with it! If Ned wanted to take me on, he was getting what he wanted. He insisted on making a childish mess wherever he wanted, leaving me the option of becoming more responsible for stopping him, or admitting to ineffectiveness. And so now I was doing my job. I was using every bit of my power, stopping him when he couldn't stop himself! He grabbed the other bataca and began to fight me.

The following dialogue took place amidst the noise of our beating each other with the pillow-like clubs.

Ned   Just stop. Just stop.

Len   I don't want to stop. I want you to clean the walls!

Ned   Never! Never! (puffing a bit). You don't want to stop?

Len   I've got to clean those damn walls now.

Ned   Oh, that's a lie. You're going to clean the wall? I just don't believe you. That isn't a wall. It feels good.

Len   You've been wanting to take me on.

Ned   You're not as tall as you used to be.

Len   Let's see who quits first.

Ned   Oh, hell, I'm not going to quit. Hey, are you really going to clean that wall?

Len   Look, at it.

Ned   I know.

Len   You won't clean it. I guess I've got to clean it.

Ned   I don't believe you. I don't believe you.

Len   You think I want to have a dirty wall in my office? You bastard!

Ned   I like it! I like it! You don't care what it looks like!

Len   I care what it looks like. It's my property.

Ned   It's not. It's your landlord's.

Len   He's renting it to me. And I want you to clean it!!

Ned   I haven't fought since grade school. Alright, I will clean it.

Len   I appreciate your taking the marks off the wall.

Ned   I was just standing up for myself.

Len   It may have felt that way to you, but you were infringing on my territory. You forced me to stand up for myself.

Ned   Yes.

Len   How do you feel now?

Ned   I'm still shaking. A little bit like it was a game. An important game to me. You really surprised me when you picked up that bataca.

Len   I was furious.

Ned   I had to stand up to you in some way.

Len   It felt to me like you were being spiteful because I wasn't taking care of you.

Ned   I wanted to hurt you.

While this session between Ned and me took place quite early in my career, before I had trained with nearly all the people I have written about in the book, I felt it was important to include. The session shows the early seeds of an undeveloped style of working–a style that is engaging and that has room for surprises. It is a style that includes risk taking with a faith that all will turn out well if the therapist can follow his or her sense of intuition as a way to work through whatever difficulties exist between patient and therapist. Much could have been explored in terms of the passive behavior of both Ned and myself that led to angry feelings and acting out. Although I clearly missed the issue several times, and had to deal with Ned's problem I finally directed the situation toward a resolution. Ned got to feel powerful and stand up to me. I did not give away power for him to feel good. I fought him as hard as I could. So in many respects while we were both acting as competitive children, we learned how to be two brothers who could feel good about each other–even after a difficult situation. An existential moment occurred in the bataca fight encounter.

Therapists will make mistakes along the road of developing an effective personal style. What is important, though, is that they keep an open mind and have the courage to risk what feels right between patient and therapist–even though, at times, it may be the working through of unresolved counter-transference issues on the part of the therapist. In this way, therapists, at least, will learn to make the best of a situation that did not begin well, and will develop their capacity to respond to the unexpected. And with continued experience, they will become better therapists.

I began developing a personal style by learning a philosophy–*existentialism*–about psychotherapy in graduate school. What I am presenting to you in this book does not come fully from the existential philosophy that I have studied, however. It is my creation and interpretation of what I learned by trial and error in the battlefield of psychotherapy.

Existentialism does not lead to a method of doing psychotherapy, but is a philosophy that has the following principles, all of which relate well to psychotherapy: (1) to be or not to be–the ability to enact all that one is at a particular moment in time, and having the *courage*, knowledge, skill, and experience to do so at finer and finer levels of discrimination; (2) people are *responsible* for the construction of their existence and "condemned" to freedom of choice in doing so; (3) there is a magical construction of emotions; (4) living the precise moment of being that one is experiencing; (5) adding meaning to one's existence; and (6) each moment encompasses *all* the possibilities of human existence within the limits of nature and circumstance. Existentialism allowed plenty of leeway to develop in whatever directions I chose. For example, how could I be interested in psychoanalysis and body therapy at the same time, and see them both as valid new directions for me?

Psychoanalysis becomes existential for me in this regard because I think more clearly and am able to interpret and respond to the moment more lucidly, while increasing my sense of personal presence by doing the above at closer and closer approximations to the here and now.

Body therapy deals with my being on different levels. Through existential awareness I can further develop physical being and expressiveness. For example, sensations may increase in the pelvic areas, tightness may be released from the shoulder areas. My feet become more firmly planted on the ground, and I can walk and move in ways that keep energy flowing through my body more naturally. I develop a more natural style of breathing.

(I would affect my ability to be or not to be.)

So bits of the truth exist in each of the therapies. For example, let's look at the *magical construction of emotions.* People construct their emotions to produce magical outcomes when reality frustrates their wants.

Transactional Analysis talks about *rubberbanding,* which means that people return to early feelings, get stuck in these feelings and live their current lives based on these old feelings. They call these old, stereotyped feelings "rackets." Chronically angry persons make their anger rackets into a way of life. People can learn to live without the anger racket, and thereby experience a new, more satisfying life. Albert Ellis, in Rational-Emotive Therapy, has an A B C D E method of challenging irrational belief systems that produce anger, depression, anxiety. My study of any of these therapies would thus be a furthering of my existential interest in dealing with the magic of emotions.

All the therapies are certainly within *all* the possibilities of human existence.

With this base I went about creating a way of doing psychotherapy with an openness to possibility that was responsible for the most meaningful personal changes in my life as well as an increasing therapeutic potency that helped me to help patients live more positive lives. I found that the more possibilities I incorporated into my existence, the greater the chances of beneficially affecting people. Once they were living positive, well-balanced and wholesome lives people could rejoice in their *freedom to be.* Many have said that they never knew they could feel that good.

The more I learned the better chance I would have when dealing with chronic patients, whether it be the trickster methods I learned from Milton Erickson, or using the aroused techniques of Walter Kempler or Albert Ellis. I have a particularly good feeling about reaching people who were previously regarded as hopeless cases.

The personal growth skills of Bob Martin, James Simkin, and Erv and Miriam Polster are a beauty to watch and experience. Martin Grotjahn helped me learn how to deal with narcissistic patients while Jack Rosberg stimulated ideas that helped with character disorders. Bob Goulding and Mary Goulding taught me how to provide an environment for redecision while tuning into the particular injunctions people were still paying attention to, such as, *don't be close,* or *don't exist.* Once people have made the decision to disobey an early parental injunction, they are then free to carry it out.

From George Bach I learned to structure situations that helped people use their aggression in ways that lead to positive action.

Stanley Keleman taught me how to tie in the existence of the body with the existence of the mind, and how to lead patients to create a new physical reality for themselves.

From Harold Greenwald I gained many insights about working with rebellious patients.

From Carl Whitaker I gained the permission to intervene in ways that often appear bizarre and outrageous to the patient's conscious frames of reference, but have such primal familiarity and impact that the patient's mind is likely to reverberate for weeks en route to the acceptance of the primal facts of that patient's existence. To do this kind of work I also learned compassion from Carl Whitaker.

From Wilfred Bion I learned about the impeccable abundance of enriched personal humanity.

Bill Ofman gave me the existential philosophical base from which I began to develop all else. So the first part of the book in a sense will start at step one. And that step is how the concept and actualization of an *existential moment* help me first and foremost, to do affective relationship therapy. Within the context of the authentic relationship I use many of the different methods that I learned from the therapists discussed in Part II of the book.

A very basic notion of the book is that authentic healing derives from an accumulation of authentic moments between patient and therapist, moments wherein the therapist is being genuine and unguarded. In a sense an existential moment is a refinement of an authentic moment, in that it is not only genuine, but of the quality of being that is likely to make a significant impression in affecting change in people. Within the flow of a relationship that is authentic, both patient and therapist will benefit, ultimately to the point of liberation.

This book is particularly intended to facilitate a liberation in the therapist. I hope that each reader of the book will be enhanced in developing a *free floating, intuitive, and empathic style of working, with increasingly accurate levels of clinical judgment.* I hope that the book will be an *inspiration for each individual to pursue a uniqueness in the development of a personal sense of being that will manifest itself in the artistic practice of a psychotherapy that will make a difference in peoples' lives.*

I

The Existential Moment

THE EXISTENTIAL MOMENT: In Part I of this book the existential moment may be defined in terms of encompassing as full a sense of being between patient and therapist as those two human beings are capable of experiencing. The focus of the moment, as it is applied to relationship therapy, deals with authenticity and the vulnerability that comes from two people facing each other as equal (I learned how to use authority over the next 40 years. General Howard, in the early 1990's invited me on two occasions to give workshops in authority and leadership to cadets at West Point. He was Supt. of Instruction participants in the human race involved in the joint venture of living.

However, the concept of the existential moment has broadened as I myself have grown. Thus there is an additional focus in Part II of the book: how the existential moment encompasses a variety of methods of therapy and personal styles used by experts in those methods of therapy. Within this context, the existential moment is defined as the unique, spontaneous actions and personal therapeutic methodology on the part of the therapist as they affect change in patients. This may include direct or indirect methods: when patient and therapist make a meaningful contact with each other; when patients make contact with alienated parts of their personalities; when patients come into contact with the environment in new ways; or when patients' minds are opened to a new way of experiencing themselves, others, the world. Existential moments may range from those that are touching or moving and influential in a positive manner, to those that are of such impact they turn peoples' lives around. Each of the moments enhances the quality of being of the patient in answering the question, "To be or not to be?"

THE EXISTENTIAL MOMENT

An interpersonal existential moment is a moment when two human beings drop any facades they may have presented to each other, capturing whatever exists within themselves and in relation to each other. This is not a moment that can be experienced by a reflection upon the moment, such as "now I am aware of . . . ." By the time both patient and therapist become aware of what they wanted to reflect upon, the moment would in most likelihood have passed. This is a moment that combines both the raw animal in humans with the compassion that is one's own humanity. It is a moment that is right on time.

Existential moments may occur when a person integrates alienated parts of his or her personality so there is a togetherness with self. While such moments can be seen in a variety of forms and therapeutic modalities, most of this chapter and the earlier parts of the book focus upon the interpersonal existential moment, primarily because this has been the most neglected and is at the core of all therapy.

In such moments both patient and therapist possess mutual respect for each other while maintaining a mystical feeling that feels spiritual in nature as a result of such an enriched contact.

Although there is much that is complexity in an existential moment, there is also a naive simplicity that gives the existential moment its beauty.

These have been moments that made me begin to realize there was something different, special and healing in them–apart from whatever else might be going on between a patient and myself during a therapy session. Here is an example of one such moment.

I remember going into a group as a co-therapist. The group had been meeting for about six months. One member of the group was in his late forties. He kept swinging his right arm, making a muscle, and letting everyone in the group know that he would punch anyone trying to get too close. Although this was only my second session in the group, there was something about this man that touched me deeply. I sensed this man's emotional starvation to be almost more severe than I could imagine. My instincts told me that he was bluffing about punching anyone. All I could feel was compassion for him. This compassion moved me to get up off my chair when he was swinging his arm and almost without realizing it, gently put my arm around his shoulder. At the same time I began to tell him that I could really sense his pain in being isolated and that even though he pretended to come across like a big mean ole bear, I could sense he was just a little pussy cat inside–and that I really liked him. He cried like a baby. He said, "I've been waiting twenty years for somebody to do that." I said, "You didn't make it easy!" (group laughed). That was the turning point in our relationship and in his relationships with other group members who were also touched by the moment. Both he and they were willing to make closer contact with each other.

Existential moments aren't necessarily moments that leave people teary; however, it happened this way for me on several occasions. This was particularly moving for me because I had a great deal of difficulty feeling at that level. I was not the type to cry or get teary easily. Many people, especially men, just isolate themselves, mistaking this isolation for freedom. They sublimate their feelings and harden themselves to such emotional starvation until they die of heart attacks, strokes, or other illnesses.

In this situation I had noticed a consistency of moments that not only captured the reality of the patient at that split second, but also the reality of the therapist. Those moments did make the critical difference in establishing a healing therapeutic relationship. A patient and therapist may experience one existential moment, and after awhile, another, and then another. Soon an authentic relationship will be developing and it is this authentic relationship which many existential therapists view as the healing ingredient in therapy. This authentic relationship, then, is but an accumulation of existential moments. Such moments leave both patient and therapist feeling truer about themselves and about their relationship. There is a double connection–with self, and with significant others. It is this connection that can either be a useful adjunct to many therapies of today, or be the basis of what I view as existential psychotherapy.

The raw desire, fear, anguish, love, anger, sadness and joy of therapist and patient may be experienced in a relationship. This moment is not a reflection upon a person's awareness, but is the capturing and expression of one's being at precisely the moment such passion becomes one with consciousness. There is no pre-meditation, no therapeutic strategy, no technique–only real being; the true expression of oneself as subject at precisely the moment that person experiences self. (Throughout Jean Paul Sartre's work, he referred to subject, object, etc.) When therapist and patient do this with each other, there exists for brief moments a subject-to-subject relationship. This is different than an object-to-subject relationship whereby the therapist views the patient as an object to be worked with. ALTHOUGH THE SUBJECT-OBJECT PART OF THERAPY CERTAINLY HAS ITS VALUE, IT IS THE SUBJECT-TO-SUBJECT TOUCHING OF TWO HUMANS THAT IS HEALING. Yet, as I stated before, it is often the most overlooked because it calls for greater degrees of vulnerability on the part of both therapist and patient. Part of the problem in experiencing existential moments is that most people have been successful in staying oblivious to themselves. A therapist who is continually evaluating what he or she is doing and what the patient is doing will be very aware of the therapy process but will have a hard time becoming free enough to experience an existential moment. Part of the therapy might be no more than therapist and patient enjoying talking to each other for pleasure's sake. That is one way a patient and therapist may work together.

If people are oblivious to themselves, they are not able to focus on their passions with the immediacy necessary to provide for a subject-to-subject moment that includes an almost mystical feeling–a touching of souls between two humans. Thus, many people have a great deal of difficulty in connecting with each other, whether it be on the verbal, physical, emotional or spiritual level.

This is why other therapies can use the inclusion of existential moments right within their foundation. These moments will provide patients with the opportunity to change from negative to positive lifestyles. This is not to say that other therapies or therapists do not provide such moments, but that many theoretical approaches ignore the moments in teaching a balanced mode of therapy. It has been my experience, however, that most effective therapists are providing the opportunity for patients to experience what I refer to as existential moments, possibly without being consciously aware of what they do to help people turn their lives around. One famous behavior modifier, who has written several books and given lectures and demonstrations all over the United States, said to me, "A patient said I really helped her. She said my work was fantastic. All I was aware of doing was sitting there and listening and making a few suggestions. I don't understand it." This therapist gave me the opportunity to observe on several occasions. What I noticed is that patients would light up when he looked at them a certain way. A warm smile would come over his face; his eyes would twinkle; his face would soften; and the patient would know that all was well. They were touched in this way. Even this therapist's technical errors didn't make any difference. This therapist created existential moments in his own way without using words. His words were often technical and a bit dry, although his particular technique is quite useful in many ways. THUS, I BEGAN TO FIND THAT *EXISTENTIAL MOMENTS OF CONNECTION* HAPPEN IN ALL EFFECTIVE THERAPIES, BUT MORE BY CHANCE THAN BY DESIGN.

Incorporating the concept of the existential moment into other methods of psychotherapy will reduce the possibility that the aspects of healing provided by an existential moment will be left to chance. This inclusion will help those therapists to connect more often with patients.

Therapists must know how to be authoritarian when called for, usually in the beginning of relationships; in many cases it is necessary to maintain the therapeutic level of authority throughout the course of therapy. The reverse of taking an authoritarian stance is also true, however. There are benefits to be gained from the development of an equal relationship between patient and therapist. Flexibility is often vital in order to maintain therapeutic authority while pursuing an egalitarian therapeutic relationship. Both authority and equality can exist side by side, or with the focus more on one than on the other, depending on the situation.

The inherent inequality of a patient coming to a therapist for help is difficult to overcome. However, surmounting this problem marks the difference between therapists being helpers or healers. It is only when human equality is at the forefront of the relationship that the therapeutic experience may be healing in both human and technical terms. The problem arises because patients have traditionally thought of doctors as godlike figures who know how to fix their ills. The last thing they may consciously be aware of looking for is equality in the therapeutic relationship. They are more likely to be in search of therapists who can cure their problem or who can promote a cathartic release that will feel good. In turn, therapists may have some unconscious fears about giving up all this power patients give to them. There is a type of security in such a relationship, although that security may be more of an illusion than a reality. I can recall two different stages in my development as a therapist. During the first I didn't have very many skills. I would tell people how I was reacting to them, but had a tendency to feel that being privy to more therapeutic technical skills would help me be more helpful to patients. This, of course, was true, as I found out with further study.

Yet, I found another type of problem that would get in the way of existential moments once my techniques became more proficient. When I was effective, I would get a euphoric feeling, as would the patients. Sometimes they viewed me as omnipotent and I chose to act that way. (To remedy this inflated ego issue, I have been carrying a little purple elephant with me that isn't impressed one way or the other by what I do.)

The question then becomes what happens to patients if the primary purpose of both patient and therapist is to feel elation without a connected and authentic relationship between them? The problem becomes one of whether the work is personal or not. In most cases patients have been willing to overlook the issue because they feel better. They may be used to giving away power. Therapists may feel an illusion of safety in relating to others in this manner. Neither has a need to disturb the omnipotent balance between them. The therapeutic artistry that helps patients feel better or solve their problems may be beautiful to watch, but without the personal touch, it only gets half the job done; that is, existential moments are not included as the more human half of the therapy between patients and therapists. However, such piecework doesn't necessarily help patients get connected in relationship. In addition, an inherent inequality between patients and therapists may be perpetuated. THE WAY OUT OF THE DILEMMA IS FOR THERAPISTS TO CONTINUE THEIR PERSONAL GROWTH EXPERIENCES UNTIL THEIR TECHNIQUE BECOMES INTEGRATED IN THEIR HUMANITY. AT THIS POINT THEIR INTERVENTIONS WILL BE STRATEGIC IN THAT THEY SPONTANEOUSLY COME FROM THE HEART. IN THIS WAY THERAPEUTIC TECHNIQUE WILL BE TEMPERED WITH ENRICHED HUMANITY. THE TECHNIQUES OF DIFFERENT THERAPIES AND THERAPISTS CAN HELP PULL PATIENTS THROUGH SOME TOUGH SPOTS. THE TRUE MEASURE OF THE THERAPIST'S ART IS APPROACHING THE ART FROM AS DEEPLY BASED A HUMANITY AS THAT THERAPIST MAY HAVE REACHED.

WORKING WITH CHILDREN

I am often asked whether the existential moment applies to working with children, and if so, how? A few examples follow. The common thread in these examples is that the children had an innocence that adults lack. They did not have to work through all the interference that adults accumulate in the process of growing up. They were raw humanity, and in most cases much easier to touch and be touched.

A very cool, isolated, and passive mother that I was working with asked me to see her five-year old son. She complained that the boy manifested her characteristics and was being beaten up at school. The boy was shy and clung onto his divorced mother during our first session. When they returned for a second session I remember that he had somehow touched me so that I wished I had a little boy like him. (I did not have any children.) His behavior indicated that he sought a close male relationship. When his mother asked if it were all right to leave the room he agreed. He came close and I asked him to sit on my lap. I hugged him as we talked. When we went to the waiting room after the session he ran up to me and kissed me good-bye. His mother was surprised. She said he rarely was affectionate. This affectionate moment between us helped the boy become confident and realize his lovableness. A few weeks later his mother reported that he wasn't being pushed around at school and that his teachers thought he had changed.

The existential moment was my telling him that I wished I had a son like him, and what I felt to be his unspoken message–that he wished I were his father.

I remember seeing a mother and her five- and seven-year-old daughters in family therapy. The mother and her husband were separated. The seven year old girl responded to her mother as if she were afraid to breathe in the wrong direction. Another situation arose between the five-year-old and myself. This girl was cute as a button and had been used to running the whole show, with total disrespect toward anyone else. She would do things such as throwing food she didn't like in her mother's face. Frankly, for the first few sessions I wasn't sure what to do with this little ball of power.

I set a few rules for the safety of both children. They enjoyed fighting with batacas, the purpose of which was to express their aggression toward each other in a safe way. However, the five-year-old kept breaking the rule that she was not to hit her sister in the face with her shoe. She was told that was a dangerous thing to do. She absolutely refused. She went on swinging her shoe at her sister as if I had not mentioned the rule. Finally, I got so frustrated I felt the only way I could stop her was with physical restraint. I grabbed her and held her by her feet and wrists while she flailed away, screaming at the top of her lungs. The battle persisted for some thirty-five minutes with both the little girl and myself using every bit of power and energy we had in the struggle. She would not quit. It was important for her to learn to deal with limits but I didn't realize it was going to be so difficult to teach her! She gave it her all, to the point where she excreted gas. She was screaming for her mother to help her about mid-way through the session. To take care of what I sensed to be the child's fright at the situation she had created, I told her mother to pat her head and tell her she loved her. At the end of thirty-five minutes she fell asleep, totally out of energy. I felt like doing the same thing, but was still in the midst of a therapy session with the mother. At the end of the fifty-minute hour, I went over to wake the five-year old. She grunted and looked very displeased to see me. I gave her a big kiss, telling her that I still loved her. She looked stunned. She didn't seem the forgiving type–at least not so soon. Her only response was another grunt. However, this battle between two people was the turning point in the therapy. *At some level she appreciated me for caring enough to set the limits.* That battle was the existential moments, and a turning point in the therapy. The problem with being selfish is that it does not work; the selfish person winds up getting short-changed, but this usually only leads them to the wrong conclusion–that they must be more selfish. Thus, the little girl had cut off her needs for contact because she knew she would not get them met anyway.

After this session the little girl began to compromise, but the process was a slow and tedious one. She wasn't used to taking other peoples' needs into consideration, but she felt enough for me to give it an honest try.

On another occasion, I was working with my five-year-old's sister, the shy seven-year-old. She and I were having fun with each other. I can remember an existential moment that I enjoyed very much. I had just moved into a new office that had not been decorated. The seven-year-old said that a picture would look good over my fireplace. I agreed, but suggested that since I did not have one, I put her on top of the mantlepiece instead. I told her she looked great up there and that she was much more interesting than an old picture. She could move in all different positions. Then I told her I wanted to hire her for two days a week to sit on top of my fireplace. She suggested I ask her mom. It was clear she did not like the idea, but was reluctant to say so. I called her mom in and made my offer. Her mom and I laughed, while she did not know whether to take this absurd sounding proposal seriously. Finally she said: "Take me down off this fireplace. I don't want the job." We both laughed and hugged each other. We played. We had fun. The outcome was that she used her power in relationship to me and her face glowed when she did so. She felt quite proud of herself. My love for her continued to grow until she felt very special to me, and I was able to convey that feeling to her. Her feeling of being special helped her to become more confident, and it showed!

While working with a four-year-old girl who looked as intimidated as anyone I have every seen, but who had the hidden strength of a forty-two foot long mouse, I experienced an interesting series of moments. Cathy kept her face buried in my chair. She would not talk or react. I told her I wanted to play with her as it would be a long hour if we both just sat around. She couldn't have cared less. However, after a bit she became restless and banged her feet one after the other. This was the first action she took in my office. I felt this might be an opportunity to connect. I banged my feet down one after the other. She banged her feet to the rhythm of one, two, three. I did the same. Now we were creating different rhythms, and seeing if the other could match the rhythms. Before the session was over we were both dancing joyfully around the room, beating to different rhythms, having a great time! I was meeting Cathy on her level, having childlike fun. Having childlike fun is also a primary adult pleasure in life, so it did as much for me as for Cathy. I found that when I began to temper *my* self-interest, which was to enjoy the hour, by caring about this little girl who was hard to care about, the situation turned out to be good for both parties. We were both doing exactly what we wanted to do and neither felt any resentment toward the other.

I have given examples about working with children in this first chapter because it is the human qualities that go into the makeup of existential moments. Children are less removed from their humanity as a result of their newness to the world's conditioning process. For the most part they find it a bit easier than adults to reach out in a *fresh way* and touch.

SELF-DISCLOSURE

One of the important facets of existential moments is the therapist's sharing his or her own experience. Such sharing is closely related to self-disclosure, which reminds me of my first meeting with Dr. Sidney Jourard.

I was a graduate student when Sid flew in from Florida to give a workshop on self-disclosure to a group of marriage and family counselors. I remember the group asking him very personal questions. He would not answer any of their questions but kept asking them to ask him another question. Why was this man who wrote two books about self-disclosure and transparency refusing to answer any questions? The more he refused, the angrier became the audience. After his evening presentation, there was a party where he drank a lot of beer and belched very loudly several times. People kept looking at him belching and wondering about this strange man. I liked him. The message he was sending was that he was not about to let himself be raped in the name of "self-disclosure." He said he felt we needed to know more about privacy and proceeded to talk about privacy instead of self-disclosure. People need private space and should not be expected to disclose themselves to people with whom they are not intimate. I was eager to learn, but the workshop would be over Sunday morning. I told him I wanted to buy an hour of his time. He replied that he would not sell me any of his time but that he would talk to me about whatever I wanted at his cottage for the weekend. I had nothing like what I expected in terms of a conventional therapy session. It was a beautifully sunny day, and we chatted on the porch over a bottle of wine. He was one who would just talk to people. When I told him I wanted to experience him as a therapist he told me he had nothing to teach me. I was a little slow to pick up that paradox, as he was indeed teaching me something–how to talk to people in the same natural way in which he was talking to me. He disclosed personal things which he felt were appropriate in the context of our relationship. I enjoyed myself on the two occasions I was with him and was quite saddened to learn of his death a few years back. There was an easy flow about him. I began to balance self-disclosure with privacy and the feeling of just talking to people as people, that is, without the therapist-patient barrier. Sid was very helpful to me in learning one side of the paradox of being a therapist–that two people should probably talk to each other as two people would normally talk to each other, and that this authenticity of relationship would be healing.

However, as I also experienced differing degrees of intensity in relationships, I realized that a *therapist's vulnerability* was a factor in regard to self-disclosure. I experimented with Sid's ideas about self-disclosure by being more vulnerable as my relationship deepened with patients. I began to see that vulnerability on the part of the therapist was critical in helping patients to let their humanity unfold, and in reaching the kind of existential moments that go right to the heart and or guts of people.

Within the context of an authentic relationship, such vulnerability and gut-level sharing has helped patients delve deeper into their inner experiences. Patients are able to go to their core levels with increasing frequency, and gradually can begin to experience the full range of human emotions. They can begin to move in the direction of *unity;* of becoming one with themselves.

Such *unity* is an ever-increasing process of growth throughout people's lives. It is a process whereby people continue to integrate the alienated parts of their personalities. At first unity leads to the formation of an identity, and integrity. Once patients can maintain integrity, this unity can lead to *creativity.*

Unity can be experienced in the quality of peoples' responses. The quality of people's responses (authentic, unity, enriched humanity, etc.) will either (1) facilitate growth in themselves and those with whom they come in contact, (2) have no effect at all, or (3) have a detrimental effect. In the case of therapists, the *quality of their responses* are of even greater importance because these responses are the nature of the therapeutic business. When the quality of response is full, it is more likely that patients will experience an existential moment.

The quality of response of therapists are contingent upon the degree of *unity* or harmony those therapists have achieved within themselves; and further, upon their ability to act on what they have integrated in terms of their personalities. So, therapists must have unraveled enough truths about themselves so they do not fall victim to their own problems (although this process of working through one's countertransference is a lifetime job). It is hoped that therapists will continue their search in a spirit of openness so they will not only be able to maintain integrity, but also to help patients create new realities for themselves whereby patients can live fuller and richer lives. So a *basic goal of an existentially-oriented therapy is the reduction of duplicity (failure to be behind one's words)* in people. Stated positively, the pursuit of a wholeness or unity of self. Therapists must be able to reduce the gap between their inner sense of being–of who they are at the very center of their guts, and of who they represent themselves to be to the world and to themselves. In other words, they must be able to reduce the false images they have of themselves so they will both accept themselves and then present themselves as they are. When therapists and patients lie to themselves and others often enough that they lose themselves. They lose themselves on two counts: first, the ability to be centered–to be who they are and speak from their guts and second, to possess enough self-knowledge so they have a foundation from which to create freer, happier and more meaningful realities for themselves. It is only with the reduction of duplicity that therapists and patients will learn to experience existential moments–moments whereby they are in non-conflicted integrated contact with themselves and with others to whom they are relating. This is not to say that they will never have internal conflicts, but that they will have worked through enough conflicts to become familiar with their own process of what they are doing, and be able to increase the levels and depth of honest contact with self and others.

In order that existentially-oriented therapists may help facilitate patients in their pursuit of unity, therapists may want to understand three basic phases of being and then bring these phases into balance in their lives. The three phases of being refer to Keen's (1970) adaption of Sartre's existential philosophy as expressed throughout one of his major works, *Being and Nothingness,* Part 3, (New York: Philosophical Library, 1956), chap. 2.

The more these three phases of being come into harmony with each other, the more unity will occur and the more often patients and therapists will be able to experience the existential moments that are healing.

People may experience their being on three levels. Although the three are separated there is a constant interaction among them. It is when the balance among the three levels of being becomes disjointed that patients may get into difficulties with self, others and reality.

Ernest Keen (1970) deals with the three phases of being in the following manner:

A. *Being-in-the-world.* We are, first, in the sense that we are desire, fear, thought, etc., of something that is implicitly seen as outside ourselves. This way of being entails an experience of oneself-as-subject: I desire a steak; I fear a germ; I think of an idea.

B. *Being-for-myself.* We are, second, in the sense that we represent what we are to ourselves. This aspect of our being entails the experience of oneself-as-object. We reflect upon *our desires, fears, and thoughts,* name them, judge them, reason about them, and have feelings about them. Furthermore, I am a 'me' to myself, with certain attributes and characteristics. With dispassionate detachment, I can, upon reflection, do everything to myself that I can do to the world. The content of this process is a second activity of being.

C. *Being-for-others.* We are, third, in the sense of presenting ourselves to others, anticipating what others are thinking or feeling about us and guiding our externally observed behavior so as to have a certain kind of effect on others, to make a certain kind of impression.[1]Keen, while still referring to the three modes of being, comments that there are three kinds of data that feed into experience: "(a) the data of the world that is implicitly referred to 'my' point of view, (b) the data of myself as I objectify myself for my own scrutiny and (c) data as fed back to me through my interpretation of other interpretation of me."[2]Each of us, therapists as well as patients, deals with the three modes of being in whatever way seems to make most sense to us; however, the implicit problem in all three is *the lie*. Let us look at a few examples of the ways in which people lie, thereby preventing themselves from experiencing existential moments.

From early childhood we learn what it is that pleases Mommy and Daddy. We learn what they want us to be in the world. How can we get what we want when facing more powerful adversaries such as parents, and others as we get older? Lying is a choice that may equalize our power. We may learn to read into what people want from us and learn to live up to their expectations. We may feel this will help us to avoid loneliness, emptiness, conflict, and anxiety. We hope this will ensure that people will like us. The problem with all this is that one lie begets another. Soon we have a complex network of lies built up over the years which we are in a position of having to defend. So, *lying for* others leads us to begin to lie for ourselves. Each of us has a self-concept. We may feel that we are "good" boys and girls, and later will become "good" citizens, husbands, wives, etc. If we know what people expect of us and deceive them into believing that we are who they expect and want us to be instead of who we really are, we may get to feel guilty–to feel bad about ourselves. We may then begin to lie-for-ourselves to escape facing the consequence of our lies, lies that will ultimately lead to inner conflicts. This may leave us feeling that our guts are rotting away and we don't know what is causing the problem.

In order to maintain a "good" self-image, people may live up to this idealized self as opposed to paying attention to their own thoughts and feelings. Once we have an idealized image we feel guilt if we do not live up to it. We may attempt to avoid guilt by doing good works. Those works or intentions may lead to self-torture. We may develop expectations of ourselves that we can never fulfill, thereby continuing to torture ourselves, unless we do not continue along the path of self-deception and give up the image of who we should be.

In addition to lying-for-others and lying-for-oneself, a third type of lie involves *misrepresentating the world* to oneself. We attempt to avoid anxiety of unpleasant realities by perceiving reality in a way that may be more palatable. However, distortion of reality may leave us closed to experiencing life to its fullest. We may make ourselves dead in the process.

Keen comments that "lying-in-the-world" is a way of not facing reality. For the child to experience him or herself-as-subject in a way that does not permit true self-expression is to begin on the road of alienation. The question is not whether the child should feel free to act out spontaneous feelings because murderous or suicidal impulses in action are not good. The question is whether these impulses and feelings are experienced as subject; whether this fact of life, which impinges upon one's "being-in-the-world," is integrated into the interaction of the individual's three phases of being or lost in the morass of interferences that come from various sorts of lies.

The resulting loss of openness to experience yields a loss of contact with this aspect of reality which in turn, yields a loss of ability to bring it under the control of conscious choice, that is, to see options in what to do with feelings. Frustration is inevitable under these circumstances, for one does not know what one wants or where one is going. As in the cases of shame and guilt, frustration may remain as a conscious experience without the particular lies that underlie it being at all apparent. One is therefore left with vague feelings of unhappiness with all sorts of lies-for-oneself and lies-for-others covering up that aspect of the given that is not being faced.[3]Let us pause a moment and look at how the three types of lies may affect a relationship. If people lie for others, or lie to please others when their consciences tell them that their behavior is not in their best interests, they will build up anger and resentment toward others, or will wind up feeling depressed. In either case, they will have a desire to withdraw from other people. Those who lie to please others lose their integrity–their sense of being centered in themselves, and may prove to be emotionally unreliable. They may not take care of their own needs and may not have the self-support necessary to gain support from others in a relationship. These people tend to be referred to as mediocre people by others, and do not see themselves as winners in life. They are viewed as either survivors or losers by others, depending upon the extent to which the person engages in being for others.

Lying for oneself, or misrepresenting the world to oneself, leaves a person responding to fantasy rather than reality in relationships. Such people are more interested in maintaining their self-image rather than bringing real joy and creativity to their lives. These people struggle to make their relationships work, but tend to claim it is the other person's fault when the relationship doesn't work. When the next relationship doesn't work, it again is the other person's fault. The merry-go-round continues, and these people have a great deal of difficulty facing themselves in a way that will permit them to put their awareness into action to change their lives and make their relationships positive. These people tend to deny honest confrontation on the part of the other person. Their denial leaves them feeling justifiably correct and scornful toward the other. Their relationships fail when the person on the bottom end of the relationship gets to a point of feeling as if they are going to suffocate.

The third type of lying, *lying in the world,* leaves people attempting to use their relationships to provide a false sense of security in the world. The world is a place where we are faced with the unknown. We are thrown into the world naked, and to some degree that reality never changes. However, the discomfort that people experience from such unprotected exposure leaves people feeling that if they could only find a secure relationship, the answer to their insecure world will be over. These people tend to engage in all varieties of destructive behavior. Manipulation and control may appear on both sides of a relationship. What begins as a quest for a false sense of security through a relationship may turn out to be the very thing both people feared most–a relationship in which both parties cannot continue to survive and to grow in productive ways–a relationship that ends up in the divorce court.

An awareness of unity to help reduce lies is critical if people are to become whole persons who are able to relate both to themselves and to their relationship partners. If this unity is not approached, and if the three modes of lying become the way of dealing with the three phases of being, the negative consequences may start people enroute to the therapist's office.

On the other hand, a unity and balance among the three modes of being, and a reduction in lies to ourselves, others, and about reality will help bring about a togetherness within each person necessary to continue the mission in life–that of becoming a whole person. In this way they increase their opportunities to engage in permanent and meaningful relationships with others. It is when therapists can deal with themselves in this way that they can engage in sustained and authentic relationships with their patients. It is in the context of such a therapeutic relationship that patients may learn to carry their learning over to people other than the therapist.

While therapists are talking with patients about what concerns those patients, therapists may use the time to assess the balance patients are able to maintain among the three modes of being. While patients may be telling a story about their difficulties, it is these same difficulties in relationships that patients will also manifest in the therapeutic relationship. Patients' tales of woe are usually a sneak preview of the kinds of issues that therapists may at another time choose to respond to in the therapeutic relationship.

One such sneak preview can be seen with Jerry, a patient who was going through the trauma of his second divorce. The following is a dialogue that took place between Jerry and me. The example shows the existential approach in terms of the therapist's dealing with the *semantics of responsible involvement on the part of the patient*. The patient caught himself in a variety of the three modes of lying by partaking in irresponsible involvement. So the therapy must redirect the focus to help patients get back to the core of themselves.

Jerry	I had great difficulty ending the relationship with my first wife because I felt put upon (victim position), and yet I found some way to rationalize or excuse her actions (lying to oneself about the nature of reality). I stuck around much longer than I was comfortable doing. I stuck around even though I'd say I wasn't entirely willing to stick around (irresponsible statement–Jerry wasn't doing anything he didn't want to do.) Finally I became so disgusted with that relationship that I walked out. Then, with my second wife, looking back at

this point, I'm sure the relationship was over, for all practical purposes, at least three or four years ago. I kept telling myself that I was in love with her and that I could work it out, and she kept becoming more and more angry each time we had a verbal argument. (Jerry was lying to himself about the nature of his reality in order to try to keep a dead relationship going.) I wanted to hang on because I felt the need to be loved. I guess I kidded myself into believing that she loved me more than she did.

Me So you would change reality around in your head to make it look like you wanted.

Jerry Yeah. I'm sure I did. I kept saying I loved her and I needed her and I wanted her back. The more I said that, the more she wanted to go the other way.

Me You said your reason for hanging on was that you needed to feel loved.

Jerry I needed to feel loved, and for some reason I did not want to start a new relationship.

Me How come?

Jerry Well, I'd say there are several reasons–first of all, by a religious background, I felt that marriage without divorce was a desirable thing– and of course, I had been through one divorce. Even though I was divorced, there were certain things that were said within the Church that let me know other people in that church did not approve of the fact that I was divorced.

Me So with the cultural, societal, and religious values that were a part of your past, you boxed yourself in. (This is where Jerry felt it was important to lie to himself so he could lie about the nature of his reality to others–so he could be how they expected him to be–so he could adopt their values instead of creating values that fit his reality. Also, Jerry has a low level of self-acceptance because he does not fit his image of a "good person"–someone who can live by all the values of his church.)

Jerry

I must say that my experience in business was confining. I found that to get ahead, you had to pretty well be the "happily-married" person. Also, the store managers who worked for me often had extramarital affairs that cost the company money. Consequently there was a great deal of pressure brought to try and keep these people from having extramarital arrangements. And if they got into them, then it was well known that it was not approved, and it could cost them their job. From the economic pressures, the business pressures as well as the religious and social pressures, I learned that first, I should be married and second, there was no excuse for not being married.

Me

All these factors made it difficult for you to end a relationship.

Jerry

Ya, because I have had all these things as teachings. It's kind of like being in the military service. They do all this close-ordered drill to try to imbreed into the person that orders are to be taken without stopping to question whether or not the order is correct. I have had this stuff drilled into me for so long. And of course the other part was the insecurity I had grown up with.

The preceding example is included to show how duplicity with oneself, reality, and others, can lead to the destruction of interpersonal relationships.

You can see from this dialogue how Jerry deluded himself and why keeping himself apart from reality worked to his detriment. Each of the lies helped Jerry box himself in and make his world tighter and smaller. Jerry used his past religious teachings in a neurotic way–to cop out on being true to himself. The problem with these lies is that the liar eventually loses himself.

All one really needs to know is oneself and the rest will fall into place. In whatever area of life, relationships are dependent upon how much unity exists within patients and how well they are balanced among the three modes of being. For it is this unity and balance that people call forth when attempting to respond as authentically as they can at any given moment, and it is this unity and balance that ultimately results in the creation of existential moments.

Therapists who respond with unity will help patients to develop a therapeutic relationship that has mutual respect; that is, a relationship that has integrity and may later help facilitate the creation of new realities. This kind of relationship may help patients regain any loss of integrity through participation in a relationship that has ever-increasing levels of equality.

The kind of relationship that I am describing between patient and therapist hits at the heart of the matter–that is, two people, in a room, facing each other superceding the facade of doctor and patient, although the reality of this paradox remains. The primary issue is that two people are being real with each other. It is within this context that other therapies, in which therapists are more clearly viewed as doctors, may be practiced with a more human touch.

Both therapists and patients surely must endure the commonalities of being human. They must endure the anguish of not really knowing how other people will respond to them. They must endure the anxiety of living in a world that is quite unpredictable. They must live with the fact of their existence–that they both were born, will live and will die. They must individually figure out how they will respond to the limits of life and death, and how to deal with the issues of their absolute freedom and responsibility in response to a determined set of facts. Each has a particular set of parents, a unique socio-economic background, different educational experience, etc. Both must grapple with the issue of how to create meaning in their lives, and how to relate to others, if that is part of how they choose to add meaning to their lives.

Although the focus has customarily been on the therapist being the healing agent, and the patient being the one with the problem to be solved or healed, such a focus may tend to either ignore or obscure the fact that both are in the situation of existence in the world together. Quite possibly the therapist may have learned to survive in the world by maintaining a one-up position over others, if that therapist's humanity hasn't developed to a level where he or she can do otherwise. Yet, while it appears that such a therapist is in a superior position to the patient, might not this situation be viewed from another angle? Although the patient is the one who complains of hurting, doesn't this patient display strength by a willingness to share personal difficulties with the therapist? A difficulty may arise if the patient's strength has come from learning to play a different game–that of being inferior (although this also applies to patients who act arrogantly to cover up feelings of inferiority). The issue may very well be that both therapist and patient are wearing masks. Both may be equally skilled at their respective roles. Thus, the contest may really be an equal one from the start, although neither may view it that way if they keep the self-images they have chosen. In such situations, being genuine in an equal way becomes critically important because the hoped-for result of therapy cannot be achieved unless both give up their roles. Patients are often reluctant to give up their roles unless therapists do so first.

Therapists should approach patients with humility for two reasons. The first and most valid is a humility that grows from therapists' compassion for humanity as a result of their equal participation in the world. If therapists have not reached such levels of compassion within themselves, however, they may still approach patients with humility for a second and more strategic reason: therapists may want to approach patients with the same humility one would show to an opponent who is equally good at playing chess. In these cases both therapists and patients are masters at maintaining the unequal relationship as a way of maintaining interpersonal distance and self deception.

While it is true that each mode of therapy is healing in many respects, it is also true that this concept of equality based on a deepened humanity may strengthen other modes of therapy. Sometimes this takes place even though there is not a direct focus on equality. In these cases the humanity of the therapists has matured to a level where it just happens no matter what kind of therapy they are doing. In other cases, it might be well to intentionally focus on equality. Otherwise both therapist and patient might perpetuate the false images they have developed of themselves.

It is when therapists and patients are able to be genuine with each other, when both drop any facades they are maintaining and share in the reality of the human condition, that a more enriched healing takes place. It is such a process that paves the way for the deepest of existential moments at the gut level, and it is the successive accumulation of these existential moments, when therapists and patients are genuine with each other, that helps to form the authentic relationship. An authentic relationship, composed of existential moments, when two people are genuine with each other, and experiencing the reality of the human condition with humility in a mutual way, is healing at the deepest levels.

I view the "human condition" as one in which people are complex in themselves, and in relationship to others as well as environment. They are imperfect and are left with relationships that leave people wanting. They must learn to live in the world of reality by giving up idealized infantile wishes about what reality should be and by giving up idealized images of what relationships should be. They must realize that satisfaction must first come from within, and then satisfaction can come from relationships with others. They must not count on others to satisfy all their needs, but must learn to accept the nature of reality, of others, and avoid punishing them for not meeting unrealistic expectations. People must learn to live with the anxiety that is aroused by the knowledge, either conscious or unconscious, of impending death–of non-existence. They must learn to live with the anxiety of not being able to control the free responses of others, and of being in a position whereby the subjective responses of others may at any time be more hurtful than they would like. To fully experience being alive, people must open themselves to experience as much as they dare–joy, sadness, fear, anger, love, affection, and empathic and spiritual concerns. It is when such emotions travel from the realm of the intellect and reunite with the body that people increase a zest for life! They must learn to deal with both cutthroat competitiveness and a sense of social cooperativeness based on human concern. They must struggle with the realization that they are condemned to absolute freedom, must understand the construction of their existence, and witness the anxiety that such awesome responsibility brings to them. They must cope with self-deception which keeps them from realizing their full potential and must assume their full power in responding to the world in a responsible way. Peoples' honesty with self and others, and their ability to act autonomously in choosing to be honest, all affect the ongoing process and the outcome of their lives. Their choice of awareness level provide them with options from which they may choose to either limit or stretch their boundaries. People are not an entity unto themselves but live in relation to the world and to others. It is their way of choosing to relate that determines who they are and how limited or expansive they may become. Such contact with self, others, and environment may alleviate some basic human solitude–the stark naked aloneness of the human condition. Contact–action–connectedness–these are all keys to how man may create meaning in his life–a life that moves toward a balance with itself and in relation to others and environment. Peter Marin, a writer, poet, and educator, says:

> Wholeness of vision rests upon more than good will; it depends, in part, upon the previous experience of relation: at least some small sense of connectedness that remains in the flesh as a sense of what is possible. Unless we have tasted, however briefly, the grave delight of a wholeness felt as the natural state of things, we cannot know precisely what is wrong with the fragmentation of vision or how to set it right.[4]

As Marin indicates, experiencing wholeness of who one is and the human condition is related to wholeness of vision. Yet, the wholeness of this vision is limited by past experience in relation to self, others, and environment. The sense of connectedness as experienced by the flesh, to which Marin refers, can be increased by therapists who have already widened their horizons. This is how therapy gets tied into a deeper reality–by the levels of connectedness therapists have experienced and their ability to make such options available to the patient via the avenues of experience, freedom, choice, and assumption of responsibility. Such connectedness and freedom of choice of the individual may permit that individual to develop his or her power to the degree that he or she can move "from the privacy of relation to the community of action–and still keep intact the ground of all meaning; our moment-by-moment connection to live."[5]

This is, as I see it, the reality that exists for both therapist and patient, and unless it is fully acknowledged between them, they will be less than whole in their relations. The human condition can only be preserved in therapy if the therapist is willing to be genuine. It is the building of a therapeutic alliance with a patient that is based upon such authenticity of relations that provides for the deepest levels of healing.

The kind of relationship that I am describing between patient and therapist can be something spiritual. Yet, when I attempt to describe a relationship that touches and expands the depths of human existence, that touches at the grass roots of the real issue–the issue of life or death or balance between the two that is chosen by a patient, it is extremely difficult to present more than a vague picture. Words do not do justice to such an experience.

A therapist does not pursue the spiritual at the expense of the real, however. In fact, it is the dogged pursuit of the real that allows one to experience the spiritual. The following example may illustrate what I mean.

A woman came to me for a double session after her grandfather died. When she began talking she moved me deeply and I found myself beginning to cry. I realized that I had never said goodbye to my grandmother who had died some thirteen years before. I was surprised that this just happened. When we talked about our respective grandparents she and I had a common experience. She and I were both our grandparent's favorite. Each of our dead grandparents had given us that unconditional positive love that provided us with a self-love and deep inner strength. Somehow we both knew we could reach back in times of trouble and tap the inner strength and love that came from the love transmitted to us by our grandparents. It helped us both deal with our insecurities. While we were sharing this existential moment she and I were also relating to each other as our respective grandparents had related to us. That special kind of love left us feeling that our souls were touching. We made a contract. If either of us were ever to become lost inside we would call the other and the other would remind the troubled one of how really special a person he or she was to the respective grandparent. At the end of the session, I wrote her a check for two sessions because I felt she had affected me as much as I affected her.

For those moments an enriched equality of relationship and mutual love existed between us that left me feeling both touched and re-vitalized. She never cashed the check, saying that it was worth far more to her hung on her bedroom mirror where it continually reminded her of how special she was to her grandfather and how our souls had touched!

It is the sharing of the therapist's weaknesses, fears, desires, lies, vulnerabilities, and methods of controlling others that makes him or her believable. It is his or her willingness to look at personal weaknesses while with patients that creates an atmosphere of equality between two humans. Without a therapist's willingness to share, that therapist only makes a pretense about the equality of two humans. The therapist is privy to special knowledge about the patient. However, when a therapist admits to a weakness, that relationship takes on a quality that makes a search to the core of human existence possible. The equality of the relationship and the therapist's sharing of him or herself helps to demystify the term psychotherapy. The therapist's own openness to this process provides a growth model for the patient. Rather than being a charlatan, of which many initially-misunderstanding patients may accuse the therapist, the therapist is doing the most loving thing he or she can do–providing living proof that the therapy process works as the patient can see the therapist's honest confrontations with self that will make it easier for the patient to unravel whatever truth emerges, while the patient also feels accepting of and good about him or herself. Such an accepting environment provided by the therapist creates a climate in which the patient feels safe and free enough to choose appropriate behavior in the context of that patient's current reality. When patients can see themselves making changes, one step at a time, to take control over their lives and create the best life they can, life becomes hopeful.

ENDNOTES

[1] Ernest Keen, Three Faces of Being: Toward an Existential Clinical Psychology (New York: Appleton-Century-Crofts, Meredith Corporation, 1970), pp. 27-28.

[2] Ibid.

[3] Ibid., p. 50.

[4] Peter Marin, "The human harvest," Mother Jones (December, 1976), p. 38.

[5] Ibid., p. 52.

REFERENCES

Keen, Ernest. *Three Faces of Being: Toward an Existential Clinical Psychology.* New York: Appleton-Century-Crofts, Meredith Corporation, 1970.

Marin, Peter. "The human harvest." *Mother Jones,* December, 1976.

2

From Theory to Style: Developing an Existential Point of View with William Ofman, Ph.D.

ALTHOUGH THIS IS a book about existential moments and the applicability of these moments to a variety of therapies (one of which is existential therapy) to increase their healing capacities, these moments would not have been apparent to me if I had not viewed therapy, reality, and the human condition through the eyes of existential philosophy. The problem I had in doing this, however, was that existential philosophy was quite removed from the pragmatics of psychotherapy. Most of the existential writers, therapists and philosophers have remained distant from existentialism's practical application. However, two therapist-authors have existential ways of viewing the roots of therapy that are similar to my own, and I will quote Drs. Kempler and Ofman extensively to help to lay out a philosophical format from which I will build a mode of practicing psychotherapy.

But first I will share some of my viewpoints. I see people as undetermined in a deterministic world. Of course, it is a matter of degree and a matter of emphasis, but people are free to choose their existence and capable of transcending themselves in response to deterministic limits. The problem is that people lie to themselves about the degrees of freedom that they have with which to choose their lives, thereby creating much of the technology for their own misery by establishing a false set of limitations.

My approach to consciousness is phenomenological in that it is based upon immediate experience. My therapy is concerned with the "here and now." I view the central issue of people in terms of being or non-being. The basic question is "to be or not to be?" I feel that while people are responsible for all that they choose, they are also responsible at a moral level to choose responsibly so that their choices will be beneficial for both themselves and society in its entirety. Such choices come from a deepened humanity that has a spirit of compassion, fellowship, kindness, and consideration for others.

Existentialism is a hopeful philosophy because it makes patients aware that they can have a response. Their choices count, and they can choose new alternatives that will at least give them a sense of integrity, and at most be responsible for freer, happier, and healthier living. Even if people cannot change their physical and environmental situation, they nonetheless can determine their response to that situation. I remember Dr. Victor Frankl who spoke at a California Personnel and Guidance Convention in San Diego, California, talking about a woman who was going to be raped and used by the Nazis before being sent to her final destination–the gas chamber. While many prisoners chose to ignore the reality that was before them, this woman, while dancing nude at the request of the Nazis, began spinning around towards a guard, grabbed his gun, and shot him–at which point she was machine-gunned to death. Not a happy ending, but she died on her terms–and not the terms of those who would attempt to deny her the integrity of choice. She had the courage to be. She had the courage to respond. The fact that people are free to choose their existence and cannot escape from doing so is liberating! It is a hopeful philosophy–a philosophy and a therapy that gives the vote to the people.

An existential view gives a feeling of freedom to the therapy. The primary question with which therapists deal is To be or not to be?

both in themselves and in their patients. Existential therapy views the problem as the quality of being manifested by the patient. By "quality of being manifested" I mean enriched versus impoverished; i.e., that patients are able to experience themselves as deeply as possible as opposed to cutting themselves off from experience of self and others, while creating meaning, joy, and zest for living that come from paying attention to their inner nature as a basis from which to choose. Such a philosophical perspective is no excuse for therapists to avoid learning as many techniques and skills as they are able, so they may combine therapeutic artistry within the context of an existential framework, while being primarily interested in the patient's quality of being. In this way they will be able to communicate in a pragmatic way with patients. They will be able to help patients with immediate problems until patients develop a perspective that allows them to examine the quality of their being and their lives.

Although I never had the opportunity to meet Fritz Perls, I've heard the stories that therapists tell about him. Most of the stories center around his responsiveness, or his being all that he could be at any given moment. I began to wonder what made him so unusual that other therapists would continually talk about him. Some say he was a loving man. Others say he was a cold and cruel man. He used four-letter words which many people found offensive. He believed that helpers were con men who kept people dependent and immature. I began to think of him as a man of action rather than words.

A man told me of his first workshop with Fritz. He said that he went before the group to sit in the "hotseat" and Perls dismissed him, saying, "You are a good little boy. Go away." The man said he felt crushed and could not understand why Fritz said that. In retrospect, he realized Fritz helped him break through his good-little-boy behavior (as opposed to saying his thoughts and feelings) to make a decision to live differently.

Dr. Jim Simkin, a gestalt therapist who worked closely with Fritz, told me about Fritz working with a woman who "was convinced that he knew the answer to a question she kept asking him. He confronted her dramatically, once, with: 'What, and rob you of the pleasure of finding out for yourself? No, I like you too much to do that to you.'"

Both stories contain a quality of free responsiveness by Perls. They were existential moments in that they created an experience between himself and the significant other or others. He did not reflect upon the moment but captured the fullness of his being through his responsiveness. Needless to say, his responses were controversial.

These stories and other experiences that happened to me along the way made me wonder what it was about certain people that affect others so beneficially.

While a graduate student finishing up my dissertation, I was invited to a Christmas party at Dr. George Bach's house. Dr. Bach is a clinical psychologist and co-author of several books, one of which is *Creative Aggression,* which he co-authored with Dr. Herb Goldberg. When I met him he came up to me, put his arm around my shoulder, and in a playfully aggressive manner that took me somewhat aback, asked me who I was and what I was doing. I told him I was a doctoral student and in a very serious voice told him I was doing a dissertation on "the Effects Of Systematic Audio Tape Feedback upon Both the Counseling Relationship and Educational Attitudes." Well, George, in his German accent and with a mischievous look in his eye said,

> I have got a great way for you to do your dissertation. Have people take off all their clothes, get under the sheets and masturbate. Tape the sounds of the masturbation as well as the groans. Then the next session, play it back to them on the tape recorder. You will cure them of all their sexual hangups!

Then George scampered off to mingle with the other guests.

I stood there for five minutes thinking about what he said. I was flabbergasted! I knew he was a famous therapist and there must have been some purpose for what he said, but the more rationale side of me said, "That sure was a crazy thing to say." Nevertheless, I remembered the response some ten years later.

The next time I saw George he was making a presentation at a California State Psychological Association Convention in Oakland, California. This was three years after his party. I introduced myself and he remembered me. I was smoking a cigar. He suddenly backed away and in a rather loud voice told me, "Don't blow that cigar smoke in my face." I was left there with a dumbfounded look on my face.

Three years later I met Dr. Bach again. I introduced myself. He reached up and touched my face saying to me, "Len Bergantino, what have you done to yourself!?" Just as instantly as he spoke, I said, "George, I've gotten handsomer." This time George backed away a bit surprised as I carried my end of the load and made it an equal existential moment.

Fritz Perls was a gestalt therapist. George Bach is an exponent of behavior modification. They both did the unexpected. This is what made me begin to think that one did not have to espouse the doctrine of existentialism to be an existentialist. An existentialist's world can be composed of as many possibilities as that person can handle. In terms of practicing psychotherapy, therapists can integrate as many therapies as are useful for them in terms of their personal growth and conjointly useful for their patients.

Both the stories about Fritz Perls and George Bach show two men who were interested in being all that they could be at each moment. However, for the purposes of theory building let us take a look at Perls' response–dismissing the man in his first therapy group experience. Perls reached the impasse in a hurry. The man was frustrated and had no cognitive understanding of what was going on. It was this frustration, however, that motivated him to continue his search for self in a way that permitted him to make a new decision about his life. Perls would take these kinds of risks–that is, that others would be disappointed or angry with him. He would say or do things that would actually put his being or his presence in the way of inauthentic behavior. He often put the patient in a position of having to relate authentically. And as this man told me, once he got a taste of relating authentically, and not as a good little boy, his entire life changed. Fritz was not afraid to be outrageous in confronting people.

Fritz's dismissal of the man led him to understand that others might experience him that way. Fritz was fully behind his words, and often put action into his responses. Such responses would make people who are more interested in keeping their self-images intact, no matter how inauthentic those images might be, find it difficult to deny the reality Fritz presented them. The kind of response made to the man was the kind that he will remember for a lifetime at the gut level. The psychic pain that his way of being in the world brought him was driven home in such a way that he could feel it intensely. Such gut level responses are important because they reach people at the primal level. They have depth, passion, energy, vigor, power and purpose. This type of response is particularly useful with hardened people who let more tempered responses roll off their shoulders. Such responding takes a great deal of caring by therapists because they have to be willing to risk responding in full, wherever that response may take them. So while Fritz's response to the man may have appeared cruel, hostile, or even destructive, when practiced by someone who has a sensitivity for working at the impasse level, it can paradoxically be the most caring and loving thing a therapist can do.

Such a response may be particularly useful with patients who are often considered to be chronic, or so entrenched in a self-destructive lifestyle that therapists inwardly may feel like giving up on them rather than risking what it takes to make the kind of impact that will rattle them at the gut level–perhaps enough to eventually motivate them to do what they need to do to turn their lives around in a positive direction.

I quote Dr. Walter Kempler directly as his quotes add an elegant depth to the issues with which I am dealing.

> The task of therapy is to arouse (remind) forgotten desires; to fire up abandoned conflict; and to keep all combatants at the front until everyone wins.[1]

> Regardless of the number of family members and irrespective of the many things happening at once, the therapist, with himself as the starting point, selects as the other point the greatest obstacle to resolving that current conflict, and engages it.[2]

> Psychology has moved along, perhaps into its own adolescence, and now considers the reciprocity between mother and child. More than that, it now strongly suspects that reciprocity in relatedness more than such things as kindness, caring and generosity, carries the greatest influence on human behavior.[3]

> When the conflict and struggle are insufficient to complete the process, another ingredient must be introduced. Fulfillment is replaced by grief. Then, the path from desire to calm is: desire-conflict-struggle-grief-calm.[4]

Crying, shouting, hating, screaming and aching silently, are all parts of the necessary total work to be done.[5]

By keeping his arousal in his work and directing it to the person who arouses it, the therapist brings reality to the therapy and authenticity to his relationships with the various family members. Additionally, his exemplary behavior sets the optimal tone for family conversations: an atmosphere of courageous self disclosure. And, most importantly, for each family member towards whom he may from time to time direct his personal message he offers the chance to stand on equal ground and to feel significant.[6]

I will face everyone with whom I choose to share my time as a significant other, whether they like it or not.[7]

Selecting the most evocative comment is learned directly from personal experience with the person. If reasonableness leads to passive understanding, it is avoided. If encouragement motivates action, it is offered. If confrontation gets the necessary responsiveness, then confrontation it is.[8]

Although Dr. Kempler is a well-known gestalt family therapist, his position is clearly in the radical existential camp. Dr. Kempler and I first met in 1973. We did not hit it off very well. He said that what bothered him about me was that I treated him as an equal and we weren't. I thought that he was pulling a one-upmanship trip on me and became angry, for it was a severe blow to my false and inflated self-image. That was another one of those comments that I never forgot. On a few occasions I have had patients who were deluding themselves that they were my equal, who became angry at me when I told them they were not. What I began to see was that Dr. Kempler did treat me as an equal by telling me we were not equals. He treated me like a significant other. What I had not taken into account was that he had about twenty years more experience. I had discounted him by not acknowledging the deeper levels of truth he had reached in himself at that time. So what I began to see was that even the pursuit of an equal relationship was paradoxical. I learned to treat people as my equals when they were my equals and to treat them as significant others--even if that meant treating them as less than equals–until they became my equals. Of course, if and when they were more than my equals, sooner or later I trained with them. Sometimes it took my ego a few years to integrate the power of such responses; that is, before my own disharmony among the three modes of being was discomforting enough to pursue change. Kempler puts it well when he says,

> Such changes are not easily achieved. One must go through the rigors of hell each revealing inch of the way, experiencing the loss of treasured traits and valued virtues as though it were death itself. There are no volunteers. Everyone who goes is forced, either by an already existing unbearable pain inside himself, or by family, i.e., a significant other with whom he cannot live and cannot live without. And, as a rule, without a family to inspire the task, unbearable pain within is dealt with largely by denial, desensitization and social achievement.[9]

I can remember some classes I took with Dr. William Ofman while pursuing a doctorate at the University of Southern California. Dr. Ofman's classes were the building blocks of my knowledge of a radical humanistic existential view of psychotherapy. He was an exciting and stimulating professor. I heard that he was an unusual man. One never knew quite what he was going to do and there was really no way to predict how one would do in his class. One semester he would give 100 multiple choice questions as an examination and the next he might give three all-encompassing essay questions. I began to feel anxiety before I even met him. I was interested in controlling my destiny–particularly the pursuit of my doctorate, and I was getting the feeling I was going to be graded on the quality of my being as opposed to the quality of my work. Dr. Ofman's classes forced me to deal with the anxiety of existence from which I had been trying to escape during my entire life. I was forced to learn to deal with the unpredictability of others and the existential dread of now knowing what was going to happen from one moment to the next. After I started doing therapy in this way, one of my patients once said that I would take him right to the hairy edge!

When I first began studying with Dr. Ofman, I was too self-controlled, to say the least. I over-rationalized and had cut myself off from most of my feelings. Coming from this background, it was very unusual for me to experience some of the things Dr. Ofman did in class. I was a bit obsessive in trying to figure out what he was doing as opposed to experiencing what he was doing. He would tell people to go fuck themselves. He would yell and scream and swear at students, hold them on his lap, hug them. I managed to do well in the first two classes I took with him, but in the third class I did an eighty-five page paper in which he gave me a B+ for the course. The only comment on the paper was "Not quite enough." I was quite angry about the B+.

This type of experiential learning was valuable, but not easy!

Ofman views therapy as an engaged struggle in which both therapist and patient strive toward a genuine dialogue–an I-Thou relationship. He further states that,

> Reality, responsibility and radical authenticity are the issues that are engaged in this relationship and are the very fabric of therapy. These are the subjects that I attempt to activate and realize in the work. Indeed, that is the work: the approximation and attainment of these goals, and the reaching for mutuality, which is the essentially healing act, the therapeutic happening. The mutual engaged encounter cannot, must not be merely spoken about (though, at times, that cannot be helped, it seems); it must be incarnated in the hour. It must be real between us, not merely discussed.[10]

> Attention to the other implies my momentaily becoming a 'zero' and thus, permits me to respond. Because I have no room or time to go into myself and process the information through an ideal-image system, thus maintaining a distancing between me and you and between me and the world, I simply respond directly and immediately.[11]

> There is no rule, image or mythology at all that one should live up to as a humanistic existential therapist save the following: . . . to be free, to be all that one is, to pay attention, to take the transaction and life seriously, to 'get wet' by the other, and to respond. The only things, perhaps, that the client has a right to demand of the therapist (and his lover, his spouse, or true friend) is his full response. And in a deeper sense, that is impossible also; either the therapist chooses to respond or he does not, and the client will then know him by the quantity and quality of his responsiveness. Nevertheless, the content of the response is unwillable by the therapist in any authentic sense.[12]

This last commentary provides the basic premise for which humanistic existential encounter therapy may be practiced–that the relationship as it unfolds between patient and therapist is the same relationship that has unfolded between the patient and significant others throughout that patient's life.

Ofman quotes Kempler when he said,

> Manifesting presence means self-disclosure, often frightening or embarrassing. It means responding with words, thoughts, feelings, and behavior as is, rather than as they should be . . . . It means returning to an encounter, with all attendant concerns about doing so . . . Manifesting presence means action. It may mean a vigorous confrontation; it may mean a watchful silence. But whether it is warring or waiting, it is deliberate; it is active. It is not mere words.[13]

When viewing the problem from an interpersonal perspective, in an existentially oriented here-and-now working style, the patient's problem is the problem that exists between the patient and the therapist in their relationship. Therapists must begin to see how and when the relationship between themselves and patients begins to falter, both in terms of what the therapist as well as the patient is doing. When the patient learns to deal with the therapist more effectively, that patient can learn to deal with life and other relationships more effectively. New interpersonal skills may be carried beyond the therapeutic encounter.

> If clients can solve their interpersonal problems with the counselor, the clients can solve their interpersonal problems in the real world–unless the reality of the clients' problems are such that they are unsolvable. In this approach, however, counseling is not viewed as the solving of personal problems but as the acceptance of responsibility for how clients choose to construct their existence.[14]

So what we have to this point is an existential therapy that is based on both the therapist's and the patient's ability to engage in a genuine, equal, and authentic relationship. It is within the context of such a relationship that existential moments occur. However, as existential moments may be quite difficult to capture, there is much to know regarding the makeup of the creation of these moments.

One type of knowledge the therapist must learn, without letting it interfere with the therapist's responses, is to *pick up the ongoing process* of what patients are doing at the moment in terms of here-and-now behavior.

One of the most difficult transitions on the road to becoming a competent psychotherapist is in learning to discriminate between what patients are saying and what they are doing. For example, if a patient in a group were complaining about his wife abusing him, the therapist should be able to spot the process of complaining as the symptom, while only secondarily paying attention to the content of what is being said. The therapist might respond in an I-Thou manner (concept of Martin Buber who wrote *I and Thou,* 1970) to the patient by saying, "Your complaining really turns me off. I get sick of hearing you." This would force the patient to treat the therapist as a significant other at that moment. The patient would learn to make contact with the therapist. The patient would learn to talk to people instead of talk to himself in front of people. When patients learn to do this they would no longer need to complain because they would be involved in satisfying and nurturing relationships. From a theoretical point of view that is, at least, "picking up the process" and dealing with it is therapeutic.

Another way of dealing with the process of complaining would be for the therapist to suggest an experiment that would exaggerate the process and make the patient integrate that process so it would be recognizable. (When I began to integrate experiment with existential theory I began to integrate gestalt therapy with existential therapy.) The therapist might suggest that the patient go around to each member of the group and complain. At this point, if the therapist wanted to use the group as a microcosm of the world, the therapist might suggest that each of the group members react to the patient.

The process through which the patient acts out problems may in itself cause a problem. For example, if a patient talks constantly about how a spouse is annoying, that process of complaining is likely to affect the patient adversely. Consequences are labeled problems when the real problem is what the patient is doing in the here and now. The patient must come to realize that a complaint is an attempt to get other people and the environment to support the patient, rather than the patient directly stating what he or she wants. The process of telling people what you want is self-supporting. Once patients become aware of what they are doing, such as complaining, and they are given options to enhance the contact (intrapsychic or interpersonal), they then have the option of choosing to do something that will bring them support instead of frustration.

When working with patients, it is important to make the resistance larger than life. In the above example, the resistance is the complaining. Therapists may pick up what patients are avoiding by focusing on discrepancies between words and body language in addition to discrepancies between what patients are saying and what they are doing. When therapists offer experiments that help patients to become more aware of their process, they afford patients the opportunity to experience themselves more deeply. When therapists add fresh input into the situation, it helps to prevent patients from floundering while they are learning to stand on their own two feet. Such input becomes one form of therapeutic artistry, in providing the proper balance between frustration and support.

Once the particular behavior has been identified, such as complaining, see what effect it has on the patient. For example, does the patient feel depression, anger, sadness, etc.? The therapist may then want to focus on what the patient is doing with that particular feeling.

Is the patient letting it flow? Is the patient ignoring it? If the patient is ignoring it, what is the continued aware process of how the patient is stopping him or herself from feeling? To increase patient awareness of his or her own process, the therapist might suggest that the patient teach the therapist how to become depressed, angry, etc. Another approach would be to have the patient make the therapist the target. For example, if a patient is a complainer, the therapist may suggest the patient complain about the therapist or someone else, using the empty-chair technique.

The empty-chair technique is a gestalt therapy process whereby the therapist suggests that the patient address the problem directly, speaking to the absent person or to that part of self currently alienated. For example, if a patient had a dream about a house the therapist might ask the patient to be the house. The therapist might ask the patient to put his wife in the empty chair and tell her what he doesn't like about her, then ask the patient to play her role. The therapist focuses on the point where the contact between the two sides breaks down and uses creativity to add a new ingredient so the alienated parts of the patient's personality will come together. This is often referred to as closure.

When concerning themselves with process, therapists may do both themselves and patients a disservice by prematurely concerning themselves with therapy outcomes. Clinical judgment determines when to flow with process and when to give input toward outcome. Such concern removes both patients and therapists from the immediate experience of the awareness continuum.

An inappropriate response would be for therapists focus on the content of the patient's complaint by saying, "Tell me more about your dissatisfaction with your wife." This would only lead to a boring and nonproductive event for both therapist and patient. Of course, there are many intricate issues involved in the facilitation of awareness.

RESISTANCE AND THE FACILITATION OF PROCESS AWARENESS

The existential view of awareness is that it is neither good nor bad–it just is. Awareness falls in the realm of a relative value system which gives humans the freedom and the possibility to define their existence.

All this sounds correct in theory, but in practice both therapists and patients must be sensitive to the issue that something quite different may happen. Why do therapists attend to some levels of awareness and not others? Are therapists critical, judgmental, curious, interested–do they possess all of these attitudes at one time or another? Each of these qualities is involved in the determination of what a therapist chooses to become aware of.

Most therapists and patients have an image of how people should be in the world. Patients' images may have more to do with cultural, societal and parental teachings than the pursuit of authentic being. Therapists may be more concerned with the image of a perfectly authentic being than with the give and take between therapists' images of where patients ought to be going and the reality of where patients are in their lives.

The danger in the facilitation of awareness is that although patients may become acutely aware of what they are doing and how they are doing it, they may begin to close up and feel less human. Patients may begin to feel that at each level of awareness there is something they need to change about themselves. A paradox of therapy is that patients may find that mapping out a project of change for themselves may only guarantee their remaining stuck. Patients must come to accept themselves in terms of who they are before they can creatively and realistically restructure their existence. If this "self-downing" process isn't resolved, the therapy may be severely hampered.

It becomes important for therapists to attain enough self-love to be able to respond in nurturing ways to rebellious and self-critical patients. A self-critical patient teamed up with a therapist who has trouble not being critical of self or patient makes for a rocky start. Therapists' personal growth and self-nurturance become important in helping patients turn the corner and become self-accepting. This is where therapists' humanity must be joined to their therapeutic skills. Only then will they be able to deal with the question of how therapists can help patients move from rebellion to autonomous free choice. All patients have differing degrees of passive behavior. They are ambivalent about change. If patients were clear about wanting to change they would not need therapists. What happens to patients who refuse to accept therapists' suggested experiments? What happens if patients are not straight about rejecting therapists' suggestions? Do therapists punish these patients? Do they stop working with them? Can they find a way to creatively go with the rebellious behavior until patients supersede an impasse?

Patients often only see two ways of responding to therapists–rebellion or compliance. Yet, a third option exists–responding with free choice (autonomously). The lack of seeing this third choice leaves patients insecure, with a sense of not being able to use their full power to choose freely. The question becomes, How do patients get to see the third alternative when they may have lived their life believing only two choices exist?

Therapists may deal with such situations by respecting the intentions of patients. Therapists need to go with such patients, not against them. For example, therapists might say, "NOTICE HOW POWERFUL YOU FEEL WHEN YOU IGNORE MY SUGGESTION. WOULD YOU BE WILLING TO TELL ME TO GO TO HELL, THAT YOU ARE GOING TO DO IT YOUR WAY?" THERAPISTS MUST BE ABLE TO MAKE SUCH RESPONSES FROM A SUPPORTIVE AND NURTURING POSITION, OTHERWISE PATIENTS MAY ONLY RESPOND TO THE CRITICAL SOUNDS OF THERAPISTS' VOICES. Another way to deal with the issue is to focus on what they are saying. For example, "I can see why you wouldn't want to stop drinking. It has become a way of life for you. It would be very difficult to stop. I can understand your not wanting to suffer that inconvenience." After a series of such responses patients may begin to argue with therapists about why they really should stop drinking. The reasons come from within themselves, and not from therapists.

When patients begin to feel all right about rebelling and know they are not going to be punished, they may be willing to consider experimenting with new behavior at another time. Patients need to feel safe in rebelling, otherwise, they may just continue to defend rebellious behavior, or go back to being compliant, without ever learning to make autonomous decisions. Respecting patients' intentions by stroking the rebellion (e.g., I can see why you would want to do such and such) allows them to integrate alienated parts of their personalities. Once rebellious patients have gotten through this process they may learn to consider what they have become aware of in themselves as strengths–something they can use to their advantage as opposed to using them to torture both themselves and therapists.

To do effective therapy therapists must be able to balance respecting patients' behavior and choice of lifestyle, and cutting through self-destructive patterns. Respecting the behavior does not mean reinforcing craziness. THERAPISTS NEED TO DO ALL THAT THEY CAN TO REDUCE THEIR OWN DUPLICITY IN ORDER TO PROVIDE A SAFE ENVIRONMENT, EVEN IN AGGRESSIVE CONFRONTATIONS.

It is impossible, however, for therapists to have perfect unity among the three modes of being. So the issues of *power* and *control* do exist between patients and therapists. In these cases it becomes critical that therapists be willing to examine their behavior in front of patients so patients may see that therapists are trustworthy. Patient perceptions that arise from scared-child feelings are different from covert manipulations that are the result of therapists' projections.

Awareness and process issues are particularly important in therapies such as gestalt therapy and transactional analysis where a lot of creative experimentation may be suggested. The issue in these cases is appropriate versus inappropriate leading of patients' experiences by therapists. This therapeutic skill comes with maturity and a sensitivity to both the patient and the self of the therapist, so that the "I" or integrity of the therapist does not get lost in the "I-Thou" relationship. Some therapists focus on inner conflicts of patients almost exclusively and others focus on the authenticity of relationship between them. To provide an optimal therapeutic relationship, a marriage between awareness of process and authenticity is required. The therapeutic structure allows two people to pursue an equal relationship, while simultaneously providing a relationship whereby patients will respect therapists for their skills and pursuit of authenticity. Both the pursuit of an equal relationship in therapy and its inequality in some respects can be appreciated. Of course, this is a difficult balance for therapists to maintain–and this is clearly what this book suggests therapists do to the best of their abilities.

Therapists who work in an authentic manner are self-disclosing human beings who share their pain and inadequacies and risk maximum engagement with patients. Therapists should offer patients the opportunity to utilize a new awareness in relationship to therapists rather than act as if patients were responding in a vacuum. Therapists are not perfect. Patients do respond to therapists as well as their inner conflicts. For example, if a patient is feeling a pressure to be compliant, the therapist should ascertain whether the therapist's behavior is sending messages such as "try hard, hurry up, please me or be perfect"[15] to the patient. Therapists can check this out by asking patients directly as well as taking a step backward to look at their process. They can also pay attention to their body pace and rhythm. If they feel they are going at a faster rate of speed than is their natural pace, they are most likely sending messages for patients to adapt to them. Such problems, of course, can also originate with patients.

On the other hand, if therapists ascertain that they are innocent of sending such messages, they may look further for inner conflicts with patients. When therapists are open about such problems, patients are then able to separate their problems from the therapists'. Of course, it is unrealistic to expect therapists to entirely avoid dumping their problems on patients, and it may even have some value in that patients will have to deal with other people's problems every day. So if they deal with therapists' doing it, in a relatively safe environment, they have a better chance to learn how to take care of themselves. When patients can take care of themselves without letting themselves suffer unjudiciously, they are in an excellent position to begin expanding their capacity for love, friendship, and a generosity of spirit based on human compassion. For the most part, at this point, they will not be the victim of therapists' duplicity.

Therapy is a difficult business in that there are two sides to many truths. Oftentimes, what is right in one circumstance will not apply in another circumstance. For example, some therapists feel that awareness should not be made aversive to patients, otherwise therapy will only retrain patients to avoid further awareness. However, other therapists believe that when patients are partaking in behavior that makes therapists want to punish patients, therapists must consider their options carefully in working out a delicate balance between punishment and its avoidance, balanced by nurturance.

When therapists do respond punitively to patients, they should talk about what happened between them so patients will have the opportunity to understand what they have just experienced. This will help patients clearly see the negative consequence of their behavior.

STRETCHING THE BOUNDARIES

There are many polarities in the therapeutic process–love-hate, intimacy-distance, contact-withdrawal, etc. For therapists to help patients stretch their boundaries, however, therapists have had to have stretched themselves. Also, they need to be willing to risk being where they are, trying new approaches, and being courageous with their patients. By courageous, I mean for therapists to act on what they intuitively know to be high quality response even though they may be accustomed to holding back.

THE PROBLEM IS THAT MANY PEOPLE, INCLUDING THERAPISTS AND PATIENTS, PREFER TO AVOID THESE POLES AND TEND TO STRUCTURE THEIR LIVES TO REDUCE THE ANXIETY OF LIVING IN AN AMBIGUOUS WORLD. PEOPLE ARE VULNERABLE TO THE UNPREDICTABLE RESPONSES OF OTHERS, AND AS A RESULT DO WHAT THEY CAN TO REDUCE THAT UNPREDICTABILITY. PEOPLE DEADEN THEMSELVES TO MAKE THEIR WORLD APPEAR SAFER.

I have found that in order to stretch my boundaries, I had to begin to tinker with my way of being in the world. I had to re-examine the forms and structures I had established to make my world appear safer. Some of these structures took the forms of an absolute value system and parental "shoulds" which I had then integrated into a personalized self-torture system. I had to get in touch with my instincts again. Having taught psychotherapy, I have found that most therapists must make similar journeys if they are to be able to reach polarities and provide a deeper relationship with their patients.

In addition to a willingness to risk, I found that many therapists have difficulty when they responded to images of how therapists "should" respond. For example, therapists feel they must demonstrate unconditional positive regard toward patients. Yet, this in turn may only lead to unconditional positive disregard. For example, does the therapist respect the patient enough to share the therapist's anger or annoyance with the patient's behavior, and if so, is the therapist willing to stay and work it through?

Therapists may have difficulty expanding their intimacy boundaries with patients if therapists are unwilling to also be distant when that is what they are experiencing. Those who don't distance themselves, and force themselves to remain in contact longer than they want, run the risk of burning themselves out. For example, there are times when I tell a patient that I enjoyed being close, but I need to back up a bit now. Ironically enough, telling this to patients would usually put me back in contact with them. If patients do not appreciate the paradoxical nature of the situation, therapists may wish to tell patients that they are making contact by holding their distance–taking the space they need for themselves.

When I take care of myself in this way, patients learn to take care of themselves. We both survive and are able to receive energetic nourishment through a contact that we both desire. When I took risks and told patients I wanted to withdraw, I found it more pleasant to make contact. WHEN I BECAME FREE ENOUGH TO FOLLOW MY OWN EXCITEMENT–WHETHER IT BE INTIMACY OR DISTANCE, CONTACT OR WITHDRAWAL, LOVE OR HATE–I FOUND THAT I COULD WORK A FULL DAY AND HAVE AS MUCH ENERGY AT THE END OF THE DAY AS I HAD AT THE BEGINNING. MY ENERGY AND EXCITEMENT INCREASED AS I DISCARDED MY FORMS AND STRUCTURES AND ACCEPTED THE REALITY OF THE MOMENT. UNTIL I BEGAN DOING THIS I USED TO FEEL BURNT OUT AFTER DOING FOUR OR FIVE HOURS OF THERAPY PER DAY.

One problem I had to overcome was feeling guilty for saying what I wanted when patients would claim I wasn't caring enough for them. Of course I had unconsciously set it up that way to limit the freedom of my responses. My range has increased considerably once I stopped feeling guilty. The therapist's range of responsiveness is important to provide a wide experiential brand of therapy for patients.

Taking control of whatever emotions or images hamper freedom to respond is an extremely important factor in therapy–and movement in that direction will be responsible for both therapists and patients enjoying more enriched lives. For example, if therapists tend to be always angry or depressed, they need to nourish themselves so that their emotions will flow from their humanity rather than from inauthentic feelings that are usually mistaken for authenticity. When emotion flows from humanity, therapists and patients will enjoy rich experiences. Then therapists will be able to reach for the polarities from a loving, nurtured, and safe place within themselves. The safety from within will help therapists to take more risks in reaching the polarities in the context of their work.

Bill and I–An Experience With My Therapist

A few months after receiving my doctorate from the University of Southern California, I began therapy with Dr. William Ofman, an associate professor at the University of Southern California and a clinical psychologist in private practice in Beverly Hills, California. I have learned from the teachings in his book entitled *Affirmation and Reality: Fundamentals of Humanistic Existential Therapy and Counseling.* He would describe himself as a radical humanistic existential therapist.

Initially, my major conflict with Bill was my self-imposed desire to be independent. I wanted something from Bill, yet at the same time I hated to acknowledge that I wanted anything from him. He could always deny my wants and that would make me feel bad. His attitude was that only by accepting my feeling of dependency would I be able to transcend it. The immature parts of my personality needed to grow up. The only way I could help them grow was by respecting my needs. He felt it was important for me to not judge what I needed, but to accept reality and say, "Yes, that's what I need–period–end of report."

I was frustrated in many of my endeavors. I was an ambitious man who would always push to reach my maximum potential and be frustrated when I didn't get immediate results. Bill said, "You'll always be frustrated if you try to lift a two-ton weight and don't expect it to be heavy." I learned about unrealistic expectations.

Whenever I said that I was stuck or that I didn't know, Bill would urge me to stay with the deadlock and to examine it. I learned that, "I don't know" means, "I don't want to look."

The issue of accepting responsibility for my feelings arose when Bill asked me, "How are you saddening yourself?" I told him that I sadden myself by being dependent on others for approval and then depress myself over their responses. My assumption of responsibility gave me the option to do otherwise, that is, to learn to take control over the process of how I produced my depression. I began to see that existential therapy may be viewed as the semantics of responsible involvement. That is, the responsibility I assumed for how I chose to live as determined by the responsibility I assumed for freedom of choice in my language. For example, if a patient hardly ever takes a stand by using the words "probably," "maybe," etc., I would say, "Will you or won't you!" I remember feeling guilty about my strong resistance to change. I learned from Bill that resistance is working. Whenever people begin to look at how they set up their lives, they have ambivalent feelings. What people do has usually brought them much good as well as the pain they confront. Resistance is a natural part of what goes on. Such an attitude on the part of the therapist casts the therapist as an involved partner, engaging and struggling with patients, while being supportive of their feelings. I learned that I would resist most when Bill would get close. When I felt threatened, however, he would respect my feelings and back up a bit.

I was having difficulty in a relationship with a woman I was dating at the time. Bill clarified what was going on. I told him that I didn't feel any better. Bill said, "Why should you? When we clarified the situation it was even worse than it looked at first." I learned that it was important not to let patients escape the consequences of what they were doing–even if that realization was painful. It may very well be that pain which would be a motivating force for change by patients.

I didn't know if I was capable of helping Jim, a patient of mine, since we were both stuck in emotionally similar situations. When I told Bill that I shared that with Jim, he felt that I was teaching Jim what being human is all about and that was the best and most valuable therapy I could do. His comment helped my confidence grow. I saw that it was all right for me to be honest even when I was a disappointment. I did not have to be perfect. I found that easier to accept than I did when I first started doing therapy. Therapists often have difficulty dealing with their insecurities and I found that just airing them was a valuable approach.

Bill said, "I feel suckered into pleasing you, yet I know my obligations are not necessarily to please you–but to explore and heighten your sense of awareness." I had a difficult time when Bill didn't let himself be suckered into pleasing me. I felt a gap between us. Separation! Anxiety! I had been attempting to avoid feeling this sense of separateness. Through this important experience I was able to later hold my ground with patients who wanted to have a false sense of closeness to avoid experiencing the aloneness of the human condition. I had to learn to differentiate between the closeness that came from genuine human contact and manipulative attempts to create an artificial closeness to relieve the existential anxiety of being thrown into the world alone.

Many of Bill's responses made me realize that being myself was my most important therapeutic asset. Although I used outside sources as models, each person helped me to build from the inside. The whole vista of psychology existed within me–if I dared to look and To Be! It is a tricky issue to help patients learn about their inner selves, especially when many people seek therapy for the exact opposite reason–to learn from without. For therapists who are learning, the process is to flow with the unconscious so the creation of technique will come from within.

Although Bill and I were not friends at this time, I wanted more from him than therapy and supervision. Later, the issue of friendship would surface with some of my patients also. I asked Bill to go to a football game with me. He refused, while expressing appreciation that I asked. I felt hurt; I wanted him to be my friend. He said, "I understand that you want my friendship, but I want to be your therapist. I do care about you, but I don't want to spend more time with you. I have things to do on my own." This response was important in several respects. He didn't allow me to trick myself out of feeling a sense of loss. It was positive that my want of intimate human contact was increasing. As my want increased, I was able to transfer the want to other people in creating the kind of world I desired.

A second issue was whether I would socialize with my own patients. Having an existential point of view I left the door open for a situational response. The first time a couple of patients that I really liked invited my wife and me to dinner, we accepted. It was a bit strained. We were not yet friends and yet our acceptance to dinner made them mistakenly assume this meant we were. They cancelled their next two sessions because "something came up." But it felt like an abuse of the therapeutic situation. They didn't express any open discomfort in the session about the social situation. I began to see that people would be reluctant to pay for a therapist's time if they mistakenly assumed a false role of friendship. I then adopted a policy of no socializing with patients, due to my inability to correctly assess each situation on its own merits. After being in practice for a few years, I began to sense the difference between my concept of an intimate relationship and relationships that were really intimate. In relationships that were mutually-based, I found that I could successfully accept a social invitation, or be both friend and therapist. As a therapist, I treated an old girlfriend as well as one of my best male friends. It actually worked to their advantage because I had a very strong affection for both. As I learned, however, if therapists' unconscious minds are not yet flowing freely enough to make an appropriate judgment, it's best to use an automatic no.

I remember bringing a woman to a session to meet Bill. It was an enlightening dialogue, to say the least.

Me   Bill, I want you to meet Sharon.

Bill   I met her, now what do you want me to do with her?

Me   (Stumbling) I just wanted you to meet her.

Bill   I met her, now do you want me to take her to bed or go out with her? Come on, Sharon, let's go!

At this point I took a realistic look at my agenda for Sharon. I had brought her with me to change her behavior without realizing that's what I wanted. My experience in doing marital therapy has taught me such occurrences are common. Most couples come to marital therapy with hidden expectations about changing their partners without modifying their own behavior. I began telling Bill how much Sharon was growing. He asked me if I was going to marry her conditionally, on the promise of her growth. I realized how foolish it was to build a relationship on the secret hope that a spouse will change. This covert non-acceptance of My wife at the time was a cause of problems between us. I learned to be more straight-forward about what I wanted from her, and to negotiate compromises that were good for both of us.

There came a time in our work together that Bill told me he felt close, friendly, equal, and warm with me. The feelings were mutual. I was beginning to notice that the more of these experiences I had with Bill, the more I sought them with others outside of therapy, and the more intimate I could be with My wife at the time.

Bill did not encounter or confront me as a primary way of doing therapy. He would be confrontive when it flowed naturally, on occasion, but for the most part he said, "What I do is not always the most direct way. I believe that when you are ready to engage me, you will. It takes time before feelings are real between humans . . . and I'm all for being like human beings with each other." I found this to be a very interesting option as a way of considering the naturalness of human responses. In other words, existential moments would come in their own good time in whatever way they chose to arrive.

Our relationship was growing closer. Existential moments were happening more frequently as our conversation gradually evolved into a directness that felt warming.

Me	I dig your affection, your liking, your love for me.
Bill	(choked up) You have come a long way. You're so much more of a human being! Less stilted, less uptight, more confident–it's fantastic to see you like that.
Me	I feel distant (the issue between us).
Bill	I don't.
Me	You were talking about your therapy rather than how you are with me. I give to Caesar what is Caesar's, but I want you to share yourself with me. I was thinking about you and me.
Bill	I broadened it.
Me	Yes.
Bill	I feel a little embarrassed . . . and inadequate to respond. Yet, I feel moved by you.

Our talking to each other in this way was an accumulation of low-keyed existential moments that were gradually and naturally forming the basis of an authentic and healing relationship. One of the most touching moments I can recall came toward the end of our work together. Bill and I were discussing a recommendation for the licensing examination.

Bill wrote, "If, at some time in the future I needed a therapist, I would choose him."

Me   Wow–that's heavy!

Bill   I want it to be there.

An equality had developed between us. It was not in concept that Bill was treating me equally, but a mutuality of feelings that came out of my growth and a deepening of our relationship together. His statement also made a tremendous impact, for I both felt very self-confident and for the first time I could remember, began to use my full power when relating to others. It was an existential moment and a return to full power to someone whose power had been denied throughout life. The full value of *affirmation* and *reality* was experienced with the *return of a denied integrity.*

Me   It feels right between us now.

Bill   Right! (In a soft, loving voice) It's between us.

My experience with Bill left me with the feeling that two people in a room, struggling to be with each other in a very human way, was the basis of psychotherapy. An authentic, loving, and intimate relationship that is grounded in a deepened reality can be healing to a patient–as it was to me. The therapy consisted of increasing numbers of what I later came to refer to as existential moments that helped us to make the healing relationship a whole experience. The most healing aspect of the therapy was the ongoing existential situation between us, and dealing with that situation.

Existential moments, and moments that were not quite as impactful or centered, took place between us. Sometimes the moments were fully grounded in reality. At other times the moments may have come from each of our childlike belief and feeling systems. However, at all times, the existential moments were based either on what was authentic or what both of us believed to be authentic at that moment in time. Of course, there is no such thing as perfect authenticity, so one can ask no more of a therapist than to call it as he or she sees it. Looking at the overall picture, our relationship became increasingly genuine. The value of our existential moments together was that they helped to create a sustained healing relationship. The moments add up. The moment totaled to a relationship that became equal. When the relationship felt and was equal to both therapist and patient, Bill then gave of himself beyond the limits of the therapeutic hour. The existential moments were based upon equality, respect, authenticity of relation, integrity, assumption of responsibility, increased awareness, and the ensuing willingness to be in reality. However, the basis was the freedom of both Bill and me to respond to each other in ways that left us both more fulfilled in terms of an enriched humanity. This relationship moved me so that it provided a solid foundation and became the building blocks from which I approached the doing of psychotherapy.

I want to show how some of the ways of thinking about therapy that I have been describing began to take a stylistic form for me early on in my career. At this time I had a very quick eye in spotting the patient's process. I was quite provocative in order to get to feelings, but I had a difficult time sharing feelings myself. I had a very good sense of what was in accord with the patient's natural flow of excitement, and what might be blocking that excitement, and accompanying actions. I was a bit harsh and hardened in myself, which left me covering my softness with a tough-guy stance. However, with a patient such as the one I am going to describe, I believe being tough may have been an advantage, because as I became softer and mellower and began to work more from my heart, I found it much more difficult to say the kind of things that would help patients who had so much stubborn self-hatred reach a natural state of being. And she was the kind of patient that would not have responded to a less forceful therapy.

Yet I think a critical ingredient in my being able to work in this way was that patients never doubted my sincere interest in their well-being, and in what I was doing. Early in my career I was not able to openly demonstrate the warmth, but as you will later see in the case with Alyson, it was lurking back there somewhere and she responded to that part of me, which I wasn't even consciously thinking about during the first session.

Alyson

Alyson was an actress who initially sought therapy because she was having difficulty in her career as well as with her husband John and a daughter, whom she treated in the same manner that she behaved toward herself.

From a therapeutic point of view I was interested in helping her turn around a process of self-torture, and torture of other people in her presence, which was making her life miserable. She was stuck in a process of continual anger that she perpetuated by turning her anger and aggression inward, and passively outward, with a voice quality and tone that would turn my stomach.

While she had an underlying sadness I was too busy running away from my own sadness, to pursue this avenue with her. I did feel that if she either became openly instead of covertly angry, that she could reverse the process. Another option I went for at times was to ask her what she wanted, assuming that if she could ask for what she wanted and get it more of the time she would have less reason to be angry. She was so lost in her self-torture system, however, that she did not know what she wanted, and this was part of the problem that kept her lost to herself.

The following are segments of taped interviews of the last part of our fourteenth and beginning of our fifteenth sessions. I felt Alyson had a tendency to distort what was happening between us so I requested she tape the session and listen to it between sessions.

Alyson   I'm sitting here *thinking* how my anger is turning on me . . . (she shouts to herself) . . . stop that!

Alyson alienates herself from her anger. She describes her anger as something outside herself that is turning on her. While she actively turns it inward, all that comes outward is *thinking*. I begin to poke and provoke, hoping for a reverse explosion.

Me   I feel very comfortable with you turning your anger on you. (I am implying that if she wants to get me she isn't doing it).

Alyson	I know. I'm well aware of that. I'm trying in my head to reverse the process.
Me	I can imagine that as long as that's what you are doing, I'll continue to feel comfortable.
Alyson	I don't know whether to . . . My reactions want to throw something at you.
Me	You mean it's not Alyson who wants to throw something at me? (sarcastically) Tell me about it.
Alyson	I feel like I want to throw something. I can see where the tears get involved. I can feel it all turning to tears inside.
Me	(I experienced her as being emotionally more honest with herself at this point and was much more empathic in my response. I felt touched at this moment. This was conveyed more by my presence in the room than by my words). You can feel yourself turning into tears.
Alyson	I can feel the anger turning into tears. I feel angry at your smugness.
Me	(This was a difficult point for me. On the one hand she just expressed sadness. On the other she took it right back to her anger at me. I sensed she was on the verge of explosion. I chose to go in that direction.) You are getting the kind of responses you deserve (giving her a bit more smugness).
Alyson	(Goes back into thinking) Yes, that's right. I'm sure you're right. I've got to turn my process around. I've got to get it going back the other way because I still, my social side won't allow me to pick up something and throw it at you. I'll tell you about it.

Me You are going to break out of your head by telling me all the strategy you are going to use to break out of your head by thinking about how you are going to break out of your head, by planning, thinking strategy. (I am attempting to make it not worth the effort for her to stay in her head.)

Alyson I don't want it to be that but it's like the ultimate game to me. I don't know. I don't know how to tell the difference yet. I'm looking for that.

Between the end of this session and the following session, which took place two days later, Alyson spent time going over the tape. During this next session, the following dialogue took place. It was a pleasant surprise to me, as I had not seen the results that took place in the session. Oftentimes patients put things together between sessions if therapists are willing to let them stew a bit, and not succumb to the urge to make everything better by the end of the session. Alyson came in vibrant, alive, excited and exciting. I had never seen her that way before. And she had almost forgotten what it was like to be that way, it had been such a long time.

Me You really look bubbly.

Alyson I've been waiting all day to see you. I almost called you yesterday. I called to apologize.

Me Why?

Alyson For my behavior. I'm not sure why I do it. I think I was trying to punish you because I was hurting. I had time to think about it. Time to feel things which was even better. I can't understand what's happening.

Me Tell me more.

Alyson   I think, I don't think. I feel, there's been a . . . I've been trying to–I'm all jumbled up inside–that was the word I used, things like that and I couldn't figure out what it was. Now I think I know what it is. I feel I'm *alive*. I've forgotten what that's like. I don't think I knew. I shouldn't say that. Maybe I knew when I first met John, that kind of thing. It's an excitement and I was attributing it to you, and somehow, that scared me. I don't think that's it and I was trying to balance it–whatever you want to call it. I was trying to get back into balance so it wouldn't . . . but it's been going on all day; once I realized that's what it was.

Me   You've been feeling alive all day.

Alyson   Yes!

Me   You look it. You look alive.

Alyson   I feel it. I really do.

Me   Your face is red and your eyes are sparkling.

Alyson   I've been waiting to see you all day to tell you.

Me   And you look great!

The breakthrough was Alyson's permitting herself to feel alive. Excitement was happening with her and in turn, with me, from the moment she set foot in the office.

While the warmth and caring I felt for Alyson didn't come across in my words, they must have been more evident in my nonverbal responses. When discussing the previous session, Alyson referred to my kindness.

Alyson   I got out of here before I started crying. I thought you wanted me to cry and I wouldn't cry. I wouldn't

> give you that. I couldn't deal with your kindness at that moment.

Me   I feel touched and warmed by you.

Alyson   It's nice to be able to say it and feel that it is really communicated.

Alyson was a very perceptive woman. It took me a bit by surprise when she said that she felt I wanted her to cry. Perhaps the part of me that was saddened and touched by her came through as loudly, or more loudly than my words. Perhaps I was coming more from my heart than I had realized. Her struggle was certainly one that touched me, although I had much difficulty being demonstrative about it.

Alyson   In our last session I was trying to put distance between us. I felt you were getting too close. So I thought, I'll put you in your place. But I didn't know that when I did it. It wasn't until I thought about you. It was your reaction. I thought, "What have I done wrong? I expected a good day. I came out and was feeling miserable. Just terrible. In fact, it lasted until John got home and I said, "Don't even ask me. It's just a bad scene."

While I was not with Alyson when the changes took place, my speculations are as follows: Alyson felt strong feelings that she was either incapable of dealing with or was running away from during the first of the two sessions presented. My provocative way of working pushed her feelings to extremes that she was then forced to deal with. While she was experiencing those feelings during the session, mostly what occurred to her was that I was the cause of her misery. However, as she and her husband were both bright and perceptive people, when they listened to the tape, she, for the first time, became aware of her role in causing her miserable feelings. I believe this left her feeling hopeful that she could change the outcome of therapy, of her relationships and of her life, by behaving differently. I think this excited her so much that she became very appreciative and this is why she was so positive at the beginning of the second session. She could see light at the end of the tunnel!

In future sessions she was able to turn her aggression outwards and feel all right about herself while doing so. When she put her self-critical strategies aside she was able to maintain higher levels of intimacy and vitality with me and in other relationships.

Characteristic of my particular brand of existential therapy was a bluntness of style as well as a vitality and intensity. I had a patient whose commitment was as strong as my own. With such a dual commitment I felt a nonspoken permission, even request, to rattle things up a bit at the deepest levels. Further, while my responses were authentic, they were also strategic, but that strategy was not planned. It just flowed from what naturally came from within me.

I HAD AN INTUITIVE TRUST THAT SOMETHING POSITIVE WOULD HAPPEN WITH THE INTENSITY OF MY RESPONSES. THIS INTUITIVE TRUST WAS VERY IMPORTANT FOR ME, BECAUSE OFTENTIMES IF I HAD STOPPED TO THINK ABOUT WHAT I WAS SAYING, THE OUTRAGEOUS QUALITY MIGHT HAVE INHIBITED ME FROM RESPONDING. I was not sure if something positive and natural would happen during or after the session if I stayed on course. Often people need a while to sort things out and put them together in a new way. Alyson did this between sessions. WHEN I RESPOND WITH THE INTENSITY that I used in the first session, I RATTLE PEOPLE AT THE PRIMAL LEVEL. I believe this is the greatest asset of such a style, if it is done with a genuine caring and concern for that patient's well-being. Otherwise patients will not feel the necessary spirit of good will. WHEN PATIENTS FEEL GOOD WILL FROM THERAPISTS, THERAPISTS CAN BE OUTRAGEOUS AND MAKE AN IMPACT THAT MAY LEAD TO PERMANENT CHANGES IN MUCH SHORTER PERIODS OF TIME. Another important issue is that I am often not sure exactly what will happen, but have a sense that if I am committed to follow through with whatever happens, and the patient is willing to do likewise, all will be well.

THIS CASE PRESENTED THE RAW SUBSTANCE OF A PERSONAL STYLE OF DOING THERAPY, AND FURTHER TRAINING AND THERAPY ADDED POLISH AND SOPHISTICATION, IN ADDITION TO A VARIETY OF EFFECTIVE OPTIONS. AFTER A TIME, THEY TOO, WOULD BECOME PART

OF MY NATURE. THERAPIST MAY WANT TO CONSIDER AN OPEN-ENDED DEVELOPMENT OF THE THERAPEUTIC USE OF SELF AS A WAY OF LIFE, AND IF THEY MARRY SOMEONE WHO IS OPEN TO SUCH A JOURNEY!

ENDNOTES

1   Walter Kempler, Principles of Gestalt Family Therapy Printed in Norway by A. S Joh. Nordahls Trykkeri, Oslo, 1973, p. 70.
2   Ibid.
3   Ibid., p. 64.
4   Ibid., p. 68.
5   Ibid., p. 74.
6   Ibid., p. 75.
7   Ibid., p. 75.
8   Ibid., p. 118.
9   Ibid., p. 78.
10 William Ofman, Affirmation and Reality: Fundamentals of Humanistic Existential Therapy and Counseling (Los Angeles: Western Psychological Services, 1976), p. 179. Copyright © 1976 by Western Psychological Services. Reprinted by permission.
11 Ibid., p. 186.
12 Bid., p. 144.
13 Ibid., p. 119, quoting W. Kempler, "The Therapist's Merchandise," Voices: The Act and Science of Psychotherapy (Winter/Spring 1969-1970), pp. 57-60.
14 Len Bergantino, "A theory of imperfection," Counselor Education

and Supervision, June 1978, p. 291. Reprinted with permission of the American Personnel and Guidance Association, 1607 New Hampshire Ave., N.W., Washington, D.C. 20009. Further reproduction is prohibited without written consent from APGA.

15 Hedges Capers, and Taibi Kahler, "The miniscript," Transactional Analysis Journal 4 (January 1974) p. 33. I have since learned to ask, "What will you do?" "Will do" is action-oriented. "Want to do" hooks good intentions with commitment to action.

REFERENCES

Bergantino, Len. "A theory of imperfection." *Counselor Education and Supervision.* June 1978, 286-293.

Capers, Hedges and Kahler, Taibi. "The miniscript." *Transactional Analysis Journal* 4, January 1974, pp. 26-43.

Kempler, Walter. *Principles of Gestalt Family Therapy.* Printed in Norway by A. S Joh, Nordalhs Trykkeri, Oslo, 1973.

Ofman, William. *Affirmation and Reality: Fundamentals of Humanistic Existential Therapy and Counseling.* Los Angeles: Western Psychological Services, 1976.

3

The Liberation of the Therapist

WHEN I SPEAK of the therapist becoming liberated I am referring to a feeling tone in the context of the general atmosphere that pervades the entire profession of psychotherapy as well as its public image. The image is a traditional one, that implies a basic conservative "don't make any waves attitude" with "good" psychotherapy. Of course, there is much that is traditional and conservative that is "good" psychotherapy; however, what I am beginning to sense is that some colleagues are becoming more interested in maintaining their professional images as a means of self-protection than they are in doing authentic, contact-oriented, effective, and stylistic psychotherapy that results in the kind of existential moments that help people change their lives for the better. The image of the profession among its members and the public tends to be an anchor that in many ways can impede therapeutic pursuit of a free-flowing artistry. While traditions are valuable in giving psychotherapists roots, those roots and traditions must not begin to feel like handcuffs that get in the way of a natural and intuitive style of practice that is tempered with clinical judgment and responsibility.

I hope that this chapter will help psychotherapists feel a greater degree of freedom within themselves and help them as well as the public actively support a spirit of liberation for action-oriented and responsive therapists–therapists who, through good judgment and a commitment to responsible involvement with patients, will be willing to experiment with the unusual when other methods of reaching their patients have been blocked.

Such a viewpoint is not less, but more demanding upon therapists. What is being demanded is that therapists avail themselves of the human encounter, but not limit themselves to it. While authenticity of the moment and in the relationship is certainly a valid existential framework from which to begin therapy, it is also the framework which avails itself to the open-ended search for personal growth and therapeutic methodology that will be most effective in affecting patients. It is also hoped that while therapists learn to make an impact, they will do all that they can to develop their uniqueness as both human beings and therapists; for it is this uniqueness that will help therapists develop a personal style that can make psychotherapy a most rewarding and creative endeavor. In essence, such a view of psychotherapy means that therapists must be extremely well disciplined to be able to know themselves and their patients well enough to risk the unconventional when it is called for.

Therapists need to be able to give themselves the freedom to respond. It is difficult to know what those responses will be, but as they come to trust their intuition, the empathic understanding that comes from an ever-deepening appreciation for their own and their patients' humanity along with a continued commitment to be there through thick and thin with their patients, will help them develop a liberation of spirit so necessary to practicing the art of psychotherapy.

Therapists might be light and funny at one time and serious and intense at another. They may confront patients directly or talk to them indirectly, or use a variety of therapeutic techniques. All the options are open. It is in this sense that all therapies and therapists are existential, no matter what they contend their philosophical leanings to be.

While therapists are responsible and committed people, they are not obliged to abuse themselves or be abused either knowingly or unknowingly by patients. It is also important that therapists do the best they can in getting their message across without letting patients push their countertransference buttons. It is this broad range of responsiveness that is most likely to take patients and therapists to existential moments and the accumulation of those moments which culminate in authentic and healing relationships.

Many issues are involved in developing a liberated spirit when doing therapy. Are therapists able to maintain their identity and separateness in relationship to the patient, or are they unwilling to risk being a disappointment to patients? Are therapists willing to be honest with patients about therapists' wants? Are therapists able to intervene in ways that do not leave their energies depleted? Can therapists refuse to give a false sense of support so patients will learn to stand on their own two feet? Are therapists willing to respond with the range of emotions they feel while working with patients?

I can remember several instances when these issues went through my mind. I remember a physician came to see me late one evening. I had seen his wife for several sessions and she described him as a person whose moods varied between anger and depression. He entered with two bottles of beer in his hands, offering me a bottle. Although it was my first meeting with him I knew I needed to do something to change the mood–or it was going to be a long night for both of us. I thought that if he could improve the quality of his time with me he would also learn how to do it with whatever or whomever he was depressed about in his daily life. I said, "Ordinarily I would deal with the transference issue, but I am thirsty and tired–so just give me the beer." I thought this might jolt him out of himself, but it didn't. He looked surprised for a moment and then went on to tell me how depressing his life was with his wife. The beer was a mistake! I only did it once in 42 years of clinical practice.

I saw the problem differently. He was depressing to himself How could I help him to not be depressing to himself? I said,

> Look, I have been doing therapy all day before you came in. You have the audacity to come in here and tell me depressing stories. Let me make it perfectly clear–I consider the basic purpose of therapy is that of having the therapist have a good time. I am not having a good time when you tell me depressing stories.

Needless to say, the patient flipped from a depressed state to one where he was angry with me. We got through the anger in about five minutes and were able to spend the next forty minutes relating in a positive way. Both of us felt good. However, when his wife came in the following week she said she was having trouble relating to her husband because she wasn't used to his being so cheerful!

Another man was very bright but had blocked his creativity and his ability to have fun. There was a garbage can over his voice that made him feel like he was sinking through my floor into the pits of hell. I thought to myself, this guy is deader than a doornail. Maybe he would wake up if I could bring out the entertaining side of him. He said, "I see your game. You want me to entertain you and you want me to pay you on top of it. That will be the end of our therapy." I replied, "You are very bright to figure all that out in two sessions. It takes most people six months. However, I can't understand your objection." I was having a good time right now playing out the role of the charlatan of which I was accused. I knew I had him against the ropes. I paused just long enough. Then I said, "After all, though you are entertaining me and paying me for it, I am also entertaining you and teaching you how to entertain yourself. That's a lot, considering how boring you are with me." The word boring caught his attention and he realized I wasn't trying to take advantage of him. His wife had precisely the same complaint about him.

I look for the most creative option that rises within me at the time. A lot depends upon continually being in touch with my unconscious flow. I find that I can best have fun and get the job done when I am paying attention to what is happening between us and then dealing with my desires in reaction to the patient. Sheldon Kopp comments on this particular way of paying attention when he speaks of Reich's manner of dealing with patients. ". . . he begins by ignoring the content of the patient's complaints in favor of focusing entirely on the style in which they are being presented."[1] Of course, many therapists, including one of my mentors, Dr. Erving Polster, feels that content must be wedded to process to make the transitions a bit easier for patients. That is what I did when I tied entertainment to the boredom the man's wife complained about.

Dr. Kopp goes on to say,

. . . the therapist is instructing by indirection, helping the patient to unhook from his old stuck ways, opening him to the possibility of new ways of living (whatever they might turn out to be). The perverse guideline for the instruction is "Be where they ain't."

For the patient who begins with immersion in his own history, the therapist must draw him back again and again to what is going on in the here-and-now. The hysterically emotional, overly impulsive patient must be slowed down to stopping and thinking over what he is doing, while the obsessionally paralyzed thinker can be met with non-rational responses which finally get him too upset to hold back any longer. Patients who are initially too hard on themselves are to be treated gently and indulgently while self-sorry whiners must be confronted with harsh demands which leave no quarter for excuse making.

This phase can be really hard work, calling for a great deal of self-discipline on the part of the therapist. Ironically, it can be a great deal of demonic fun as well. There will, of course, be present the corrupting temptation to simply be clever and manipulative, to succumb to the healer's power trip. I find that the best protection for my avoiding the charlatan in myself is to keep aware of the patient in myself, to renew again and again the image of myself as "the wounded healer."[2] While I am talking about liberation and authenticity of response–culminating in existential moments–I also consider the differing shades of authenticity. For example, the appropriate response may be as tricky as it is genuine. Being tricky and authentic can be two sides of the same coin. Being an authentic trickster will not destroy the patient's confidence if the therapist's heart is in the right place. This viewpoint opens up the world of existential therapy to a wide variety of possibilities and methods of doing therapy.

Adding the trickster side to the quality of the therapist's being helps that therapist to facilitate the patient's ability to engage in growth experiences while they both enjoy themselves. They come to appreciate that both therapist and patient have a collection of imperfections that are part of being human. Kopp is able to laugh at himself when he says,

> My fantasy image of my newly-bearded self was that of an amalgam of a ferocious wildman, an untamed shaman, and simultaneously that of an older, wise prophet and archetypal father. I loved it when a patient said that I looked like a Santa Claus for the bad children.

Such humility is important when pursuing an equal therapeutic relationship.

An occurrence that was both daring and authentic took place in a class I was teaching for school counselors. One student was a punitive, out-of-touch robot, and he used words to intellectualize, to avoid contact with members of the class. I saw the basic purpose of each of my classes as that of helping people be with people in an existential sense such as I have been describing. It was from this premise that the course content took shape. I told this man "I don't want you to say another word as long as you remain in this class. I have no desire to be in your presence when you do what you do." I was a bit surprised myself to hear what came out of my mouth–telling a man not to talk for the remainder of the graduate school course, yet, at an intuitive level there was no question at all about doing what I did. I have learned to have a great deal of faith and trust in the intuitive and unconscious processes that may initially appear to be absurd.

At first, the class was outraged that I made such a request. The man, to my surprise, did not appear to be as outraged as I thought he might. At some level he sensed that he needed to do what I asked. However, the class felt that I was treating him like a grammar school student and abusing my power as a graduate school professor. I felt the limits should have been set for this man when he was in grammar school. At the last group session I told him I wanted him to talk to me. He was much more in touch with his feelings, the process of what was going on between us, and the group process. Again I was a bit surprised that he was sending me such appreciative vibrations. On top of all that he did an excellent term paper. I gave him an *A* for the course. His willingness to get his feet wet with the others and his courage moved me. The requirements of the course were that he learn how to deal with people and he had done so. He was living proof to me that it's not where people start that counts, it's where they finish.

In making what I view as a liberated response, that is, a response that may be initially viewed as intuitive or absurd, I had to be *willing to be a disappointment.* Patients' conscious minds, which are usually in command of their self-destructive behavior patterns, are often less than receptive to surprises. Patients might either not understand or pretend they didn't understand, as if understanding were the only thing that mattered. However, as long as I could pick up the disappointments and deal with them, the situations could be worked through in ways that were beneficial. Picking up patients' unexpressed disappointments in the absence of magical cures is also an important part of patients' having the opportunity to work through the infantile wishes that remain with them. If therapists miss the subtle cues of the scalp hunters (patients more interested in proving that whatever the therapist says or does won't help them in helping themselves), those patients will probably terminate therapy prematurely, which would be neither to their benefit nor in therapists' best interests.

Paramount to being able to respond in a liberated way, is that therapists must learn to feel secure within themselves. Such security will help them to discriminate what is genuinely helpful from responses that only appear to be helpful.

I remember supervising a doctoral student who was dealing with the issue of help. She was seeing a patient who was suffering from the beginning stages of multiple sclerosis. The patient complained that he was unable to find employment due to his physical condition. He felt it was difficult to make friends, especially of the opposite sex, since his physical condition made him a poor marital prospect. He wasn't sure whether he would be better off committing suicide.

My student felt stuck in her work with this man. I asked her what she was doing. She said, "I'm trying to encourage him–to help him–to motivate him and to make his world better for him." I sensed from what she was saying that this man was into playing a heavy game of "poor me" and that the payoff was having my student work her butt off trying to rescue him. I asked her to role-play the situation with me. I would play the therapist and she would play the patient.

Student   (Playing the patient) Things are just awful for me. I have multiple sclerosis. I don't make friends easily. Women don't like me. I'm probably better off killing myself.

Me   I don't know what has kept you going this long. (My student was stunned–and I paused for about 30 seconds.) You know, your self pity turns my stomach. I can see why people don't want to be around you. I have a hard time being around you too. Your reality is a bit difficult to swallow, but you certainly could learn how to be with people in a way that they would find you attractive.

Student   I can see that I was stuck because I felt so inadequate. Whatever I suggested, the patient came back for more self pity. It's so hard for me to feel helpless, powerless.

Me   That is a difficult issue, to learn to feel secure enough within yourself to avoid the panic of not being helpful.

During a group therapy session one of the women in the group told a man she wanted to help him. He said, "Let's go to my place after the group and fuck. That's what I really need and would be most helpful." The young lady began to think about exactly how helpful she wanted to be.

The following is another example of how a therapist can try to be helpful without being so. I was feeling hurt, frustrated–just terrible. The woman I was dating for quite some time had broken up with me. That same day a whining patient came in with the same type of heartbreak. I felt helpless to be helpful. The patient was really pressuring me out of his own desperation. The conversation went like this:

Patient   You've got to think of a way for me to feel better, or make her come back to me.

Me   How should I know? I'm in the same situation. The way I feel today I can't even manage my own life.

Patient   Well, you oughta know. You're the doctor!

Me   Oh, because I'm the doctor I shouldn't be allowed to have my own dilemmas in life. I should have the answer to your problem. Hell, I'm having enough trouble trying to figure out my own.

Patient   Well, how can you help me?

Me   Maybe we will just have to struggle through this period together and find our own ways. Then again, developing the ability to find your own way may be useful to you.

The issue between the patient and me was the same as existed between him and his wife. She was alienated by his dependency, and his inhuman punishment of her for not being able to rescue him from life. Therapists should not subject themselves to such abuse, particularly when they have their human needs. Therapists need to be treated as people, too, and it is not unfair to deal with patients in a way that lets them know about therapists' human foibles, despairs and dilemmas. By not being helpful in this situation, which was an authentic sharing of my life, that patient was given the opportunity to learn to stand on his own two feet. Although the patient's wife did not go back to him, nor did my girlfriend go back to me, he did learn to create a reasonably good life for himself by tempering his passive behavior and learning to maintain more reciprocity in relationships.

Edward Smith paraphrases Helmuth Kaiser when he says,

> The universal psychopathology is the attempt to create in real life the universal 'illusion of fusion' (the illusion that one is not alone but is fused with others). The universal

symptom is 'duplicitous communication' (failure to be "behind one's words"). The universal treatment is straightforward (nonduplicitous) communication.[4]

One such experience took place while I was working with a bright young writer who was having difficulty establishing a relationship, and who, due to his fear of losing other people in relationships, would rarely get to the point. He would talk in circles to keep me listening to him. I responded by saying, "I feel drained. I am going to space out–to pay attention to anything in the room–or to my fantasies, but I will not pay attention to you while you remain dead." He got angry, telling me as a therapist I was there to help him and that he did not think I was being helpful. I told him that I was interested in life producing, arousing, engaged dialogue with people, and that I could not see how listening to him die would be helpful. The moment between us changed from death, to anger, to engaged dialogue. I have found that blunt responses often are the key to shaking things loose at the primal level.

Although blunt responses often reach people who otherwise might be difficult to reach in shorter periods of time, there has been a lack of acceptance of such responding. Havens makes an interesting comment when he says, "Everyone fears leaving the apparently secure base of objectivity and rationality. At the same time the objective, rational approaches favored by both descriptive psychiatry and psychoanalysis restrict our capacity to deal with the irrational forces that are most feared."[5] However, in addition to dealing with blunt responses that come from a combination of intuition and unconscious flow of the therapist, a further issue becomes therapists' use of anger, if that is what intuitively arises from the unconscious flow of awareness. Havens, in describing the work of Eugene Minkowski said that although Minkowski went as far as to live with a patient so that he might understand how the patient saw things, Minkowski instead grew alienated and couldn't imagine why the patient would continue to engage in such self-destructive behavior. He found that the patient was not only infuriating, but contemptible.

The central question then became whether familiarity led to contempt and a loss of objectivity and authority. While Minkowski found this to be true, he also found that it was built up again when he became spontaneous. When Minkowski lost his temper with this whining, obsessive, and irascible patient, the two became closer.

Existential therapy extends an invitation for expressiveness on the part of therapists. However, Havens suggests that two criteria are important: *being* and *staying*.

Havens felt that

> The critical tests are only two, however difficult they may be to pass conclusively. Has the therapist tried to be and stay; more specifically has he practiced the phenomenological reduction and translated his empathic experience? Second, has he had success in this, as measured by affective responses to the patient, but been blocked?[6]

Then, for example, just because therapists are angry is not sufficient reason to express that anger unless "the goal of expression was to reach or remain where the patient was."[7] Havens felt that more was needed than the therapist thinking about staying. The desire to stay must have been demonstrated to both the therapist and the patient. Therapists must have learned that they desired to stay through the thick and thin of the struggle with the patient.

So the genuineness of therapists' interest must be demonstrated. It is the genuineness of this interest, or desire, that demonstrates a *commitment to stay*. It is with such commitment that therapists are able to expand the spontaneous quality of their *being* with patients; and that such can be done within the overall framework of a loving and caring therapeutic relationship.

The basis of encounter or emotional confrontation then comes from the therapist's desire to stay but not being able to stay under present conditions. Thus, the need for change in the patient, the doctor, or both, is the need to *stay*. Havens puts it well when he describes the existential method as seeking to provide a relationship that is so valuable to both patient and therapist, that they are *willing to change to preserve it*. It is when the therapist fails to be empathic and exclude conclusions while trying to stay with the patient's immediate conscious state that emotional confrontation becomes a necessary part of the therapeutic relationship. Without such confrontation, Havens felt there would only be an understanding therapist and an immovable patient.

Havens describes the process when he says, "Being and staying as ends in themselves, the commitment to accepting appearances, translating and extending our shared grasp, 'keeping looking,' the willingness to confront and change–all these outline a clinical technique or method."[8]

Minkowski's use of anger means that the patient now had to either decline what was being presented or empathize with him. Patient and therapist changed roles. Such changing of roles provides the basis for an equal therapeutic engagement. It is the exchanging of subjective and objective roles that provides the basis for both patient and therapist changing as a result of engaging in the process. The therapist was now presenting the objective material that called forth the empathic capacity of the patient. Such a method of working is valuable in that it both helps the patient deal with narcissistic behavior and helps the therapist to have a channel with which to release feelings that might otherwise continue to build into a more and more furious state.

Havens describes the pitfalls of the existential method as two. The therapist may be condescending. The countertransference may flow rampantly as the vigilance against the unconscious is given up. When distance is so reduced between patient and therapist, the opportunity for a rational perspective may greatly be reduced.

It is my feeling that a balance must be achieved here, or therapists may reinforce a bit too much craziness on the way to working through the relationship difficulties. The balance can be achieved when the therapist responds fully with one part of his or her being, while another part looks over the shoulder to monitor the process. It is only in this way that therapists may reduce the blatant unconscious distortions that Havens feel are a natural consequence of the existential method.

While Havens comments upon the split between existentially-oriented psychiatry and psychoanalysis, I think both schools have missed something of importance in their perspectives. Existentialists feel that the distance between patient and therapist that results from a psychoanalytic reflection creates countertransferences that a successful empathy would reduce. They further feel that psychoanalytic ideas of what constitutes a mentally healthy person become part of that countertransference. I believe, however, the psychoanalysts' feelings about what constitutes a mentally healthy person come more from what is grounded in nature than from preconceived ideas, and I further believe that this is an existential distortion that would not be made when looking at excellent analysts' work. Such a split between the camps does not take the whole human being into account. We are both object and subject. To think of ourselves any differently is to pander the nature of human beings themselves. And while existential psychiatry sees all judgments about others as countertransferences to be avoided, I believe that such judgments are only natural for humans. And if they be psychoanalytic judgments I see nothing wrong with this. The judgments may be dealt with openly within the context of being and staying described by Havens. This would provide a more comprehensive method of therapy for a complicated human race. For example, I might yell at a patient to stop what I consider to be crazy and outlandish behavior. (I use the word crazy in the same context a lay person would use. I don't hold back my use of it because I am a therapist. Patients know what I mean.) The patient either at some level knows and acknowledges that it is crazy and outlandish behavior; or the patient argues back with me until both our viewpoints are different; or the patient refuses my assessment of the situation either demonstratively or passively. In any of these situations there is the opportunity to work things through with the process of being and staying. In addition, I do not make private judgments about patients that I do not share with them. Everything is out front. In this way all parties have both the best chance for growth and the best chance to protect themselves if need be. The irreducible attitudes that seem so objective may be met with confrontations that produce fresh objectivities between patient and therapist. Or, if the attitudes are based on a natural flow, it is more than attitudes we are talking about. It is the working through to become in accord with nature. Such a method means that it is not in the therapist's private world that countertransference will be resolved, but in the meeting and contact of two human beings; namely, patient and therapist.

Sharing those thoughts, ideas, feelings and attitudes which therapists hold about patients, with patients, and a willingness to risk with patients in this sense gets at the heart of the matter. That is, that existential moments must come from within us before they can occur!

I have quoted Havens extensively because many of his theoretical formulations provide the basis for my definition of existential moments. For example, Havens says, "If the accidental bonds are important to treatment results, any procedure that systematically enlarges those bonds (or reduces the points of separation) must have comparable importance. It is not too much to claim that this is the specific goal of being and staying."[9]

I feel that Haven's concept of staying can be refined. He speaks of staying in terms of therapists becoming empathic in their here-and-now way of responding to, engaging in, and entering into their patients' world. He also intimated that therapists' responses would only come after a studying the patient's world for some time. I redefine staying, or commitment, as I prefer to think of it, in terms of therapists' commitment to be with the patient through it all, and that patient's willingness to make the same commitment. If that commitment is made clear from the very beginning of therapy, therapists need not wait to respond. Such a therapeutic working alliance is crucial to effective therapy. Otherwise, therapists may be out of balance; they may be more for others (pleasing patients) than they are being-in-the-world (being solid therapeutic citizens who get the job done). An example was with John, the man who had the machete strapped to his leg that I wrote about in the prologue of the book. My vigorous confrontation with him, even with his paranoid schizophrenic diagnosis, established a trusting relationship right from the very beginning. We both permitted ourselves to feel the fundamental reality of our existence.

When both therapist and patient are able to allow themselves to feel the fundamental reality of their own existence which is the human condition–without facade, while they are in touch with each other–existential moments occur in the healing relationship. The major importance of such a viewpoint is that patients will learn how to deal with the ups and downs, the nitty gritty of a relationship, where they might ordinarily cut off their relationships (or limit them) in their lives outside therapy. The authentic relationship between patient and therapist provides the opportunity for that patient to weather the storms of the battleground until the patient is able to develop a relationship that is both intimate and loving with the therapist. When this has happened, patients will not only have had the experience of a variety of healing moments (as with the other therapies I will mention), but they will have had the experience of those healing moments within a relationship that has been genuine and progressively equal on both sides–a relationship that has allowed patients to get to a place where they are able to love and be loved by another at increasing levels of intimacy while they do not hang onto unrealistic expectations of how other people should behave in the world.

Although patients may surely come to therapy not believing they are equals of the therapist, the presumption of equality by the therapist helps patients to see that they, too, have power. They come to feel good about using their power, just as they see the therapist use his or her power. Both patient and therapist have the power to respond freely. Both can steer the therapy session in a direction. Both have rights. Neither patient nor therapist has to live up to stereotypes of what the other should be. Both are free to choose and define their own existence with each other. They are only limited by the surroundings of their environment. The rest is up for grabs. They can create a new existence for themselves at each moment.

The relationship may very well begin with the therapist being more able to mobilize energy and vitality while working than the patient. However, after a series of frustrations and supports of what is vital and life-producing in patients, they may slowly give up inauthentic behaviors that leave them half dead while they still manage to walk and talk. Each bit of excitement and energy they can mobilize creates a desire for another ounce of excitement. The idea is to get them addicted to life, not death. The therapeutic task is to turn around the entire conditioning process we have been exposed to since our birth. We have been conditioned to become robots to one degree or another, who fit into the existing order of things and who will not upset anybody's apple cart. However, under the cloak of morality many have been deceived and then gone on to deceive themselves. This process is not irreversible. Once we gradually begin to experience what it feels like to live again—the world of joy, excitement, energy, intimacy, and love may become ours. We can give up the manufactured feelings of anger, depression, and anxiety and get on with the business of life. We can make ourselves well enough to deal with the authentic emotions[10] that accompany the human condition, even if they be sadness or grief at times.

Milton H. Erickson, M.D., is a responsive and liberated spirit who has been an inspiration to me. In the following example, described by Jay Haley, Dr. Erickson got to the heart of the matter in one session.

The presenting problem was a fourteen-year-old girl who had developed the idea that her feet were much too large. The mother came alone to Erickson and described the situation. For three months the girl had been becoming more and more withdrawn, and she didn't want to go to school or to church or to be seen on the street. The girl would not allow the subject of her feet to be discussed, and she would not go to a doctor to talk to him. No amount of reassurance by her mother had any influence, and the girl was becoming more and more seclusive. Erickson reports: "I arranged with the mother to visit the home on the following day under false pretenses. The girl would be told that I was coming to examine the mother to see if she had the flu. It was a pretense, and yet the mother wasn't feeling well and I suggested that an examination would be appropriate. When I arrived at the home, the mother was in bed. I did a careful physical examination of her, listening to her chest, examining her throat, and so on. The girl was present. I sent her for a towel, and I asked that she stand beside me in case I needed something. She was very concerned about her mother's health. This gave me an opportunity to look her over. She was rather stoutly built and her feet were not large.

"Studying the girl, I wondered what I could do to get her over this problem. Finally I hit upon a plan. As I finished my examination of the mother, I maneuvered the girl into a position directly behind me. I was sitting on the bed talking to the mother, and I got up slowly and carefully and then stepped back awkwardly. I put my heel down squarely on the girl's toes. The girl, of course, squawked with pain. I turned on her and in a tone of absolute fury said, 'If you would grow those things large enough for a man to see, I wouldn't be in this sort of situation!' The girl looked at me, puzzled, while I wrote out a prescription and called the drugstore. That day the girl asked her mother if she could go out to a show, which she hadn't done in months. She went to school and church, and that was the end of a pattern of three months' seclusiveness. I checked later on how things were going, and the girl was friendly and agreeable. She didn't realize what I had done, nor did her mother. All her mother noticed was that I had been impolite to her daughter when I visited that day. She couldn't connect that with the daughter's return to normal activity."

It seems self-evident that this technique is based upon a hypnotic orientation. As Erickson put it, "There was no way for the girl to reject that compliment about her feet, no way to dispute it. 'If she would grow her feet large enough for a man to see.' The girl couldn't tell me I was clumsy; I was her mother's doctor. She couldn't retaliate in any way. There was nothing for her to do but accept the absolute proof that her feet were small." It is not unusual for Erickson to use hypnosis to arrange that a subject have an idea he cannot reject, and in this case he achieved that end without hypnosis in a social situation.

The examples of John and of Dr. Erickson's work show the value of immediate responsiveness. In Dr. Erickson's case it resulted in a one-session cure. However, one may naturally ask why I use Dr. Erickson's case as an example of existential therapy. I do so because Dr. Erickson was a liberated therapist.

In *a truly liberated* therapist, strategy that flows from therapists' unconscious minds is also legitimate. There is no use in therapists' tying their hands behind their backs for the love or pursuit of any theoretical way of viewing the practice of psychotherapy. Obviously Dr. Erickson had that commitment to stay as part of his own personality, and as that was the case was able to do what he did strategically on the first session–in that patient's best interest. So there are times when being strategic is in the best interests of patients.

In a sense this use of strategy is closer to the psychoanalytic way of viewing things because it does make objects out of patients and there is a detached, reflective quality. However, existentially isn't this also part of what people do with other people? Why should such behavior be excluded from the normal realm of human behavior because of prior existential theory? That is, the theory that only the subject-to-subject touching of two human beings is healing as taught in the radical humanistic existential camp. It may be the meat and potatoes of therapy, but it is not the all of it.

Furthermore, Dr. Erickson did not find it important to wait to fully understand the girl as a psychoanalyst would; he just acted, based on his unconscious and intuitive understanding of her. He was an authentic trickster. He put something over on her to accomplish the task of restoring the girl to a more psychologically healthy state in the shortest time possible.

Let us look once again at Keen's definition of being-for-myself.

> We are, second, in the sense that we represent what we are to ourselves. This aspect of our being entails the experience of oneself-as-object. We reflect upon our desires, fears, and thoughts, name them, judge them, reason about them, and have feelings about them. Furthermore, I am a "me" to myself, with certain attributes and characteristics. With dispassionate detachment, I can, upon reflection, do everything to myself that I can do to the world. The content of this process is a second activity of being.[12]

Transporting Keen's description to psychotherapy, therapists naturally make objects out of patients as part of the therapeutic work. It is important that patients be approached person-to-person, with a spirit of equality in the relationship (although there are times that it is important to be authoritarian within the context of an equal therapeutic relationship, such as Dr. Erickson did in the previous example). But it is also important that therapists be able to make reflections so they will be able to make accurate judgments. This balance between treating the patient as a subject and as an object will help therapists in two respects. They will reduce the amount of countertransference to patients. Or, therapists who wish to respond by using countertransference material in reaction to patients' actions will be more likely to capture passionate therapeutic moments while at the same time they have reflected upon and made a judgment about what they are doing. This balance, when it is down to the split second–is the type of response that is most valuable. Therapists may respond as passionately involved significant others while at the same time being objective.

I can remember the first time I met a well-published existential psychiatrist. When he found out I was doing straight existential therapy he referred to me as a soft head. My immediate reaction was that he must be a hard head, and that as long as I was being and staying, I couldn't understand why he would say what he said. Later, I happened to get interested in transactional analysis. I began to see that in the pursuit of my only goal at that time–the goal of authenticity–I was watering down my clinical judgment. I was not aware of finer discriminations. That is, patients would respond with different ego states, such as critical parent, nurturing parent, adult, scared child, and rebellious child. They would engage in repetitive script behavior, such as doing something "over and over," "never," "always," "open-ended," etc. (An example of "over and over" script is Sysyphus, who rolls the stone nearly to the top of the hill before it falls, and has to begin again.) Patients would manifest certain injunctions such as "don't be close," "don't be successful," etc. They would have certain inbred commands, referred to as "drivers," such as "please me," "hurry up," "try hard," "be perfect," and "be strong" that would motivate their behaviors. They would come into self-destructive and repetitive game behavior that is out of awareness from one of three game positions–victim, persecutor, or rescuer–and then switch to one of the other positions. I do my best not to reinforce script behavior, while at the same time I do my best to respond potently in ways that make a difference in patients' lives. Learning to think clearly about scripts, drivers, games, etc., while still being able to respond fully took a bit of doing in moving from a soft head to a balanced head. Yet without these kinds of judgments, existential theory might dilute itself in practice beyond a point that is productive for both patients and therapists. I will talk more about the wedding of transactional analysis and existential theory and practice in a later chapter.

Therapists may choose to state their judgments spontaneously as part of the ongoing process of being and staying, or they may choose less threatening ways to reach patients. While it is important not to cheat the patient of authenticity, it is also important to know when to give the raw spontaneity as opposed to a more tempered response.

The following interchange may provide the reader with an example of the subjective-objective process of which I speak. Albert is a very bright attorney who knew how to play with paradox and could laugh at himself while still being able to integrate what was happening. He prefaced my response with a long-winded tale of woe about how he was being victimized.

Me	Whether it's true or not doesn't make any difference. I get a charge out of seeing you pretend to be suffering when you unconsciously know all along that you are the one with the whip! (Although this was said in a slightly humorous and spontaneous manner, my objective judgment was to avoid buying Albert's victim position.)
Albert	Suffering comes so naturally to me. My people have been suffering for 2,000 years (he is Jewish) and my mother was the best yet (getting playful). How can you evoke guilt if you don't suffer–and guilt is the basis of control. But you don't let me get away with anything. (He says this in a patronizing way. He is fast enough to put a percentage of his maneuvers right by me.)
Me	That's because I'm a guru! (Playfully provocative and spontaneous while still making the judgment about his patronizing behavior.)
Albert	So what! I'm a genius! (Albert acknowledges his power and brilliance, something he earlier denied in the same session.)
Me	Be a genius–you asshole! Be a genius! (Said affectionately, spontaneously, while making the judgment to stroke Albert's acknowledgment of his brilliance by implying he is an asshole when he doesn't.)

Albert	Be a guru–asshole! (He needles me about the times I water down my potency in the sessions.)
Me	That will teach me to mess around with a genius!
Albert	(A bit maudlinly) Thank God for gurus, otherwise how would a genius like me find himself?
Me	Your thanks has been well received on two counts. (Such a blatant acknowledgment of the power he has so graciously given to me reminds him that the power rests within him. Then a more serious flash comes from my unconscious mind. I choose to say it.) A self-enclosed system can be dangerous for you on the occasions when you are mistaken. Check it out more with others. Include them in your life. You will have a more loving and powerful existence.
Albert	I'm afraid to let others in because they would think I'm a fool.
Me	You are a fool. Now that you know that you have nothing to fear!
Albert	Duh! (Playfully)
Me	Don Rickles is a fool and a genius at the same time, too.

So in this dialogue I am being, but almost in a zen way. I am responding to whether Albert is fully present on each response, and when he isn't, I am making a judgment about that and responding simultaneously in a playfully condescending way that helps him to resume his own power. I enjoy working in this way, particularly with people who can appreciate the nature of paradox and then integrate for themselves.

Such objectivity and the use of strategy as it flows through the unconscious in a non-strategic way, leave therapists with even greater degrees of freedom in meeting patients that they might otherwise not be able to relate with. This can be seen in reading Jay Haley's *Uncommon Therapy* which gives numerous examples of the spontaneous use of unconscious strategy. Although it is strategic, and certainly sounds that way from Haley's descriptions, it is not strategic in that the objectifying of patients takes place through an unconscious flow of Dr. Erickson's in which they are also treated as subjects–that is, in a subject-to-subject, person-to-person way.

In the same context of paradox, the issue of when therapists need to be authoritarian doctors is also an important question. If treating patients equally is non-productive as a means of doing therapy, then maybe the most productive thing therapists can do is to help patients regress to a childlike state so they may be reparented. (Dr. Erickson does this with hypnosis and Dr. Kempler does it through *arousal*. Both use *intimidation* to attain their goals discussed in later chapters.) Equality with patients who know no limits can be a mistake. In these instances it may be unwise to cling to existential theory and one basic premise of this book–that an equal relationship is a critical part of the healing process. It may be that such equality will be down the road a bit and that therapists can later move toward an equal relationship once the child in the patient has been mothered or fathered in a firm way. At this point they may be ready for a more mature relationship.

For true freedom to exist, patients must be able to set limits for themselves. When their grandiosity gets in the way of such limits, therapists must be able to set limits and enforce them. Haley comments on Dr. Erickson's response which are authoritarian, condescending and belittling. Yet, within the context of what these particular patients needed, they were bullseye responses. They were limit setting. They were so condescending that they were intimidating. They were intended to be intimidating, to patients who used intimidation as a way to avoid dealing with themselves. In Erickson's words,

> He came in to see me on February 26, and on April 17 he came in and very apologetically, in an embarrassed fashion, said, "I'm afraid you were right. I was hanging on to a little kid's headache. I've waited and waited. I've waited daily ever since that first day, and now I've

finally decided that I haven't got a drug addiction, I haven't got a headache."

I said, "Well, it took you a long time–from the twenty-sixth of February to the seventeenth of April–to decide that you didn't have a headache. Rather a slow learner, aren't you? There's something else. You mentioned your family not being very happy. Tell, me, what kind of misery did you inflict on your wife, what kind of miserable shrew did you make out of your wife, and how many of your six children have you damaged?"[13]

While the man did not have six children, Erickson saw fit to accuse him of damaging six.

Dr. Erickson then requested the man have his wife come in to correct some of the damage the man did to her. Dr. Erickson turned the man's games right back on him. The wife came in with the two children. Dr. Erickson went on to say,

I spent four hours telling that woman, in very impolite terms, that she was the supreme shrew and she ought to be ashamed of herself. She was appalled. She tried to defend herself. I kept insulting her. The girl and the fourteen-year old boy tried to defend their mother to me. I told the girl, "Now you stand up and turn around. How old are you, and how much do you weigh, and do you realize you look like the south end of a northbound horse?"

I turned to the mother and said, "As for you, Mother, you just think of how you've changed from a nice, sweet, pretty young girl into a nagging, quarreling, screaming shrew. You really ought to be ashamed of yourself. You're old enough to know better." After four hours of that tirade, mother finally said, "I'm not going to take any more of this insulting," and she rushed out of the office. She lived fifteen miles away. She got in her car, and you could see the smoke boiling out of the car as she pulled away from the curb. After about the time it took to travel fifteen miles, the telephone range. It was her voice, and she was panting. She said, "I ran all the way from the garage to phone you. I was halfway home before I realized that you told the truth. I was just burning up all the way until it dawned on me that everything you said was the truth. Now, when can I have my next appointment with you?"[14]

Things worked themselves out with each of the family members, but for the purposes of this book I am just interested in showing how a condescending and authoritative way of responding can be crucial in helping certain kinds of patients turn their lives around. It's hard to work with people if you don't have their attention.

R. D. Laing, Thomas Szasz, and other existential therapists claim there is no such thing as mental illness. When I bought the party line, I too, saw things from this frame of reference. However, after I was able to incorporate the transactional analysis frame of reference into a broader existential philosophical framework, I began to see things quite differently. I see behaviors that come from habits, behavior patterns that were developed during childhood, that no longer fit people. These behaviors and emotional states do indeed show a mental imbalance of one degree or another. I make judgments about each discrepancy from what I experientially, cognitively, intuitively, and affectively know to be a balance. The question then becomes one of facilitating patients in attaining a physical, spiritual, and emotional balance; a cure. Therapists need to consider treating the whole person, the symptoms, and the authenticity of relationship to make the greatest impact with a wide variety of patients. Although the authentic relationship provides the framework, each of the therapies has something to offer in the form of a cure or people wouldn't seek them out. It is worthwhile to know more and more about more and more. It is important to be able to meet patients where they are in their lives. The more therapists have incorporated into their lives and therapeutic styles, the more different types of patients they will be able to help. It is my experience and belief that all humans have some of the characteristics that compose each form of mental illness, and the more therapists can identify these traits in themselves, the more they will be able to help patients work through these troubled spots.

I have been setting up a broad framework that may liberate therapists, or help them continue their lifelong pursuit of liberating themselves by increasing their capacity to respond. I would now like to examine therapists' capacities to be outrageous, as oftentimes it is the outrageous response that helps people turn the corner.

When Dr. Erickson was dealing with a mother who complained that her eight-year-old son was becoming progressively more defiant each day, Dr. Erickson used an outrageous response to the situation. Dr. Erickson described the situation.

> As the mother told her story, Joe listened with a broad, triumphant smile. When she had finished, he boastfully declared that I could not do anything to stop him, and he was going to go right on doing as he pleased. I assured him, gravely and earnestly, that it was unnecessary for me to do anything to change his behavior because he was a good big, strong boy and very smart and he would have to change his behavior all by himself. I assured him that his mother would do just enough to give him a chance to change his behavior "all by himself." Joe received this statement in an incredulous, sneering manner. I said that his mother would be told some simple little things that she could do so that he himself could change his behavior, and sent him out of the office. I also challenged him in a most kindly fashion to try to figure out what those simple little things might be. This served to puzzle him into quiet reflective behavior while he awaited his mother.[15]

The following morning,

> Joe demanded that she prepare his breakfast without delay, threatening physical destruction of the first thing he could lay his hands on if she did not hurry. His mother merely smiled at him, seized him, threw him quickly to the floor on his stomach, and sat her full

weight upon him. When he yelled at her to get off, she said she had already eaten breakfast and she had nothing to do except to try to think about ways to change his behavior. However, she pointed out that she was certain she did not know any way. Therefore it would all be up to him.[16]

After over five hours Joe surrendered by stating simply and abjectly that he would do anything and everything she told him to do. His mother replied just as simply and earnestly that her thinking had been in vain; she just did not know what to tell him to do. He burst into tears at this but shortly, sobbing, he told her he knew what to do. She replied mildly that she was very glad of this, but she did not think he had enough time to think long enough about it. Perhaps another hour or so of thinking might help. Joe silently awaited the passing of an hour while his mother sat reading quietly. When over an hour had passed, she commented on the time but expressed her wish to finish the chapter. Joe sighed shudderingly and sobbed softly to himself while his mother finished her reading.

With the chapter finally finished, the mother got up and so did Joe.[17] Here we see how an outrageous response by Dr. Erickson in his suggestions to her helped him create an existential moment between Joe and his mother–or a series of existential moments. She was being both authentic and strategic in her setting limits. Joe managed to figure out exactly what he needed to do to change his behavior without one instruction from his mother. Also, in these kinds of stories you can begin to see the wedding of existentialism to behavior modification.

Erickson had a way to combine action with the moment, and he put that action between mother and son, where it needed to be. The mother's action was worth a lifetime of words. The boy, once he got the message that mother would use all her authority and parental power to stop him, knew that it would be best if he set his own limits. Once he got the message that limits would be set, it wasn't very hard for him to figure out who it was he had antagonized, and began making reparations. Some of the most intriguing existential moments are those that result from finding the right action to cut through to the heart of the matter. This, most certainly, was the genius of Erickson.

The additional focus on change and on cure also makes the existential philosophy I describe a hopeful one. Although authentic relationships are important, one's life work is to grapple with the life plan based on heredity and the environment. When blacks say, "We shall overcome," they are referring to overcoming what in a sense may be viewed as tragic life scripts that they have become too familiar with in being an oppressed people for hundreds of years. In a sense all people have the lifelong task of learning to choose freely options that are in accord with their inner being. The closer they come to freedom from childhood script and the rewriting of their own scripts, the more we think of them as people who have done much in terms of taking charge of their lives and doing so within a deepened humanity. Such people are thought to be autonomous. In many cases there is a conservative and politically-involved element of the profession that defines psychotherapeutic limits in such a traditional fashion that innovation and creativity in affecting patients becomes a risky business. However, professional psychotherapists must really ask themselves whether doing little or nothing to maintain a low-profile image that is not in any way controversial is really in the best interests of patients? Unless psychotherapists are willing to risk their full responsiveness with patients, those patients may only get watered-down versions of the therapeutic experience they might have had. They may never be affected in ways that will help them change their lives significantly and permanently.

The issue of sex may be important when considering the liberation of the therapist. Consider the following example:

I was recovering from an appendix operation. The surgeon told me that I was not to have sex for twenty-one days from the date of the operation. After two weeks' absence I returned to work. A woman came for her appointment. She inquired about my health. In a joking but frustrated manner I told her the doctor said no basketball and no sex, and that my wife kept asking me how many days were left. The woman returned the following week wearing a blouse that left little to the imagination. Of course, this was well within the twenty-one day era of my sexual frustration. She began by telling me her problem. I could not hear a word she was uttering. Finally, after several conscientious attempts I told her, "Your teats are taking precedence over anything you are saying today." She ran over and grabbed a beach towel I have in the office and teasingly put it around her upper torso. She replied, "Is that better?" The first thing that came to my mind was, "I don't think so." She said, half teasingly and half without awareness, "Well, what do you want me to do?" I replied, "Frankly, at this point I'm at a loss for words." She arrived for the next session in more moderate attire. Nevertheless, the issue of sex between patient and therapist as it arises in the therapeutic situation must be dealt with. The above example shows how I attempted to deal with the issue of sex in a liberated and responsive way.

Several patients have come right out and asked me to go to bed with them, but I will not do so. My position is clear. I am unwilling to have sexual relationships with patients. Besides being unethical, it is humanly immoral. At the levels of conscience and of heart it would be the same as molesting patients in a crippled children's ward. While it may appear to be a situation between two consenting adults, the therapist has the unfair advantage of patients' coming to therapy to present the crippled-child part of themselves, and in doing so, letting themselves become "hooked in" emotionally to the therapist, as they might "hook into" mommy or daddy or a spouse. However, were it not for the special situation that exists between patient and therapist, it is unlikely that patients would be so attracted to those therapists if they were to meet in a common social situation.

Touching patients is also somewhat of a hot issue these days. While touching must be done appropriately and probably should be avoided unless therapists are confident of judging the situation correctly, it can be of great value in providing the basis for existential moments, such as my use of the batacas with Ned in the prologue, or placing my seven-year-old client on the mantlepiece to make humorous contact with her. As existential moments often involve mentioning the unmentionable or suggesting the unsuggestible, touching is but a logical extension of the liberated spirit of the therapeutic relationship. It will work well, if in fact, that spirit does exist between patient and therapist. Touching will become more and more prevalent as psychotherapists begin to get into the area of body therapy (discussed later in the book). I predict that touching and body work will become progressively more valuable in helping patients become integrated sexually and emotionally. I recommend that therapists proceed with caution in this area.

Further, get the additional rider on your professional liability insurance policy to cover therapeutic touching. But do proceed if you are the intuitive type who can sense when touching is appropriate. Therapeutic touching will add a richer dimension to the therapy–even if it is only so much as a goodbye hug given to a patient in need of physical stroking.

A HOLISTIC APPROACH TO PSYCHOTHERAPY/HYPNOSIS

A holistic approach to psychotherapy/hypnosis advocates balanced living and common mental and organic sense. For too many years psychotherapy has concerned itself exclusively with the psyche. It is time that the soma be considered in relationship to the psyche. People must be considered in their totality. They must be balanced in terms of physical exercise, proper nutrition and relaxation in addition to their spiritual needs. People need a strong body if they are to have the physical strength to make psychological changes that are a result of psychotherapy. And people who have healthy bodies must be psychologically well-balanced if they are to lead happy and healthy lives. I urge those in psychotherapy to stretch the boundaries of traditional psychotherapy to also include common sense, the accumulated wisdom of the ages, to help people use their natural resources in as many ways as possible to continue to make themselves well and enjoy good health–physical, mental and spiritual.

Psychotherapy and hypnosis go hand in hand in helping patients live a balanced life. Hypnosis provides the suggestion and stress reduction; psychotherapy the working through of conflicts. In addition, the commonsense attitude of health–proper nutrition, proper exercise and proper relaxation, along with well-developed contact functions (self, others, environment)–may allow people to experience more existential moments than they might otherwise have.

PHYSICAL ILLNESS AND PSYCHOTHERAPY

Illness is something that no one looks forward to, but it is part of the process of life and death. Psychotherapy and hypnosis can help people make themselves free of disease. However, in cases where freedom from disease is questionable, or death a certainty, psychotherapy and hypnosis can begin to help patients see their illness as a friend. Patients can learn to accept their illness and establish obtainable goals. They can come to find meaning in the illness and accept the totality of the life process. In this acceptance and utilization of what exists patients can come to hear their inner voices giving them messages in more clear and powerful ways than they previously experienced.

Non-medical therapists must make clear to patients that they are only working with the psychological ramifications of physical illness and/or psychosomatic illness. *Therapists must be sure patients have seen or are referred to a medical doctor for any real or imagined physical ailments.* In addition to being sound therapeutic practice this will protect therapists against any legal charges of practicing medicine without a license.

Working with Psychological Ramifications of Physical Symptoms

Two examples of patients who worked with the relationship between their illness and themselves follow:

Patient number one was a twenty-six-year old man who complained of herpes. He said he had had herpes on and off for several years and medical intervention hadn't been able to cure him. The therapist who was working with him asked him to begin talking to the herpes. This particular work was within the context of gestalt therapy, so the herpes was in the empty chair. While the man looked kind of sickly when he began, he came into such full contact with himself--that is, between the side that was him and the side that was the herpes, that at the end of the work he was using his full power. The value he got from the work was that the herpes part of him that he had been trying to rid himself of was giving him a message. The message was that there was a powerful part of himself that he was not using. He was being much less than he could be. While I do not know what happened to the herpes at the end of the session, he looked vital and almost booming with energetic power! He had assumed responsibility for his herpes, and made friends with that part of him.

Patient number two was a forty-two-year old woman who had just come to me from her physician for her weekly marital therapy session. On this particular occasion, however, her marriage was the least of her concerns. She was very frightened about a tumor she had on her side. The doctor said he thought it was a fatty tumor that needed to be watched. As long as it wasn't growing, it was to be left alone. Knowing that she was receiving medical care *first*, I began by asking her to talk to the tumor in the empty chair. During the normal course of therapy she had a great deal of difficulty with reality. She would often make up reality as she went along. The problem with her process was that oftentimes she became hopelessly lost, she did not know what she felt.

Even though this was a fatty tumor, it was not known at that point if it was malignant. So while she was talking to the tumor in the empty chair she became as genuine as I had ever seen her. The tumor side of her was telling her that it was going to beat her unless she stood up for herself and stopped being afraid of her own shadow. After twenty minutes of rather severe confrontations of this kind from the side being her tumor, she began to deal with the tumor from a position of strength instead of a position of fear. The tumor side of her became upset, telling her that it hadn't counted on her using her power that soon or that fast, but that it was going to hang around just in case she went back to her old ways. While this woman would often sabotage empty chair work, as control was an important issue to her she did this work relatively free of any outside therapeutic interventions. Her motivation was coming so strongly from within her that I hardly had to say a word, she knew exactly when to switch chairs. But the tumor was working as effectively as any therapist I had ever seen. Its purpose, as she and I saw it, became clear. Her tumor was telling her it was disgusted about how she was living her life, and that it was going to really give it to her unless she continued to live a life that was more genuinely connected to the reality of her life.

It was only after she had come to this understanding with her tumor that I was willing to do hypnosis with her. I began by telling her to imagine the white blood cells attacking the tumor. "Imagine them in a warm fluid healing all the red raw areas. You can see the fatty tumor just beginning to become smaller and smaller. All the fatty tissue is beginning to melt away." I went on in this fashion for about twenty minutes, after which she began saying that she could feel her tumor becoming smaller and smaller.

The tumor did not grow. Her physician diagnosed it as a fatty tumor. So for all practical purposes the psychotherapy session did not have any practical effect on the actual growth of the tumor.

Several months later, when I asked the patient if she felt this particular session had been of any importance to her she said that it did. She said it made a significant difference in that her tumor was something she no longer feared. She no longer related the tumor to guilt, or anger, or not using her power. As a result of the session she had basically come to grips with these problems and felt that now she could see her tumor for what it was—a fatty tumor. She felt good about being able to generally maintain a firm sense of herself.

Both patients were able to profit from their illnesses. They were able to give meaning to their illnesses, which helped them to establish goals in their lives. In this way, they have learned to use their illnesses as a way to move into health. They accepted their life processes and moved into a more powerful use of consciousness by taking charge of their lives. They truly had an internal psychotherapist, which they used.

The psychotherapist, the clinical hypnotist, the nutritionist, and others in addition to a medical doctor, may in their special ways also contribute to the common sense approach to balanced living. They may compliment the physician in some areas and provide important services independently in other areas. Yet, each type of health specialist would do well to recommend the services of other health specialists when they are certain that patients are out of balance in a particular area; whether it be nutrition, relaxation, or physical problems of an organic nature. It is such use of common sense that will provide for the health care of the whole person.

It is with this spirit of place that I see existential moments related to *holistic psychotherapy;* that is, psychotherapy which is based on common sense, the accumulated wisdom of the ages, the nature of people and what is natural about them–and the application of peoples' natural resources in ways that will help them to remain whole. Holistic is applied to the practice of hypnosis within the context of this broader definition of holistic psychotherapy, as hypnosis is customarily practiced within the field of specialty of the practitioner (medicine, clinical psychology, dentistry, marriage and family counseling).

EXERCISE AND FUN

As part of my growth process, a woman in my group therapy training session asked me what I was doing physically to keep myself in shape. I told her I would try doing exercises, such as "An Eleven-Minute-a-Day Program," or a "Four-Minute-a-Day Program." I would follow it faithfully for three weeks, then put it off for six months, then try it again. She asked me what I liked to do. I said I liked to play basketball, but most guys my age were retired. I told her I played tennis, but I was unwilling to have to wait to use a tennis court. She asked me if I ran any faster in tennis than I did when playing basketball by myself. I said no. I began to realize that if I ran at a pretty fast pace, imagining I was on one of the teams that were to clash for the big game each week, I could have a half-hour of fun each day while I was keeping fit through exercise. The key correlation is exercise and fun. If I had to depend upon willpower I never would have made it. A grateful thanks to my loving group member, Lilliana!

I began to talk about overall well-being, physical and mental health, proper foods and nutrition and exercise in my hypnosis sessions. I told stories during hypnosis, with indirect suggestion, that had a repetitive quality. In this way people could identify with the main character in the story who repeated the same self-defeating behavior until finally one day he or she tired of it and turned a new leaf.

The politics of therapy must be considered when writing about impact by therapists. It is the responsibility of the therapist to maintain an aroused, involved, engaged and active position in life–and to respond with gusto to patients. However, whatever inspirational and creative interventions therapists may think about, the reality of the political climate is a factor therapists need to consider when making professional judgments about particular interventions. Ethics committees and a number of expert witnesses are as likely to make their decisions based on the image of the profession they feel should be represented to the public, as they are likely to judge what is impactful therapy. There are limited amounts of funds, several groups fighting to be included in national health insurance, and some therapeutic interventions harder to explain to the public than others. The image of the profession is usually protected first. Yet, it is hoped that the political climate will not dictate therapeutic interventions and that therapists will assume full responsibility in being all that they can.

Of course, things may not be relatively different now than in prior years.

> Reich (1949) declared that the therapist's work is in conflict with most of the heavily defended positions of conservative society and, therefore, the therapist will be exposed to enmity, contempt, and slander as long as he maintains his integrity. One can escape the negative sanctions of the conservative society only by making concessions, at the expense of his theoretical and practical convictions, to a social order which is in opposition to the demands of therapy. There is no doubt but that Reich went political because he believed that depth psychology requires the complement of radical politics.[18]

The politics of psychotherapy as it applies to the issue of the liberation of the therapist are threefold: (1) *Aggression castration* of both therapists and patients; (2) the medical model, diagnosis and assessment; (3) the therapist's responding in ways of a trickster-healer, or what even may be termed outrageous behavior.

Aggressions *castration* is the first major political issue. In their book, *Creative Aggression*, Dr. George Bach and Dr. Herb Goldberg speak of the "nice" psychotherapist. They feel that most therapists create a false reality between themselves and patients because they "tend to suspend or at least greatly inhibit and limit their own aggressive responses toward the patient during the therapy hour."[19] They speak of therapist' reluctance to incur the patient's anger, resistance, and possible rejection, and comment upon a study that indicates therapists will even avoid patients who openly direct hostility toward them. "Therefore, patients motivated for therapy are in a sense forced to suppress or redirect their aggressive feelings lest they alienate and lose their therapists."[20]

Bach and Goldberg go on to say that many patients come to therapy because there is a disturbance in their aggressive flow. Major distortions occur when patients were raised by parental figures who were incapable of tolerating aggressive behavior. Such children learned to either cloak their emotional reactions, primarily by denying and inhibiting angry feelings. This leads to patients experiencing depression, anxiety, fear, and guilt instead of being able to express assertive and angry responses openly. If such responses continue to be suppressed during the course of therapy, only a simulation of an authentic relationship may take place. Until repressed negative feelings have been aired, positive expression of affection if usually only a defense against underlying negativity. Bach and Goldberg say, "If the emphasis is placed upon the giving and receiving of love, the repressed negativity becomes further entrenched and will appear as resentments at the first disappointment."[21]

> In a therapy atmosphere where the therapist is all-accepting and all-loving, it becomes difficult, if not impossible, for the patients to express these kinds of feelings without at the same time feeling that they are behaving 'inappropriately' or neurotically. In turn, the therapist must feel free to share his anger at the patient without feeling that this is a breach of professional conduct. Therefore, patients also must be re-educated in terms of their expectations of what appropriate professional behavior by a psychotherapist is.[22]

Bach and Goldberg discuss the value of an aggressive confrontation approach because it helps patients deal with aggressive and angry feelings, as well as learning to be assertive in the here and now. Patients get a chance to learn by practicing in response to the therapist. "Confrontation, rather than being irresponsible or self-indulgent behavior by the therapist, is the ultimate way a therapist can take responsibility for providing the patient with an authentic relationship."[23]

While discussing the "attack therapy" of a group that worked primarily with drug addicts, Abraham Maslow commented,

> . . . what I saw last night and this afternoon, suggests that the whole idea of the fragile teacup which might

> crack or break, the idea that you mustn't say a loud word
> to anybody because it might traumatize him or hurt
> him, the idea that people cry easily or crack easily or
> commit suicide or go crazy if you shout at them–that
> maybe these ideas are outdated.[24]

Bach comments that when it is difficult for him to stay in the relationship as a result of what the patient is doing, he engages in an "occasional rotten, name-calling spree."[25] He described this as his "silly way of having a temper tantrum"[26] with people he cares about.

Bach and Goldberg refer to the therapist as a

> victim of the aggression taboos of our society. The
> therapist who aggressively confronts may be accused of
> acting unprofessionally. The typical patient expects the
> doctor to have a professional demeanor characterized
> by a controlled, even-tempered, soft-spoken attitude.[27]

They go on to say that therapists who do not live up to patients' unrealistic expectations may be victimized by patients who (1) play the part of a helpless victim who has been maliciously attacked, (2) threaten to quit or actually do quit therapy, (3) act sicker, (4) use the ultimate way of indirectly punishing the therapist attempting suicide, so the therapist will both feel guilty and have a tarnished reputation. It is no small wonder that many therapists avoid being open and direct with their patients when they fear such retaliation. Bach and Goldberg believe the solution is to have patients retrained by psychological and psychiatric professionals, who can accomplish this only by becoming real people with their patients. It is this authenticity between therapist and patient, as opposed to a collusion with patients by therapists playing out the images patients expect, that will provide for both effective and impactful therapy.

Diagnosis and assessment are the second major political issue. Nearly all of the therapists I have written about in this book did therapy with me at the beginning of the first session without any formal assessment procedures. They did not give me any psychological tests. Only one gave me a preliminary assessment interview. And Milton Erickson had me write my name, age, occupation, education and marital status on a piece of paper–which took about one minute. My style, like that of my mentors, is that of beginning to respond immediately to patients. There is no formal assessment in terms of how assessment is customarily viewed, although I do use psychological testing when I feel there may be possible brain damage. In these cases patients agree that this information will be beneficial. However, that does not mean that I do not involve myself in assessment. I believe that the art of assessment, is to both be able to assess the situation moment by moment as the therapist is engaging in a subject-object relationship with patients, while simultaneously responding as fully as possible thereby relating to the patient as subject-to-subject. Each of the people with whom I have worked have had their unique ways of doing this. My way is through the use of sensory perception where I gauge the patient's sense of presence, well-being and vitality, or lack of it, while they are in front of me. My responses are made according to this spontaneous diagnosis. I heard Walt Kempler make the comment that "therapists who spend a long time with historical diagnosis usually don't know what they are doing." Albert Ellis, writing about the characteristics of therapists, said,

> I personally know a number of RET (rational-emotive therapy) therapists, and effective ones at that, who in their manner of doing rational-emotive therapy go counter to some of the main behaviors of the majority of RET-ers. Some of them are quite slow moving and relatively passive, and tend to get a great deal of background information on clients (which I personally would rarely bother getting) before they tackle these clients' irrational beliefs.[28]

William Ofman, writing about a humanistic existential way of dealing with diagnosis and assessment feels that "testing or assessment violates the person's deep subjectivity in that he becomes an object to both himself and to another."[29] Ofman feels that therapy starts with the very first words between patient and therapist.

While the literature supports the premise that from the very beginning of therapy the patient's statements, the therapist's reactions to the patient, and the patient's reactions to the therapist's responses have both diagnostic and therapeutic value, there are conservative psychotherapists who may contend that such methods are both inadequate and irresponsible on the part of existentially (here and now) oriented therapists. While I can see how the therapists making such accusations might come to such conclusions, based on their own inability to pick up the ongoing process quickly, I feel that such contentions are absolute nonsense and must be vigorously challenged.

Wilfred Bion, of the psychoanalytic school where diagnosis and history are usually in the forefront, said,

> The more the analyst becomes expert in excluding memory, desire and understanding from his mental activity, the more he is likely, at least in the early stages, to experience painful emotions that are usually excluded or screened by the conventional apparatus of 'memory' of the session, analytical theories, often disguised desires or denials of ignorance and 'understanding.'[30]

Bion then cautions therapists who adopt his system:

> the analyst will soon find that he appears to be ignorant of knowledge which he has hitherto regarded as the hallmark of scrupulous medical responsibility. It is disconcerting to find that one is without an idea, say, that the patient has been married, or has children, or of certain events deemed by the analysand to have been of great significance. If the patient has paranoid trends and displays a tendency towards litigation it may seem to be running an unwarranted risk to be ignorant of matters that could, in a court of law, be regarded as significant and as evidence of ordinary medical care for detail. This would indeed be the case if there were not cogent reasons for not 'remembering' such detail. As it is, I think that whatever the risks may be the obligation is for the analyst to conduct the case in accordance with his lights–and not in accordance with the supposed risks to himself.[31]

Bion again refers to the example of not remembering that his patient is married. He sees this as significant because at an emotional level the patient is not married in the eyes of the analyst. Further, the fact of the marriage contract may be irrelevant until such a time as the patient says or does something to remind the analyst of this fact.

The third basic issue is the therapist who engages in outrageous behavior, or the trickster-healer. "Trickster" in my sense of the word implies one with a free-wheeling responsiveness that is inherently mischievous, sometimes harmless and sometimes hostile. The reader may justifiably ask, is that what I am proposing as "good" therapy? The answer is most definitely, NO! What I am proposing is that when needed a therapist must have the courage to be bold, and daring in his or her actions if need be. Such action comes out of an act of love, an act of caring, and while it may be bold and impertinent, if it doesn't work it is not harmful. It is an act that is born through liberated wisdom.

Such high-quality responses by therapists provide a change of context that can bewilder a patient. Such bold experiments, as those I describe of Milton Erickson, are responsible actions. They can bewilder a patient so that patient has the opportunity to include new input into his or her frame of reference, getting past self-destructive stubbornness and having an opportunity to live a happier, healthier, and freer life.

Erickson and Rossi describe one case in which Dr. Erickson used shock to *depotentiate* old behavior patterns and *transform* identity. The patient was a 24-year-old woman who had accepted a proposal of marriage from a man she loved, upon his return from the military. Although she agreed to be married within six months, she postponed the date as the time approached, scheduling a later date for the marriage. She continued this pattern until she had postponed the marriage for three years.

This woman was closely tied to her long-widowed mother, her siblings, and two spinster aunts, and in fact unnecessarily contributed all her earnings to the family. Her personal expenses were both rigidly limited and strictly supervised.

After much persuasion, a physician to whom the woman had confided referred her to Dr. Erickson. She complained of being afraid to leave home, afraid to travel without her family, afraid that her future husband would not live in Arizona, but stated that she could not give up the hope of marriage, although she kept putting it off. By this time the woman's fiance had given her an ultimatum that if she didn't marry him he was going to find another woman. At this point Dr. Erickson said that she would be married to him by September, which was in accord with her promise to marry him. Dr. Erickson had also requested that she attend the next session wearing shorts, as he commented that she was always wearing high-necked dresses with long sleeves, even in the summertime. He also noticed that her dresses were always below the knee. He reassured her that despite her fears, the marriage that she wanted so badly was coming closer and closer.

When she came to the next session it was well chaperoned. A woman was present. Erickson and Rossi report as follows:

> "Now stand up and, one by one, take off your clothes, naming each article as you place it neatly on the chair."
>
> She looked helplessly at the placid, composed face of the chaperone, then blushingly stood up, hesitated, then took off her shoes, more hesitantly her stockings, then, with many lingering movements, her dress and finally her slip.
>
> "Won't this be enough?" she asked pleadingly, looking first at the author, then looking pleadingly at the chaperone, but no response was made.
>
> Awkwardly, clumsily, she removed her bra, hesitated a moment, then removed her panties and stood in the nude facing the senior author defiantly. Thereupon he turned to the chaperone and remarked, "She looks all right to me. Does she look all right to you?" The chaperone nodded her head.
>
> The author then turned to the patient and stated, "I want to be sure you know and can name all parts of your body. I do not want to point to or touch any part of your body nor does the chaperone. If necessary I can do it, but please don't make it necessary. Just don't try to skip over anything with a name. As you name each

part, touch it with one or the other hand, since you must use your right hand to touch your left elbow. Now start from the shoulders and work downward progressively, then turn your back to us and do the same as well as you can. Now go ahead, and no oversights."[32]

It was after the embarrassment of this session that she followed through with her desire for marriage to her fiancé. As Dr. Erickson had planned, her fear of undressing in front of her fiancé to consummate the marriage was not as embarrassing to her as undressing in front of two strangers. Embarrassment was her impasse.

It was only a few weeks later that she brought her fiancé into the office to see Dr. Erickson for premarital counseling. Dr. Erickson saw each of them separately and then together. The effect was positive and afterwards the woman called long distance to assure Dr. Erickson that after much struggling she had convinced both her mother and her spinster aunts that her wedding guests would be those of her choosing and that the wedding would not be made a community affair. Over the course of the next seven years, Dr. Erickson received a Christmas card and three birth announcements.

Erickson was a trickster-healer. He was outrageous. He was bold. He was daring. He did something that might easily be viewed as having an unprofessional image. Was he irresponsible? Or was he using his full creativity in providing an act of love that came through a liberated wisdom that would free this woman to live a full life? I contend it was the latter, and that the profession of psychotherapy must liberate itself so it may flow with the kind of liberated wisdom that will free people from their inner shackles.

Although I have described a variety of responses and left the realm of existentialism open to all who want to join, it is still the authenticity between therapists and patients that provides the spirit of place for a healing relationship to occur. We have come full circle by returning to the unity of wholeness of two people in a room together–the way in which they make contact with each other.

To facilitate authentic relationships, therapists must have vitality because patients' well-being is dependent upon that vitality, and an energetic relationship is healing. To maintain an energetic relationship, therapists must have a good deal of self-love. When speaking of therapists' self-love I am referring to an acceptance of self that allows therapists a child-like freedom throughout their bodies. If therapists have been able to attain this level of freedom within themselves, they will know how to help patients attain this goal. This type of freedom and self-love in patients will motivate them toward giving up self-destructive behavior. This type of self-love is not narcissistic, and is not meant in terms of–"I love someone else"–which is a love that has an object. This type of love allows both therapists and patients the freedom to follow their energy via messages from their inner core of being. There will be a removal of self-constraints and a removal of self-critical messages. If therapists love themselves they may feel an inner strength that will enable them to choose in ways that continue to produce more energy. Although patients may initially be quite frustrated in experiencing such a process, the end result may be patients' ability to mobilize their energy, excitement, vitality, joy and love.

Vitality of therapists is a result of a continuation of the liberation process throughout both therapists' personal and working lives. It is with this continued spirit of liberation that therapists will be able to either become or remain free agents, able to reach in and touch the souls of patients. It is this spirit of liberation of therapists that will provide the environment in which existential moments can occur. Without this spirit of liberation therapy runs the risk of being a situation whereby patients may be taught to play their parts in counterpoint to the masquerade of therapists–a ballet of blind dancers.

ENDNOTES

1   Sheldon Kopp, "The Trickster-Healer," in The Growing Edge of Gestalt Therapy, ed. Edward W. L. Smith (New York: Brunner/ Mazel, 1976), p. 75.
2   Ibid., pp. 75-76.
    Ibid., p. 80.
4   Edward Smith, "The Roots of Gestalt Therapy," in The Growing Edge of Gestalt Therapy, ed. E. W. L. Smith (New York: Brunner/ Mazel, 1976), p. 14.
5   Leston Havens, "The Existential Use of the Self," The American Journal of Psychiatry, 131 (January, 1974), p. 1.
6   Ibid., p. 6.
7   Ibid.
8   Ibid., p. 7.
9   Ibid., p. 10.
10 Real emotions–such as love, joy, grief, sadness, anger, and fear are different from being in a constant state of anger, depression, etc.
    Jay Haley, Uncommon Therapy: The Psychiatric Techniques of Milton H. Erickson, M.D. (New York: W. W. Norton and Co., Inc., 1973), pp. 197-198.
12 Ernest Keen, Three Faces of Being: Toward an Existential Clinical

Psychology (New York: Appleton-Century-Crofts, Meredith Corporation, 1970), p. 28.

13 Haley, Uncommon Therapy, pp. 259-260.

14 Ibid., pp. 260-261.

15 Ibid., pp. 213-214.

16 Ibid., p. 214.

17 Ibid., p. 215.

18 Smith, The Roots of Gestalt Therapy, p. 12.

19 George Bach and Herb Goldberg, Creative Aggression (Garden City, N.Y.: Doubleday and Company, Inc., 1974), p. 68.

20 Ibid., p. 68.

21 Ibid., p. 71.

22 Ibid., p. 69.

23 Ibid., p. 75.

24 Abraham H. Maslow, "Synanon and Eupsychia, "Journal of Humanistic Psychology 7 (1967), pp. 28-29.

25 Bach and Goldberg, Creative Aggression, p. 73.

26 Ibid., p. 73.

27 Ibid., p. 78.

28 Albert Ellis, "Personality Characteristics of Rational-Emotive Therapists and Other Kinds of Therapists," Psychotherapy: Theory, Research and Practice, (Winter 1978), p. 330.

29 William Ofman, Affirmation and Reality: Fundamentals of Humanistic Existential Therapy and Counseling (Los Angeles: Western Psychological Services, 1976), p. 199.

30 Wilfred Bion, "Attention and Interpretation," in Seven Servants (New York: Jason Aronson, Inc., 1977), p. 48.

31 Ibid., p. 49.

32 Milton Erickson and Ernest Rossi, Hypnotherapy: An Exploratory Casebook (New York: Irvington Publishers, Inc., 1979), pp. 448-449.

REFERENCES

Bach, George, and Goldberg, Herb. *Creative Aggression.* Garden City, New York: Doubleday and Company, Inc., 1974.

Bion, Wilfred. "Attention and Interpretation," in *Seven Servants.* New York: Jason Aronson, Inc., 1977.

Ellis, Albert. "Personality Characteristics of Rational-Emotive Therapists and Other Kinds of Therapists." *Psychotherapy: Theory, Research and Practice.* (Winter 1978).

Erickson, Milton, and Rossi, Ernest. *Hypnotherapy: An Exploratory Casebook.* New York: Irvington Publishers, Inc., 1979.

Haly, Jay. *Uncommon Therapy: The Psychiatric Techniques of Milton H. Erickson, M.D.* New York: W. W. Norton and Co., Inc., 1973.

Havens, Leston. "The Existential Use of the Self." *The American Journal of Psychiatry.* 131 (January 1974).

Keen, Ernest. *Three Faces of Being: Toward an Existential Clinical Psychology.* New York: Appleton-Century-Crofts, Meredith Corporation, 1970.

Kopp, Sheldon. "The Trickster-Healer." In *The Growing Edge of Gestalt Therapy*, edited by E. W. L. Smith. New York: Brunner/Mazel, 1976.

Maslow, Abraham H. "Impromptu talk given at Daytop Village." *Journal of Humanistic Psychology* 7 (1967).

Ofman, William. *Affirmation and Reality: Fundamentals of Humanistic Existential Therapy and Counseling.* Los Angeles: Western Psychological Services, 1976.

Smith, Edward. "The Roots of Gestalt Therapy." In *The Growing Edge of Gestalt Therapy*, edited by E. W. L. Smith. New York: Brunner/Mazel, 1976.

PART TWO

The Impact of Existential Moments

T HE SECOND PART of the book presents a variety of therapeutic styles and how they may be implemented to create a positive impact on patients' lives. The common thread that runs through each of the different methods of therapy is the existential moment. It is the impact of these existential moments, no matter what form the therapy, that provides the impetus for change.

In covering a wide range of therapies, I feel it is appropriate that the father of psychotherapy, Freud, be discussed in existential terms. Thus, I begin this section with the question, "Was Freud an existentialist?" The wedding between psychoanalysis and the existential moment is carried further in the second part of this chapter when discussing my experience with Dr. Wilfred Bion, a British psychoanalyst.

The last part of the chapter takes the existential moment from psychoanalysis to group analysis and the treatment of narcissism with Dr. Martin Grotjahn, past president of the Society for Psychoanalytic Medicine of Southern California, and former director of the Training School of the Institute for Psychoanalytic Medicine.

4

Psychoanalysis and the Existential Moment

WHEN I FIRST began practicing I met Dr. Robert Dorn, a well-respected psychoanalyst in the community. He took an interest in me but I wasn't quite sure why. One day I asked him. He said that he thought I had an ability to integrate and synthesize that would help therapists of differing modalities better understand each other. He had hoped I would become interested in psychoanalysis, so I might contribute in this area. Bob's comments stuck in my mind for four years. Dr. Dorn is currently Professor and Acting Chairman of the Department of Psychiatry and Behavioral Sciences, and Professor of Family Medicine at Eastern Virginia Medical School.

WAS FREUD AN EXISTENTIALIST?

While Freudians tend to think about analysis as the working through of the transference neurosis, I believe that Freud offered his patients a great deal more of himself as a person than followers of the writings of Freud–who know his works well but may miss the spirit of Freud– would care to admit. It was these existential qualities in Freud that had impact upon his patients. One cannot divorce the impact of Freud's personality from his methodology, even though this is what his writings attempted to do. Perhaps this can best be exemplified by contrasting the Freudian view of the working through of the transference neurosis with how Freud actually responded to one patient who wrote about her interactions with Freud.

Psychoanalysis is thought about as the working through of the transference neurosis where the psychoanalyst is but a blank screen onto which the patient projects the kind of relationship that the patient has learned since childhood. It is customarily viewed that if the analyst is silent for the most part, making only occasional interpretations, the patient will not be able to attribute his or her own difficulties to the analyst (although analysts are well trained to know how their own interpretations may be countertransference reactions projected onto the patient as a result of their own difficulties). All in all, this is described as a very careful and meticulous process, where the more personal, responsive qualities of the analyst are not supposed to come into the relationship. In such a methodology, the primary impact of the analyst would be attributed to correctly timed interpretations.

Dr. Lawrence Friedman, a psychoanalyst and former training analyst at the Los Angeles Psychoanalytic Society/Institute, described the Freudian transference situation in the following way:

> . . . the analyst, cognizant of what is going on, does not react personally, as he very well might with anyone who is not a patient. Instead, it is his task to analyze these transferred emotions with his patient and to trace them back to their source.

> It is because the transference situation is so vital in the treatment of the patient that the analyst must maintain a neutral, objective relationship with him. The less the patient knows about the analyst as a real person, the easier it will be to fantasy about him during the analysis, and the more suitable the analyst will be

to represent the various transference figures.[1]There is a great difference between feeling loved or hated, rejected or punished by someone we do not know or by someone who is close to us.[2]This he accomplishes by establishing an analytic atmosphere, which means that he preserves a neutral, non-critical, non-directive attitude, indicating neither approval nor disapproval of the patient's words and actions.[3]Whatever his reactions, however, the analyst uses them to understand and to help the patient understand the underlying meaning of his feelings and actions.[4]I believe there is another component of the psychoanalytic process, however, that is ordinarily left out of discussions of psychoanalysis: the existential component. Furthermore, I believe it to be an equally if not more powerful explanation of the psychoanalytic process than the one that currently exists. So in answering the question, Was Freud an existentialist?, I must say that indeed he was. He was an existentialist in that he was a responsible human being and it was the quality of his being that was impactful to patients, although Freud didn't think of himself in such terms. And he did react more personally than the neutral and objective psychoanalytic method described by Dr. Friedman. Freud put Freud into the psychoanalytic process.

A very personal book called *Tribute to Freud*, written by a patient of Freud who refers to herself as HD or Hilda Doolittle, and who does not reveal her true name, discusses Freud in the same personal way in which I wrote this book, and the following passages are included to give a flavor of the personal impact Freud made with his patients. Her descriptions certainly involved more than the working through of the transference neurosis.

HD, writing about her psychoanalysis with Freud, said that "Once he beat his fist on the headpiece of the old-fashioned horse-hair couch where HD was lying and said, 'The trouble is–I am an old man–you do not think it worth your while to love me.'"[5] HD notes:

The impact of his words was too dreadful–I simply felt nothing at all. I said nothing. What did he expect me to say? Exactly it was as if the Supreme Being had hammered with his fist on the back of the couch where I had been lying.[6] While Freud may have been a detached old man in some respects, HD's words indicate that Freud had a lot more kick in him than many modern practitioners of psychoanalysis and of Freudian psychoanalysis–slamming his fist down behind HD's head while telling her, "The trouble is–I am an old man–you do not think it worth your while to love me."[7] How much more of meaningful existential moment can one create, especially considering that the Freudian method was not one that wasted words.

Dr. Martin Grotjahn read what I had written about HD and Freud and said that I left out the best part of the story, which I had not seen in the book but which I assumed Grotjahn knew from personal experience. He went on to tell me that some time after Freud had reacted so strongly to HD, civil war broke out in the streets of Vienna. However, HD came at her appointed hour and Freud himself opened the door and said, "You are the only one who came to me today." HD thought, but didn't say, "And you thought I don't love you." It is difficult to capture the emotional impact of this half-unspoken interchange on paper, but when Dr. Grotjahn told this to me I felt chills run up and down my entire body. I felt that I was back there in Vienna with Freud and HD experiencing that existential moment with them. Again, Freud the man, emerged as a very touching figure.

Freud's responses were pure responses that captured the moment. They needed no rhyme or reason, as such responses are so impactful in themselves that they jar the unconscious processes of patients, so that those patients' unconscience minds begin to provide the necessary ingredients by which patients begin to heal themselves.

The success of his methodology was Freud's ability to respond with full presence, full being, and engaged participation with his patient. Freud provided the basic ingredients for what I define as an existential moment, and in doing so has provided the basis from which each of the therapies may borrow from and once again speak to each other in helping patients.

Peter Jones, who wrote the introduction to the original copy of the book, commented:

> There is, of course, love in the relationship between HD and Freud, between the student–as he preferred to call his patients–and the master. Without it, the unreciprocated intimacy of the student would have been sterile, almost blasphemous. The overwhelming sense of the humanizing effect on both parties is reflected in Freud's words to HD in a letter written when he was eighty, the year before his death:

> What you gave me was not praise, was affection and I need not be ashamed of my satisfaction.

> "Life at my age is not easy, but Spring is beautiful and so is love."[8]So here we see another existential moment where Freud extended himself personally, and commented that he was touched by HD, and reached out to touch her in return.

Freud did not hide his authoritarian ways as evidenced by HD when she reported:

> There was the stove, but there were moments when one felt a little chilly. I smoothed the folds of the rug, I glanced surreptitiously at my wrist-watch. The other day the Professor had reproached me for jerking out my arm and looking at my watch. He had said, "I keep an eye on the time–I will tell you when the session is over. You need not keep looking at the time, as if you were in a hurry to get away."[9]I can feel the impact of Freud's words go right through my body as I read that comment. The analyst doesn't have to say much to make an impact; he or she only needs to be in tune with the unconscious and respond when it is appropriate.

Allowing fewer opportunities to respond may be an advantage, however. Patients are more likely to listen and integrate the analyst's response or interpretation if they know the analyst may not say anything for quite some time.

I began personal therapy with a gestalt therapist who appeared to be a pure gestaltist in his language talking and method of working. After entering therapy, however, I noticed that he was asking me to lie on the couch and just talk about whatever came into my mind. I began to feel as if I had been double-crossed–that I was in some sort of psychoanalytic gestalt therapy. When I asked him about it he told me he had trained for six years in a psychoanalytic orientation.

What I began to see was that lying on the couch and talking about whatever came into my mind was serving an important purpose. It was helping me to develop my own creativity, my own richness, my own humanity. It helped me to develop an uninterrupted inner flow without being concerned about the therapist. I remember telling him when I first began the process that I wished he were outside the room while I was talking. But the more I talked the more I was able to enjoy the existential moments of being centered in an increasing personal richness. This was particularly important to me because I had a built-in censor. I would edit out much of my richness and give people what I thought were the safe results. The analytic process gave me the opportunity to say it all without having to worry about editing. It also gave me the opportunity to become privy to what I had edited out. Unfortunately, one of the disadvantages of such an editing process is that the editor may lose sight of the richness of the story while worrying about the punchline. I was experiencing existential moments both in developing human richness and paying attention to my life as well as feeling the effect and bodily sensations that were going on inside me. Part of my tuning into a moment-to-moment continuum while lying down was a gestalt interjection into the psychoanalytic process. On one occasion I began to notice the green leaves and plants in the office, the painting on the walls, and the colors and texture of the furniture. This was a major breakthrough; I was learning how to experience more life and less obsessive thinking. On another occasion I was lying on the floor talking about the ambitious part of me and that part of me that wanted to do nothing. It was as if I were doing an empty-chair gestalt session while I was lying on an analyst's couch. The lower half of my body was numb. It wasn't moving at all. The upper part was struggling with the lower part and harrassing the other part to wake up. The lower part kept resounding that it was sick of the upper part pushing it. Finally the two came to an agreement, and a peacefulness came over my entire body. The pushy side agreed to allow the other side to grow at its own pace. There was a flowing feeling that made me feel as if my body were in a euphoric state of fluid motion. Another existential moment, and one which showed to me that psychoanalysis and gestalt therapy may be wedded.

Of course, what I am describing is only a small bite of the psychoanalytic process. I have not yet been psychoanalyzed, but do feel that there will be a time in my life, soon, that I will want a psychoanalysis of about five years in depth. Right now I feel that my personal needs lead me more toward working in bioenergetic therapy or other methods of helping my body energy flow at optimum levels. After that I feel my body will be able to handle my pursuit of the kind of clarity, responsiveness, and state of being I describe in talking about Wilfred Bion in the second part of this chapter. While I am certain that the pursuit of psychoanalysis in itself does not necessarily produce people with the characteristics of a Wilfred Bion, I do believe that it does have the ability to help people develop the unimpeded flow of both their unconscious, and with a little direction, the affective material from which they have cut themselves off. There are many feelings and emotions that I feel would take charge of me were I to experience them, and so I block them out. Psychoanalysis is a way for them to flow naturally into the context of a person's life. Psychoanalysis is a way of unifying one's richness of humanity and alienated affect from the past that has been prevented from entering the present, along with an unimpeded unconscious flow. This unconscious flow runs minimal risk of interruption via projected demands of therapists, when therapists are judgmental or aren't clear about any desires they have of patients. Such a process may enhance the emerging growth of life and vitality of the patient.

I recall one patient who asked me how face-to-face therapy differed from psychoanalysis. I commented that she must have a good reason for asking and that I wondered if she found it difficult to face me and do what she needed to do to develop herself. She said she did. So I had her turn the easy chair and stool around facing the wall, and begin to talk, after which I made only one or two comments the entire session. The woman was elated after the session. She was able to achieve a sense of presence or unity that she had not been able to achieve when facing me. Her desire to please me got in the way of her natural flow. By experimenting with the psychoanalytic method, an existential moment was reached in which the patient made the impact for herself. Such moments are as important as those when therapists making an impact on patients.

THE LEGACY OF FREUD LEFT US, FROM WHICH WE HAVE BEEN ABLE TO PROGRESS, HAS BEEN AN APPROACH TO THE DEVELOPMENT AND ACCESS TO THE UNCONSCIOUS, TO SYMBOLISM, TO DREAMS, TO THE FERTILITY THAT LIES WITHIN PATIENTS, AND TO A WAY OF HELPING PEOPLE BY TALKING WITH THEM. While Freud is known for all this, it is my belief that Freud the man has been too often left apart from his methodology, and that the kind of existential moments that come from the interpersonal impact of therapist upon patient may come to be viewed as an important part of the psychoanalytic process. In this way, psychoanalysis, as with all good therapies, will be providing both kinds of existential moments that are healing–the interpersonal and the intrapsychic. It is with such a balance that each therapy blossoms to its fullest potential. And, of course, in psychoanalysis as in other therapies, this is related to the psychoanalyst's development to the point of being able to provide an environment where both types of existential moments may occur.

A final comment from HD crystallizes Freud's personal impact that helped his patients change their lives, gain insight, and grapple with symbolism. She reported,

> When I said to him one day that time went too quickly (did he or didn't he feel that?) he struck a semi-comic attitude, he threw his arm forward as if ironically addressing an invisible presence or an imaginary audience. Time, he said. The word was uttered in his inimitable, two-edged manner; he seemed to defy the creature, the abstraction; into that one word, he seemed

to pack a store of contradictory emotions; there was irony, entreaty, defiance, with a vague, tender pathos. It seemed as if the word was surcharged, an explosive that might, at any minute, go off. (Many of his words did, in a sense, explode, blasting down prisms, useless dykes and dams, bringing down landslides, it is true, but opening up mines of hidden treasure.) Time, he said again, more quietly, and then, time gallops.[10]Wilfred R. Bion, M.r.c.s. Member Of The Royal College Of Surgeons The Man And The Legacy: The Language Of Achievement

Wilfred Bion was born on September 8, 1897 in Mutra, United Northern Provinces, India. He attended public school at Bishop Stortford in England. He studied history at Oxford and returned to Oxford to finish his education after the war. He then returned to Bishop Stortford to teach history. In the 1920s he attended medical school at University College London.

Wilfred Bion was able to integrate psychoanalysis with contemporary thought and make it become alive in the interchange between two people. He had the rare combination of being one of the finest theoreticians since Freud while having the ability to do psychoanalytic practice with the same quality as his writings. Much of what I have tried to do is share how it is that Bion would speak to give the reader not only some of his concepts, but an impressionistic feeling (through a particular way of writing the way he spoke) for the experience of being with him.

Bion was a Member of the Royal College of Surgeons (M.R.C.S.) and was a world-famous psychoanalyst. While living in London he felt so loaded down with honors, that he decided to come to the United States, where he was less well known. He came to Los Angeles in the middle 1960s and not many people knew he was here, nor came to him for a couple of years. Further, the antagonism of the Freudians toward the Kleiniens spilled over onto Bion, who was analyzed by both Melanie Klein and John Rickman. However, after a few years the quality of the man and his work was such that many psychoanalysts were knocking on his door, even for a second psychoanalysis. DR. BION DIED SHORTLY AFTER DECIDING TO MOVE BACK TO

LONDON. HE RETURNED IN SEPTEMBER 1979 AND DIED IN OXFORD ON NOVEMBER 8, 1979.

This chapter is different than most of the chapters in the book in that my direct experience with Dr. Bion was very limited. The experience I did have with him, however, touched me in a way that left me hungry to experience and know more about Dr. Bion and his work. In fact, I was so touched by Dr. Bion and the kinds of thoughts and feelings that what he said and did evoked in me, I wrote to him to make plans for my moving to London to be analyzed by him. I felt a terrible loss when he died at the age of 82 a short time after our communication.

My curiosity about Bion and his work did not stop with his death. I began to interview psychoanalysts who had been analyzed and/or supervised by him. Several of the members of the Los Angeles Psychoanalytic Society and Institute and their spouses helped me to complete this chapter. Their contributions helped me to write about his legacy. The last section was taken from tapes of Bion doing supervision with a psychoanalyst who was just beginning his practice at that time.

A further motivation to write this chapter was to expose Bion and his ideas to therapists throughout the helping professions in addition to those in the psychoanalytic area. It is hoped that such exposure will prompt readers to pursue his works.

My Reaction to Bion: A Clear Mind and a State of Discovery

I had heard about Bion from time to time but the rumors did not particularly attract me to see what he had to offer. I heard he was a genuis who put psychoanalysis and psychotherapy into formulations that were extremely difficult to understand. In actuality my experience with him was diametrically opposite to this. The amazing fact was that I would have such an experience just as a result of being part of an audience of about five hundred people hearing him speak and interact with other panelists.

Bion's sense of presence, and the way in which he gave of himself to a large audience, were unusual. He had a presence that I had never seen before, and evoked a depth of feeling and a clarity of mind that went far beyond what I was accustomed to experiencing. All feelings of heaviness, pain, and nausea (my reactions to what went on before Bion spoke) left immediately when he began. I felt my body and my sense of presence expand over the course of time in his presence, and there was a sense of fulfillment and satisfaction that became richer as he went on. All this was happening while he was talking about things that usually struck me as demanding too much attention. But he spoke of truths that, although difficult to understand at the conceptual level, were a part of people's primal preconceptions. The unusual part for me was that I had never been drawn to remain in this state of discovery for so long (about one hour of his speaking and each time he reacted during the course of a three and a half hour presentation by a number of colleagues, of which he was part). I experienced an extension of my capacities of thinking, attention, feeling and perception on multiple levels of awareness, both mental and physical.

I was delighted and excited. I felt wonderful to be in the presence of somebody who could evoke hope of living with the kind of richness I was experiencing. I had an inner sense that Bion was a person who wouldn't disappoint me. Dr. Bion often told Dr. Michael Paul that

> One of the painful things about living are two nasty facts. We're alone and we are dependent. The snag is that you've got to be dependent on someone. And that depends a great deal as to whether or not the person on whom you depend is depend-worthy or not.

I felt that Bion was indeed such a person.

When Bion talked, one moment flowed into another with the fluidity of Toscanini conducting a symphony. Bion had revived a quality and spirit of life that had been dead in me. I felt he was unique, that he lived his life with precision, a sense of truthfulness with himself and others, and stayed fresh and clear by not boxing himself into fixed versions of reality. The conceptual way that he said things, his sincerity, his direct way of communicating a refreshingly basic and even primal level of authenticity, and the power and intensity with which he made contact, made him unique in that his entire sense of being was different from anyone with whom I have ever come into contact. The level at which he was full in human terms and in which he could share this generosity was astounding. Furthermore, I viewed Bion as existential in that he brought psychoanalysis, in both theory and practice, into the here and now.

Grinberg, Sor, and Tabak de Bianchedi wrote:

> One of Bion's greatest merits is that he had placed psychoanalytic theory and practice in a new dimension, preserving the most valuable classical contributions of Freud and Melanie Klein while approaching them from different perspectives (or "vertices"). He adds freshness and originality to them and stimulates a new attitude in the analyst by encouraging him to abandon rigid schemes and old clichés, thus opening up new ways of psychoanalytic thinking. The richness of his hypotheses, the scope of his theories, and the flexibility of his models, together with his advice of approaching the task of observation and investigation "without memory or desire," exercise an enormous attraction while at the same time provoking some uncertainty. All this tends to increase creative capacity, common sense, and the development of intuition, helping the investigator to get himself into what we would call "the state of discovery."[11]Bion speaks of the difficulties of expressing new ideas in familiar words; and this sometimes leads him to introduce terms that are intentionally devoid of meaning or to use familiar words in his own particular way.[12]In reading Bion one often feels that the depth and strength of his ideas is equivalent to agitating the surface of the lake and altering the reflection.[13]Bion believed that Shakespeare was a genius because he had the negative capability of tolerating half-truths and uncertainty, without boxing himself in through the search for fact and reason. Conveying these aspects of Bion's work is a task that can only be approached.

I have quoted Grinberg, Sor, and Tabak de Bianchedi because their comments are representative of my experience in the following ways: first, just being in Bion's presence helped increase my creative and thinking capacities; second, my responses to him were primarily in the areas of common sense and intuition at a very basic level; and third, I entered into a state of discovery on both mental and physical levels.

In addition, I experienced my thoughts with a primitive intensity and a clarity that I didn't know was possible. Bion's way of relating was so unusual that it was for the most part out of my frame of reference.

I have not had psychoanalysis with Bion. Thus, I am basing what I write on the following assumptions: First, what I see and experience people doing is what they do. It is what they do when they do psychoanalysis in terms of the quality of their responses. It is what they do when they relate to their wives and children. It is what they do because it is where they are in terms of the development of their own state of being along the continuum of "to be or not to be." When I do therapy in this manner I make the assumption that patients will do with me exactly the kind of things that make their relationships difficult or pleasurable with others–and therefore, only replace the characters in the cast. So, in a sense my reaction to Bion is the same as me being one of the characters in his cast.

I make a further assumption that strength, power, and health are correlated to the quality of being manifested by a person. And in terms of the unusual physical and mental reaction I had to Bion, I equate strength, power, and health with the balanced quality of being exemplified by Bion in terms of clarity of mind and intuitive knowing. But most important, Bion's qualities were as pure as he was humble. He had state of being that avoided the ordinary needs for self-aggrandizement.

Friedman, when writing about primary process, said ". . . there are no contradictions, and totally contradictory forces exist simultaneously without being in conflict with each other, such as love and hate, masculine and feminine desires."[14] Bion had the ability to both understand and function, deeply and easily, with these contradictions at the primary process level.

Bion helped me tap into my understanding of what Bion would call "preconceptions" or primal kind of perceptions that made things unusually clear. I would have ordinarily filtered out these primal preconceptions in some other way at a much more superficial level of experience. Such thinking was much more accessible to me in the presence of Bion and his process. Bion was both evocative and provocative in his ability to create an environment in which thinking could occur in the presence of basic primal forces. His view of thinking was well beyond one's ordinary expectations. The therapist's abilities to both think and feel, were, in Bion's view, contingent upon the capacity to tolerate emotional experience including pain and frustration.

Bion felt that the capacity to tolerate pain was the primary basis of negating mechanisms. If a person is so busy blocking out pain that he or she cannot tolerate frustration or any amount of mental stress, then the capacity for thinking is compromised. So, for Bion, the fundamental issue was the analyst's ability to tolerate emotional experience.

Lyndell Paul, a psychiatric social worker in West Los Angeles who was supervised by Bion, put it well when she said,

> I think that's why Bion always talked about analysis as such a difficult process. He often drew the comparison between a mother and an infant. The mother is required to take in the feelings of the infant, and in a sense contain them, understand them, and give some kind of a response back. So it is a process that involves suffering when the baby is yelling and screaming, and yet, not yelling and screaming back at the baby. It involves detoxifying the painful experience, and allows for the development of the growth process. It may scream. Maybe it's cold. Maybe it's hungry. But you've got to tolerate listening to it long enough to figure out what it needs.

Her husband, Dr. Michael Paul, added, "Because if you can't stay with it long enough to make discriminations, you can't make the proper interpretations."

Bion began his presentation spontaneously by saying, "After hearing all that has been said about me and my work I can hardly wait to hear what I am going to say." This humor came from the heart and the audience felt warmed by him immediately. Furthermore, he was sincere about what he said, because the remainder of his presentation was unplanned. He delighted in his own spontaneity of what would come from within him.

On that occasion Bion was dressed in a dark blue suit and wore a black bow tie. He had an aristocratic bearing and spoke with an Oxford accent and had a refined demeanor. He was as solid as a block of granite, particularly in response to the gunfire by colleagues on the panel whose agendas for the evening appeared to go beyond presenting their views of Bion's word. Bion felt the difference between an officer in the military and an enlisted man was the officer's ability to think and respond in the line of fire. He was a World War I hero, and for a time, there was even a comic strip about him in a British newspaper. Bion viewed a psychoanalyst's job in the same way he viewed that of an officer, to think and respond in the line of fire.

The expression was creative and unusual in that Dr. Bion was able to respond so purely, combining thought with truth, responding from the heart, and making the kind of cognitive, emotional, intuitive and knowing statements that cut through an entire lifetime of cobwebs in one split second.

He continued to talk at a consistent slow pace that never varied from his center–that is, the center of his being. His presence was awesome, but in a peaceful sense. It felt like hearing a Stradivarius, but not a violin, a Stradivarius cello. While he was a complex man I found his way of expressing his thinking very simple and very easy to understand. I felt both nourished and replenished as I was continuing to learn to think more clearly by being in his presence. My head felt so clear and peaceful I thought this is how it must be when a baby is born. To put it bluntly Dr. Bion's thinking wasn't complex at all. In fact, it was so clear and simple that I believe it is wrongly mistaken to be complex due to the contamination, toxicity, convolution and network of lies existing in the mind of the listener. In fact, if Dr. Bion were teaching first grade I suspect he would have an entire class of pupils getting a grade of *A*. This simplicity also runs throughout his books, but they appear complex in that they demand a different level of attention and they do not present the reader with the answer, but evoke further thought.

I experienced Dr. Bion as being very existential. The purity of truth with which he spoke captured one existential moment after another. I felt that while I understood what he was saying, I had no need to try and remember it, because at a deeper level I knew that what he spoke existed within me and the rest of the human race. A Jungian might say that he spoke from the collective unconscious.

Bion mentioned the value of the analyst coming into each session fresh, without any remembrances from the past to cloud the analyst's mind. This would leave the analyst's mind free to continue to experience one moment of truth upon another–and to make interpretations that have a freshness that soothes the brain instead of creating the confusion the analyst tries to analyze.

While Bion may have felt that the analyst must be able to tolerate emotional experience and pain to think clearly, he provided the kind of emotional and mental nurturance that helped people to think in his presence by not having to overcome these obstacles so that thinking processes would get a chance to begin operating at deeper levels. Bion's responses and sense of presence were so impeccable that there was no need to be defensive in any way. His sincerity was so evident that it became unusually easy to think clearly and focus attention beyond ordinary capacities. Such clear thinking was much different from intellectualizers who are removed from the thinking they present. The kind of thinking that Bion facilitated was congruent with the entire being of people, both in receiving and responding. This is truly, in my opinion, Dr. Bion's most rare gift to humanity–the gift of pure thinking that is composed of cognition, emotion, intuition, and deep levels of knowing in sync with a compassion for the human condition that permits injured minds to replenish themselves with a childlike sense of freedom and joy.

In fact, my friend brought his wife and five week old baby. At 11:20 p.m. the baby's eyes were wide open and she had a clear and serene expression on her face. I sensed she knew she had partaken in a rare happening. I couldn't help but wonder what the difference might be in her life in terms of an unconscious memory of this experience. It was also interesting that at the times during the evening that I felt the most discomfort with different speakers, the baby cried or shrieked.

After the presentation I noticed Dr. Bion walking out and went up to him, telling him that being in the audience while he was talking was like having a warm bath cleanse my mind. In an instant he replied, "I enjoyed myself and I always make it a point to do that." We looked at each other as if we both knew we had more to say to each other, but that it wasn't right to say anymore then. His comment had touched upon a central struggle in my life–getting in touch with my desires and responding so I could enjoy myself in a meaningful way.

I was particularly taken with Dr. Bion's generosity of spirit with the audience. His heart was as impeccable as the rest of his being. As I told Dr. Bion, I felt privileged to know him for even a few hours as part of a large audience. I felt myself becoming a more touching person in his presence.

I concluded after that first evening that Bion was as simple as he was complex. At the personal level if one understands that simplicity of self then Bion would be very easy to understand. However, the consistency with which he responded at such a simple level would sooner or later blow wide open the framework of boxed-in realities that most people manifest. Bion was always fresh. He was always simple. People's networks of lies would be shattered as they approached more approximate levels of truth. This would leave them experiencing chaos or the existential anxiety of not knowing. It is within such turmoil that people may enter a "state of discovery."

Bion found a way to humanity, compassion, and the joy of living through variation in his pace of life. He allowed time for the connection to take place between the center of him and his consciousness.

Bion taught me about humility by example. I felt deeply touched by him in each communication we shared.

After experiencing Bion on this occasion I wrote him a letter in great depth requesting that he analyze me. Also, I sent him a copy of the reaction to him and his presentation telling him I intended to include it in my book if he liked the chapter. I was tickled by the first part of the letter and saddened by the second. He wrote,

> Dear Dr. Bergantino,
>
> Many thanks for your letter and enclosures. Thank you for what you say; this work is certainly most evocative and stimulating. This applies to the papers you sent me–which I return herewith.
>
> I am no longer in a position to offer any vacancies for analytic work of the kind that you mention. Unfortunately the pressure of time, as you indicate, is the determinant factor. I therefore am not free to choose what I would like to do from amongst the many options.
>
> I wish you well with the book that you are projecting and hope in due course to have the opportunity to read it.

Sincerely yours,
W. R. Bion

I wrote a second letter requesting that he reconsider, telling him that I was willing to assume the risk in the matter of time. He graciously responded in a clear and potent way, saying,

Dear Dr. Bergantino,

Many thanks for your letter of May 24. I am glad that you appreciate the difficulty that I have in having to say "No" to requests which are made to me. I cannot even say that I would like to embark on a piece of work when I know that it can arouse false hopes.

Sincerely yours,
W. R. Bion

I felt his "No" to be an outrage that I would have asked him a second time given the fact he already expressed that he would have liked to have worked with me, but was not free to, because of the "pressure of time." I felt that he was not happy that I had again asked him to deal with the fact that he was eighty-two years old at the unconscious level, and with the question of how long he would live. I had mentioned in my first letter that he looked very healthy.

Being gravely disappointed, but feeling a genuine warmth toward Bion, I wrote him a letter in which I said that while I was quite disappointed in not being able to work with him, if he were interested in meeting with a younger friend for lunch, I would be most interested in doing so. Also, I sent him a tape of my father and me playing Italian MANDOLIN duets. His wife told me several years later that he listened to this tape OVER AND OVER! A few weeks later Bion replied,

Dear Dr. Bergantino,

Thank you for your letter of June 28. I have had to wait until I had a chance of the leisure to listen appreciatively to your tape–hence the delay. We found it very interesting and are filled with admiration of your competent musicianship.

Many thanks also for your kind suggestion of lunchtime meeting. I do not in fact take lunch–the calls on my professional time are even more heavy as the date for my departure for England approaches. As I am not coming back I had better make this a farewell note.

With every good wish for your continued work.

Sincerely,
W. R. Bion

Several things touched me about his letters. First, the care and personal sensitivity with which he responded to me. Each time he wrote, I felt emotion welling up in me at deeper levels than I had expected from a man who I had only met for a brief while. I was puzzled, somewhat disturbed, and yet delighted that I could even feel a deeper emotional richness in terms of the way he wrote to me. I was touched by his gracious, but yet personal response, right from the comma after "Dear Dr. Bergantino,." Also, I found it unusual that his letters were typed double spaced. It gave me the feeling that he was a man from another age.

His last letter surprised me as I did not know he was going back to England. But two things struck me. "I AM NOT COMING BACK." "WITH EVERY GOOD WISH FOR YOUR CONTINUED WORK." I knew that Bion was a man who related on multiple levels of awareness. Also, I knew that I could read these levels. When I READ, "I AM NOT COMING BACK" I NEARLY BURST INTO TEARS. I FELT HE WAS TALKING ABOUT HIS DEATH, AND NOT JUST HIS DEPARTURE TO ENGLAND. "With every good wish for your continued work" motivated me to continue my search about his work with those who had been analyzed and/or supervised by him in the Los Angeles area, in addition to purchasing all that he had written.

I had given up any hope of working with Bion. But in the meantime I began to apply what I had learned by experiencing Bion on the evening of which I wrote about. I was seeing an older woman who had a very low frustration tolerance and who said she wished she could think clearly and creatively; that this had been her major stumbling block in life. I immediately thought of Bion. I used an Erickson form of hypnotic storytelling until my body pace, my sensations, and my mind began to take on the same qualities as the night I EXPERIENCED BION. I could reproduce a similar kind of experience in myself with self-hypnosis while I was working. My sense of presence began to expand and my thinking BECAME CLEARER. I BEGAN TO SAY THOUGHTS WITHOUT THINKING. I have no memory of the content of what the patient and I were saying but both of us began to respond differently than we had ever done with each other. She and I both felt that something quite unusual had happened in terms of creative, clear thinking and expanded sense of presence in the context of a more personal interpersonal exchange.

The loss of not working with Bion was looming ever larger in my mind. I wrote him another note, hoping he would get it before he left Los Angeles. I said that while I had read some of his work and doubted if I would ever fully understand the subtleties of his system of psychoanalysis, I COULD DO WHAT HE DID. I told him that were it not for what I felt to be an extremely moving primal connection between us and how he worked, and my ability to do the kind of work that he exemplified through his being, I would have been much too embarrassed to write yet a fourth letter after he had been so generous in responding to the first three. I told him I was willing to go to London for three weeks the following summer so that I would have a chance to have enough continued impact upon me that would not fade. Bion wrote back from London nearly three weeks later, saying,

Dear Dr. Bergantino,

Many thanks for your letter of August 24. I am not yet sure what work I shall be doing here, but I do not think it would be practical to attempt an analysis in the way that you suggest. Perhaps I could get in touch with you at a later date; I shall let you know my permanent address at the earliest opportunity.

Best wishes,
Sincerely yours,
W. R. Bion

I was pleasantly surprised to say the very least. I had given up all hope of being analyzed by him when I suggested three weeks. I felt his excitement ("at the earliest opportunity") in the letter. I knew that if he worked at all he wanted to work on a long-term analytic basis. I was tickled that he was considering working with me if he planned to do any work yet afraid of giving up everything I had worked so hard to build in Los Angeles. I was in tremendous conflict about moving to England for five years and then coming back to Los Angeles to start over again. However, I had decided to do so and wrote Bion a letter to that effect.

On the day I was going to mail the letter November 8,1979, I had a very strange feeling. I don't know why I decided to hold off mailing the letter for a few weeks. I consciously thought, Bion was a man of his word and after relocating would write to me soon. About two weeks after this I received a telephone call from a colleague saying that she had been informed that Wilfred Bion had died about two weeks before in London. Bion was eighty-two years old. I felt sad and brokenhearted, with a very great sense of loss.

An Analysand's Experience with Bion, with Richard Edelman, M.D.

I had lunch with Dr. Richard Edelman, a psychoanalyst, senior faculty member and supervising analyst at the Los Angeles Psychoanalytic Society and Institute. When analyzed by Bion, Dr. Edelman said that he would go into a session having a particular view of reality. Bion would say things that would leave Edelman's particular views of reality shaken; he left each session with a sense of chaos. He then told me that Dr. Bion felt the analyst's mind should always be in a state of chaos, because it is in this way that both the analyst and the patient will continually be open to fresh experiences instead of stereotypes of reality. Bion would say things that gave him a feeling that he had never been understood that well in his entire life. He said it was eerie, almost as if Bion would have to be him to understand him that well.

Dr. Edelman viewed Bion as one of the most unusual men he ever met. He felt this was primarily a result of Bion's enormous humility. He felt Bion had virtually no needs for any aggrandizement of himself. Dr. Edelman said he had always taken it for granted that everybody wants something and that Bion was the absence of that. He further described Bion as maintaining an "egoless state." Bion never implied that a patient should come to see him, or that he had anything to offer the patient, or that the patient could get something from him. In fact, Dr. Edelman said that when his wife first had an appointment with Bion she felt rejected because he made no attempt to schedule a second appointment. Bion left the responsibility in the hands of the patient. Dr. Edelman said patients often had the feeling they had to fight their way into psychoanalysis with Bion.

In describing his analysis, Dr. Edelman said that Bion would break things up all the time. Bion felt people were "saturated" with a lie and because of this, were not free to experience the moment–an existential moment if you will. One of Bion's objectives was to break up the saturation.

Bion was gentle and considerate. He would talk a lot during the session, but not challenge a person's lies directly. He would not add something from outside that could be considered to be superior knowledge. Bion believed such responses would be felt as foreign objects which would create hostility. (Bion's work with Dr. Edelman was in this respect quite different from the work described by other analysts later in the chapter in which Bion was also quite confrontive.)

Dr. Edelman said Bion created an environment so beneficial that the patient felt as though the pathological behavior would drop out without ever being spoken about. He said Bion had an attitude of well-being and health that pervaded the sessions and this attitude allowed nature's forces to heal psychological wounds. Dr. Edelman went on to describe an atmosphere of humanity, healing, and growth–"a marvelous kind of acceptance and non-critical atmosphere."

It is my opinion that such an approach prevents or at least diminishes the possibility that the narcissism of the therapist will interfere with a healing atmosphere.

Dr. Edelman stated that while there was an atmosphere of understanding and non-critical acceptance when working with Bion, and that a patient might experience Bion as *being with* that patient, Bion made it clear that he and the patient were separate people. Bion was quick to challenge any idealization of the therapist. He was quick to challenge what Kleiniens refer to as projective identification (attributing traits that exist within yourself to the therapist).

When patients showed aggrandized versions of themselves, and then projected it onto Bion, Bion would shove it right back into the patient by saying, "If there is anything in me that you see is so great, it must be in yourself." He never had an attitude of "I have it and you don't have it," or "You have to get it from me." In this respect he was quite different from much analytic thinking which states that it is important to maintain the idealization of the psychoanalyst to properly carry through the psychoanalysis.

Bion might interpret projective identification, making it clear that the patient was separate and different from the analyst, by saying to the patient, "You must think I am so and so . . . . What's the evidence?"

Dr. Edelman said Bion was against too much therapeutic zeal. By his refusal to say, "I want you to come because I have something to tell you," he did not reinforce the saturation of childhood. Bion felt the saturation of childhood was tantamount to "You don't have to think for yourself or ever develop." Bion got the message across to neurotic patients that he didn't need them, but that he was not indifferent to them. Dr. Edelman felt this was particularly important because of the neurotic's need to cling to the therapist. Neurotics want to hear that therapists need them.

When I mentioned to Edelman that he, also, seemed both humble and touching, as was Bion, he remarked that I could not compare the two of them in the same breath. I couldn't help but wonder if Bion had helped to shove this humility back into Dr. Edelman, or if Dr. Edelman was doing that with me, or both.

Dr. Edelman described Bion as having no desire to move someone from 'a' to 'b,' and that he simply provided an environment in which people moved in harmony with themselves. Yet this did not prevent Bion from using his capacity to respond by being tough as well as gentle. He had a great range of responsiveness in terms of his ability to impact patients.

A Practitioner of Dr. Heinz Kohut's Methods Comments On Bion, with Lars Lofgren, M.D.

Dr. Lars Lofgren, a psychiatrist and psychoanalyst in West Los Angeles, and associate professor in psychiatry, at the UCLA Medical School, gave me his impressions of Bion. He said that Bion never did the expected. He never resorted to standardized thinking. Everything was thought anew for the first time. When Bion was asked about the benefits of a successful analysis, he said, "increased income."

Bion took others seriously, and felt that whatever people asked him deserved great concern. He was in no way derogatory. Once, when asked about the relationship between "this . . . and that . . .," Bion replied in all sincerity, "I don't think there was any until you asked about it."

Dr. Lofgren experienced Bion as both serious and amusing in light conversation. His wife, Francesca, spent a great deal of time gardening, and when asked if he, too, liked gardening, Bion said, "Yes, but it does not extend to the spade."

While Dr. Lofgren was in group supervision with Bion, he partook in a humorous situation and was a bit apologetic for being disruptive. Bion responded, "Child play should be taken very seriously." This had the same kind of simplicity and accuracy as did his statement to me about doing what I enjoy doing.

DR. LOFGREN RECOUNTED THE STORY OF BION IN A GROUP OF PEOPLE WHO WERE AT THAT TIME IN THE PRESENCE OF THE KING OF ENGLAND. THE KING WAS PASSING BY THE PEOPLE, BUT STOPPED WHEN HE CAME TO BION. HE COULD NOT PASS BION, BUT WAS DRAWN TO HIM AS IF BY A MAGNET. THIS IS THE SENSE OF PRESENCE THAT I THOUGHT SO EXTRAORDINARY ABOUT BION.

The chapter to this point has presented a view of Bion the man and Bion the analyst. While this was presented to give an impression of Bion's presence, there is much to be learned from what he said.

Bion's Legacy: The Language of Achievement, I, with James S. Grotstein, M.D.

Dr. James S. Grotstein, a psychoanalyst in Beverly Hills as well as a supervising and analyzing instructor of the Los Angeles Psychoanalytic

Society and Institute, provided me with the following interview and helped me restructure my thinking about how I could best describe Bion's work for the purposes of this book. The focus on Bion's legacy and the language of achievement are Dr. Grotstein's conceptualizations.

Dr. Grotstein commented that Bion would come up with remarkable and unexpected interpretations. Dr. Grotstein replied to one of these interpretations:

Grotstein   By God, you are right. You are absolutely right.

Bion   On, right I am. Oh, yes I'm right (sarcastically). Yes, you want me to be right, don't you!? Oh, how right you want me to be. What you forget, Dr. Grotstein, is I'm right only because you are cooperative with me in giving me the associations that help me to formulate the second opinion about what it is you are saying. I could just as easily say, (dramatically) Dr. Grotstein, you're right! But the snag is, you don't listen to you. You would rather listen to me than to yourself.

Dr. Grotstein went on to say that Bion spoke a very special kind of language. He wanted very much not to be grasped. He wanted people to be evoked by him. His language was a *language of evocation* so we could be introduced to our own *language of experience*, or *language of achievement*, whereby we could form in our own terms those images which were evoked by listening to Bion.

On another occasion Dr. Grotstein said, "Oh yes, I think I follow you." Bion replied, "Yes, I was afraid of that."

Bion brought Plato and Kant into psychoanalysis. He referred to pure or absolute truth as 'O,' which we could never know. We can only know 'O' by its shadow–'K'–knowledge. We are trying to make a transformation from 'K' to 'O' indefinitely. We are always in the process of becoming. Bion would say, "I'm not an analyst. I'm trying to become one." About Mary, Queen of Scots, he said, "It's quite clear that Mary's problem was that she believed she was the queen, rather than trying to become one."

Becoming 'O' is becoming one's truer transcendental self. We are always evolving through 'K' towards 'O,' but never becoming 'O.' But in order to do that one must be existentially alone. One must never grasp the object, but only be evoked by the object. To grasp the object is to become the object.

Dr. Grotstein said that when Bion began the presentation about which I have written by saying, "I can hardly wait to hear what I am going to say," he meant it. He was often surprised by what he said. How much more interesting this can make the adventure of life!

Thoughts before thinking require a blank surface. The absence of memory and desire is important in order to be able to respond to one's own thoughts before thinking. To be in contact with one's inner truths, inherent truths and inherent preconceptions, one must abandon memory and desire. Bion felt this process was the key to creativity.

One must abandon all preconceptions. The analyst explores his "thoughts without a thinker," which are being elicited by the patient's associations.

Bion felt that once thoughts emerged they were a definitory hypothesis and people could pay attention to them, compare them with other ideas, inquire upon them, and ultimately relegate them to mental action.

MRS. SUSAN GROTSTEIN, WHO WAS ALSO ANALYZED BY BION, DESCRIBED HIM AS "... A MAN FOR ALL SEASONS. OUT OF ANOTHER TIME. . . . SOMETHING OF A MYSTIC. VERY MUCH IN TOUCH WITH ESP, AND VERY MUCH IN TOUCH WITH SOMETHING BEYOND THE NATURAL, OR THE USUAL IN PEOPLE."

Dr. Grotstein said that Bion would contact people by evocation and still remain separate. He would go far out of his way not to establish common ground. He was a mystic by remaining aloof. He knew the dangers of contact. He felt that people should not be in analysis any longer than they had to be. Dr. Grotstein then discussed how his analysis came to a termination. After five and one half years he told Bion in January that things were going very well. Bion replied, "March 31." That was the date of termination. When I told this story to a friend who had been in analysis for seven years, he was astounded. He had been talking about termination for the past two years, but could not seem to complete the analysis. Bion said, "One can't ever really grow as long as one is in analysis. It has to be afterwards."

Mrs. Grotstein commented that Bion did not like to nurture extended dependency. He thought the analytic experience was valuable for itself, and that it wasn't being something, but becoming or moving with your experience that was important. "I have arrived" implies a closure to the self.

Dr. Grotstein said that Bion felt impeded by his contact with others. He felt sensuous links between people joined them and kept them from becoming 'O.' This is why he always eschewed attention. Unlike any other analyst, Bion would say,

> I'm a very unimportant person who is felt to be a very important person only insofar as I may remind you of important people in your past or even your present life. In actual fact, that isn't true. In actual fact I'm very unimportant, and my real importance to you lies in my unimportance.

Part of Bion's uniqueness was in taking away his uniqueness.

I asked Mrs. Grotstein if there was any significant experience that stood out for her during her analysis, and found her reply to be quite interesting.

Mrs. Grotstein   There is nothing coming to me.

Me   Maybe that is significant.

Mrs. Grotstein   There was so much significance at times, going on in a session. I would leave and think, what was going on? There would be a sense of something having happened and not being able to bring it back the way it was. His capacity to say, "We don't only deal with what you have done wrong, what your sins have been, what have been the errors and the mistakes; there is also the other part of it, the you that has been able to make it thus far.

She went on to say that Bion's timing could be very jolting (when one was depressed.) His capacity to hold several points of view, to be able to show you the way you were thinking or feeling and then juxtapose another vertices that could really bring you up thinking, "My God, there is another side to this."

Dr. Grotstein said that Bion kept himself undiscovered. He never allowed you to grasp him as object. As a result all of us who were analyzed by him are puzzled as to what the experience really was.

I commented, "You mean it left you open to knowing you had a significant experience; not being able to hang onto it, and therefore able to continue to move with significant experiences as they happen on an open ended basis."

Mrs. Grotstein replied:

> Move close to experience of the thing in itself, or the evolution of the thing in itself. We learned to evolve with our lives and our objects, but never pinpoint and say, "This is exactly what has happened or is going on." There would be an aura and then you could get into it and feel definite about something and yet there was a vagueness because there was that openness to travel more space with one's thoughts and feelings.

Dr. Grotstein commented that analysis presumes that understanding will lead to the solution of the matter, while in actual fact that isn't the case. Psychoanalysis is a mystery story insofar as the mystery always remains. You don't find out what was. You only find out what it wasn't. The thing in itself is always undiscoverable.

He went on by saying, on the one hand the thing in itself was inherent preconceptions–the thoughts without a thinker in us. On the other hand, the thing in itself is also related to the external world.

During the analysis with Bion Dr. Grotstein went back to an area of concern about his childhood. Bion would say,

> Oh, you must remember, they are not members of your immediate family. They are members of your father's family. That isn't your family any longer. That is part of your rehearsal family. *Your childhood family is the rehearsal*

family and analysis is simply the completion of the rehearsal. It isn't the thing in itself Your wife is your permanent family, and your children are so young, they haven't yet found their permanent families. But you're not their family. You're only their rehearsal family.

I replied that such a comment would jolt my entire orientation. It would feel like a one hundred and eighty degree twist.

Susan replied,

> Bion had a way of really bringing you in touch with you, and there was one comment he made that I will never forget. Bion said, "You are really meeting and talking about wanting to get to know the most important person you are ever going to meet in this world, yourself. It is important for you to be on good terms with that person."

Susan went on to describe Bion as mystical and very religious, for he was a devout believer in the spirit of the human being becoming.

Dr. Grotstein said that Bion was a mystic philosopher and that he perceived that mystery that must always be mysterious. 'O.' As people have a great hatred of 'O,' of the uncertainty and the frustration of what lies ahead, Bion was not the kind of analyst that all people could work with.

I replied, "Then working with Bion must have been like being in a constant state of existential anxiety." I was thinking of my experience with Dr. Erickson at this time, and couldn't help but wonder how it might have been in a five day per week analysis.

The common thread between Bion and Erickson was that both left patients in a chaotic state of not knowing, which forced the kind of letting go that helped people both flow more freely with their unconscious reactions and be able to think more clearly.

Bion was well-disciplined. He showed patience and actively continued interpreting, even if the patient acted like a baby and was evacuating all over the place through the patient's words and actions. Bion referred to this discipline as *containment*.

All psychological phenomena were understood by Bion in terms of a container-contained series. Take the example of the baby, who is evacuating through projective identification, a terror of dying, and a mommy insofar as she can withstand the evacuating process and translate that into thinking about the infant's needs. Thus, she becomes a container for the infant's content. Is it a bowel movement? Is it a wet diaper? Does it need to be held? Such occurrences get translated into something other than evacuation. This makes Bion's view of the therapist's responsibility similar to that of a parent raising a child.

The container and the contained becomes a paradigm for all mental operations. Thoughts without a thinker emerge through projective identification from some permanent source and one's mind, if it is clear of memory and desire, can become a container for it to be thought about, so that all thinking would be a container and a contained series, and a transformation from the paranoid schizoid (PS) position to the depressive position (D) as referred to by Melanie Klein in her writings.

PS is the first stage of development according to Melanie Klein. We are in a state of persecuting anxiety because of a sense of helplessness. So we *attack pain, we project bad feelings into objects,* and *we split them into good and bad.* It is a process of organizing chaos in a very personal way. Good guys versus bad guys. Good breasts versus bad breasts. Then, when we get enough of a confidence in the power of the good breast over the bad breast, there is the threshold of the depressive position.

In the depressive position the infant is more and more aware of his or her own individuality, but also that mother is a whole object. Mother is neither idealized, nor terrible. She is good and bad on balance. But she is very important. So the infant becomes more realistic and more contrite about all the omnipotent expectations put upon mommy earlier in the paranoid-schizoid position. So the paranoid-schizoid position is a period of omnipotence, omnipotent magic, projective identification, idealization, whereby the depressive position is much more nearly real, much more in contact with external reality. One releases mommy to her own agenda. In a sense, Bion worked by using his power to get peoples' hands off of him, in helping them move from PS to D. It is really the acceptance of weaning, and so Bion would talk about the *transformation from PS-D.* From omnipotent mechanisms to reality mechanisms, through the container and the contained.

Depressive position doesn't mean clinical depression. It means the abandonment of one's omnipotent stranglehold on mommy. Pining for the loss of omnipotence with mommy. Pining for the loss of the womb. Pining for mommy's absence, but being more able to tolerate the absence. Dr. Grotstein said he saw this phenomena frequently with patients who get very sad and mournful during analytic breaks, rather than becoming omnipotent, or destructive. They tolerate it but there is a sense of sadness and mourning. It is the beginning of a reality orientation. It is the *acceptance of separation*. Bion would say that all thinking takes place in the container and the contained series from PS-D, and begins in omnipotence while ending in reality.

Dr. Grotstein said that Bion worked very hard and was very dramatic in that he lent himself to the role of the projections to dramatize them. For example, Bion said to Dr. Grotstein, "There's no analysis going on here. This is just plain persecution." (Bion of Grotstein). Bion's interpretation of Dr. Grotstein's state of mind at that moment was so real that he actually had the belief that Dr. Bion didn't want him to return. However, the tone of Dr. Bion's voice would change at that moment. He was never harsh, but strong. The analysand would have the feeling that there was a strong person behind him. Bion called this person the man of experience. He was an unusual analyst in his own being, but he allowed his patients to become unusual patients and to discover their own uniqueness.

When I asked Dr. Grotstein about Bion's slow pace of talking, he said that Bion would really give himself a chance to listen to himself talk. He was disciplined in this way.

I feel that it is important for a person to find the right pace between being able to listen to what you are saying while still being spontaneous enough to surprise yourself.

Another of Bion's concepts was the selected fact. A configuration is presented: an animal. It's furry. It has a tail. You begin to develop some idea of the constant conjunctions throughout the material. All of a sudden you hear a meow. *Meow* is the selected fact. It is that which makes everything clear. Then you know it is a cat. Until the selected fact is revealed it could be any one of a number of animals that are furry and have a tail.

The selected fact is finally that thing which begins to emerge which makes everything clear, but it takes patience for a therapist to listen to one's own thoughts without a thinker, one's own associations and preconceptions, and also to the evocative material from the patient. If the analyst or therapist has patience and listens, eventually the selected fact emerges to help the analyst or therapist organize the meaning of the constant conjunctions, the regular patterns.

Bion engaged in the analysis of being here now. He felt that one couldn't analyze the past and couldn't analyze the future. While he was personally hard to grasp, this was purposeful–for patients to be evoked and to know one's own thoughts. That was his analytic technique. He was not interested in patients sensing him as a desirous person because they then might be desirous of knowing him and that would obscure them knowing themselves and their own thoughts. In a sense the analysis would take place in a state of deprivation, so that all the qualities the patient would project onto the analyst would be pushed back into the patient, and the patient would be able to experience his or her own human richness.

Bion's legacy, *the language of achievement*, helped people to continue becoming the man or woman of achievement. This is a person who can tolerate half doubts and half truths. Such a person is willing to put aside the need for certainty. He or she learns to tolerate the gap until something emerges which becomes significant and meaningful. The language of achievement is evocative but not graspable. It allows one the advantage of being in the state of mystery so as to hear one's own thoughts without a thinker emerge. It is a matter of tolerating the unknown without memory or desire.

In these terms Bion's life was close to a series of uninterrupted existential moments, and his legacy–the language of achievement, is the method by which we can help ourselves to continue becoming so that we can experience the existential moments of our own existence at deeper and more meaningful levels.

Bion's Legacy: The Language of Achievement, II, with Michael Paul, M.D.

Dr. Michael Paul, a psychoanalyst and member of the Los Angeles Psychoanalytic Society and Institute, contributed the information for this section. The commentary is taken from a taped interview with Dr.

Paul, who had four years of psychoanalysis and five years of supervision with Dr. Bion.

I asked Dr. Paul about the differences between Bion's work as an analyst and Bion's work as a supervisor. Dr. Paul said that Bion would often say, "Analysis is all personal comments. Although it is generally considered rude to make personal comments, one of the problems of analysis is that it is all personal. So as a function of that it is exceedingly pro and evocative." Dr. Bion felt it was important to have the opportunity to follow a situation through its course before he would use the full capacity of his personal commentary. This is not at all intended to mean that he was impersonal when he was supervising, but that the intensity of his comments were different.

For example, a comment he would make in analysis that he would be reluctant to make in supervision might be "Oh, sure you know. Absolutely, you're right," in a very sarcastic tone. "It seems as if everything I say to you you have said already. Quite interesting, so I suppose there isn't much I can do for you. We have got a situation in which you have all these understandings as soon as I seem to give them to you. You said you've already said it yourself."

The characteristics of Bion's communication were such that direct experience was always the primary focus. Bion's goal was to break any set experience of the past or future. (In this respect his work is similar to that of Dr. Milton H. Erickson which to a large degree explains my own strong interest in both men.) Past and future were focused in the present, for Bion was a *here and now* person. But he was always precise, disciplined, and respectful to the patient.

Bion's technique was very classical in that he always dealt with the transference, but he did it in an extraordinary way.

There were no cliches and no interpretations that sounded like interpretations. Bion would say things in the course of conversation, but a very special kind of conversation. It was always related to the experience in the moment, which he would never repeat. This is what made me feel that Bion had an extraordinary ability to capture one existential moment upon another in a way so the accumulation of these moments led to an extraordinary sense of presence and fullness of being. Bion always focused experientially with the idea that there would never be a repeat of an experience. His emphasis was on paying ATTENTION.

Dr. Paul gave the following as an example of the kind of dialogue Bion would have with a patient.

Patient	Could you repeat what you said. I'm afraid I didn't get it.
Bion	No I can't.
Patient	Well, why not?
Bion	It's not repeatable.
Patient	(Angrily and forcefully): I just asked you a question. How come it's not repeatable?
Bion	I think we are now exploring what I would call hostility and I think there is no question about it as far as you can tell that what is going on between the two of us at the moment is a situation which would involve your hatred of me. If I don't do what you say and if I don't seem to be controlled by what you say, then you are capable of expressing your hatred. Apparently you have very little respect for the facts, because in fact if you were capable of apprehending the reality of the situation you would recognize that there would be no possibility to repeat anything; because the moment has changed and the context has changed and the situation has changed.

Dr. Paul then went on to say that Bion was the toughest man he ever met in his life. He experienced Bion's power and intensity. In the next breath he described Bion as a man who was extremely kind and extremely gentle.

Dr. Paul said that Bion was terribly upsetting to people who lived their lives on the basis that time doesn't move, or that change doesn't really exist. It's frightening to believe there is a world where there are no repeats.

Bion asked for evidence for nearly everything. This was not to suggest that what a person said wasn't true, but to help that person to think and feel more deeply about the experience. In this way a person would be able to cut below the ordinary names people give things and get down to the experience, so that what goes on between two people when they talk could be an extraordinary evocative and provocative experience that could lead to change. The specificity of the words and the attention paid are skills that develop such ability.

Whatever Bion said would be likely to stimulate a patient's thinking. Bion would rarely answer a direct question. His responses would be geared in some way to a particular issue which Dr. Paul believes Bion felt was an abstraction to thinking. Dr. Paul described the experience as feeling like he was having his mind operated on.

Dr. Paul gave the following comment as an example of what Bion might say to a patient to help that patient become more attentive.

> Bion might say, "I may be able to draw your attention to what I think you think and what I think you feel. You can then compare that to what you know you think and what you know you feel and decide for yourself as to whether you think they are concordant. *In order to be able to do this you have to not only be able to pay attention to what I say but also to what you say.* In this particular manner, if you wish, you could lead me astray because you could say that an interpretation was incorrect when in fact it was correct and you could say the interpretation is correct, when in fact it was incorrect."

Dr. Paul stated that Bion's method of interpretation was a very precise instrument and that such attention would lead to deeper levels of self-knowledge. Dr. Paul feels that in order to have any meaning come out of a relationship there has to be an extraordinary attention that goes far beyond what is ordinarily considered to be adequate when having a conversation.

Bion felt that attention also helped one to focus on what interferes with paying attention. He studied the phenomena that interrupt the capacity for paying attention. Perhaps this is why I found my experience with Dr. Bion to be so unusual, in that my attention was able to continue uninterrupted beyond what I felt my normal span of attention to be.

Dr. Paul went on to say that Bion viewed attention in the same way one would view an athletic skill. Bion responded in ways that helped patients learn to extend their capacity for paying attention beyond the interruptive elements in order to shift the balance of power. Interpretations were focused in such a way as to stimulate maximally, oftentimes, the evocation or provocation of the psychotic part of the personality. Dr. Paul then said he didn't know whether he could make that statement, but that he could certainly say that it happened frequently. Attention would be paid to all sorts or processes that would interrupt–the capacity to hear, to listen, to wander, to fall asleep–interruptive experiences that happen at the moment.

Bion helped people to listen to what they say when they are talking.

My Reaction to Dr. Paul's Interview

I feel that three of Dr. Bion's instruments of interpretation as presented by Dr. Paul are a major contribution in dealing with the issues of projective identification. First, asking for what *evidence* a patient has for attributing characteristics to the therapist forces that patient to become clearer about which characteristics are in the patient and which characteristics are in the therapist. This is where Bion's lack of a need for self-aggrandizement was particularly important. He helped prevent the maintenance of a false idealization of the analyst and further helped to perpetuate assumption of responsibility in patients for an evolving sense of personal richness.

Second, making the differences explicit as to what the therapist thinks and feels in concordance or contrast with what the patient knows the patient thinks and feels further differentiates "I" and "Thou" in addition to putting the weight of knowledge back in the lap of the patient. That is, Bion spoke about what the therapist thinks and feels about the patient as opposed to what the patient *knows* the patient thinks and *knows* he or she feels. Such a process helps patients come to appreciate individuality and separateness, or a lack of merging one with the other through contaminated contact that may very well prove to be toxic to patients.

Third, Bion focused the patient on differentiating the two kinds of denial that would cause problems in terms of the patient's ability to differentiate and focus attention. He did this by ending the interpretation with such a comment as "In this particular manner, if you wish, you could lead me astray because you could say that an interpretation was incorrect when in fact it was correct and you could say the interpretation is correct, when in fact it was incorrect." Such a comment would have two effects. First, it would further the patient's clarity about who is the person of the therapist and who is the person of the patient. Second, it would help the patient think even more clearly about which of the two kinds of errors that patient is likely to make, thereby reducing the possibility that either type of error will be made. This increases the possibility of the patient moving toward closer approximations of truth, manifested in the expanded sense of presence of that patient.

Bion's Legacy: The Language of Achievement, III, with Stephen E. Salenger, M.D.

This section is the contribution of Dr. Stephen E. Salenger, a clinical associate of the Los Angeles Psychoanalytic Institute. The material was taken from a taped interview with Dr. Salenger.

Giving an interpretation during the course of psychotherapy has certain dangers. Bion was aware that interpretations could stop associations and growth instead of facilitate them. He realized that psychoanalysis was an ongoing dynamic process. The moment something is added into the flow of associations by the analyst, the analyst alters the nature of the interaction between both parties. The problem with giving interpretations then becomes how the analyst will do so without stopping growth, freezing time, and re-structuring the patient's; perception along the ideas, conceptions and preconceptions of the analyst as opposed to facilitating the patient's ability to do that for him or herself.

Bion's interactions opened up space and allowed patients a view from another angle of the interaction. Bion had the ability to put the interaction into an unusual perspective, so that it caused disorientation, whereas traditional analysis would be more inclined to give an interpretation that fills up space by defining the objects, or by giving the analyst's interpretation of the experience. The emotional impact of each is quite different.

Bion had the ability to get out of touch with those things that are usually thought of as sanity, and to give them up so he could look at things from an entirely different perspective. This was a major strength–his ability to live in a space of *not knowing*, or accepting an uncertainty of living.

The capacity for patients as well as therapists to listen to something they don't know, to absorb it, to integrate it, and to form new ideas is the essence of thinking. It is not something that any of us do easily. People do not like to be disoriented. They do not like to feel stupid, nor do they like to feel that everything they have learned has to be thrown out. With Bion, everything you learned previously had to be thrown out. In this respect, I think the intention of Bion's work is again similar to that of Dr. Milton Erickson, although the methodology is quite different.

Bion would say something like, well, psychoanalytic theory is useful, but only for the first or second session. Because after that you would have to listen to the patient. What you have to listen to is not your psychoanalytic theory, the way you understand it, but you have to listen to the way the patient understands his psychoanalytic theory, which may be of a very different nature.

He felt theory is a functional tool which you have to be prepared to throw out of it doesn't explain the facts or bring new facts into view. Dr. Salenger felt that what stood out for him was that analysts need to *forget their preconceptions* about what a patient is talking about so they can listen to what the patient *is* talking about.

Dr. Salenger said Bion would ask a question that would "flabbergast me and I would be lost. I wouldn't know what the hell to say, and Bion would look at me and say something like,"

Bion   Well, what would you say to the patient?

Dr. Salenger went on to say that Bion's questions would focus on the fact that even if you understood what that patient said, what is it that the analyst would say to a patient and how would it be said in such a way that it might be able to be listened to?

Dr. Salenger gave an example in which Bion asked a simple but disorienting question in the supervision process. Dr. Salenger was seeing a manic-depressive patient in the hospital after a suicide attempt. She had taken one hundred pills, gone to a motel, taken off her wedding rings, and lay down. To her dismay she survived the experience, and upon waking was so angry that she set the motel room on fire. She then became frightened and jumped out the window. When Dr. Salenger saw her she had her arms in a cast, legs in a cast and her face was very swollen, with two black eyes. The woman asked Dr. Salenger if she could go to a Bar Mitzvah on Saturday. Bion's disorienting question to Dr. Salenger was, "Who was it that invited her?"

Dr. Salenger didn't know what Bion was getting at, but about two months later the search evoked by Bion's question *came together* for Dr. Salenger in his own mind. He concluded from his own thoughts, feelings, and intentions that the woman was in such a state of denial that she must have felt in league with God. She wanted to go to this Bar Mitzvah, this growing up. God had told her it was alright. God invited her even though she was sitting there in traction. It was Bion's question that helped Dr. Salenger put the patient's words into a new perspective. It broke through his usual thought patterns, and opened up space for new thought.

While Bion would intervene in ways that created chaos for some patients, such as Dr. Salenger, in others he would approach things more on a step-by-step basis. For example, Bion made open-ended comments to Dr. Salenger that put him into chaos, leaving it up to Dr. Salenger to come up with whatever new perspectives occurred to him in reaction to the patient.

While the manner in which he would facilitate new perspectives is a matter of degree, Lyndell Paul, a psychiatric social worker in West Los Angeles, put it this way. "Bion greatly tended to expand by going as far as he could go in one direction, and then as far as he could go in the other direction."

Dr. Michael Paul gave an example of moving from one direction to the other with a patient who might say, "I can't afford analysis." He said Bion might say, "I suppose you do have to consider that," Then he would deal with the issues involved in not being able to afford the analysis. Then the question would be posed, "Can you afford not to have analysis?" Dr. Paul felt that Bion never shifted the ground with them. He would try to cover and explore the area, but he wouldn't cover the ground for you. *He would try to help you develop the tools to explore it yourself.*

Lyndell Paul went on to say that Bion also helped to develop the perimeters of the ground by asking the reverse sorts of questions. What does it cost to have an analysis? What does it cost not to have one? This *opens a space* while at the same time widening the perimeters. There is both containment and space.

What I can deduce from the varied experiences of his patients is that Dr. Bion had the capacity to help with the building blocks involved in thinking, while expanding the perimeters of thinking. But as well, he had the capacity to totally disorient a person where letting go was the more pertinent issue.

Dr. Salenger commented that when Bion gave a presentation to the Los Angeles Psychoanalytic Society and Institute he began by saying, "None of my work is original or of much consequence, but if you are interested I will tell you about it." Dr. Salenger said he felt, "My God, if his work isn't original, whose is?" This led Dr. Salenger to talk about his view of Bion's concept of a thinker in search of a thought. While Bion certainly helped to stimulate what was unique in a person, he also appreciated the paradox that no one is that unique. Thoughts and preconceptions exist in everybody. None of us, no matter how uniquely we may deal with our space and the manipulation of knowledge within that space, is original. Everything we have is based upon something we have gotten from someone else, or is potentially pre-existing. The most that we can have is a unique way of ordering and delineating ideas. "Never original, and never of much consequence."

Bion's idea was that thinking developed as a function of the presence of thoughts. The connections between thoughts and the permutations–resynthesis–would be new, or said in a way that might be useful as a tool when an important formulation didn't get through.

One may certainly question the statement "never original, and never of much consequence," particularly in terms of a thinker like Einstein. But then according to Bion, Einstein might be viewed in terms of the way he ordered and delineated his ideas. Einstein was a humble man who could never understand why people made such a fuss over him. Bion was the same kind of man. Perhaps those who understand the paradoxical nature of the half truth "never original, and never of much consequence," have a key to the road to humility and an effective approach to the problem of narcissism as it relates to both the analyst and the patient.

Dr. Salenger wrote a paper dealing with the embryology of narcissism. It was the beginning of his work trying to understand how the character developed, and how perception developed. He gave it to Bion for review. Bion gave it back to him, saying, "It won't be published." There was a long pause and then Dr. Salenger said to Bion, "Can you tell me why?" Bion replied, "You don't split a log with the thick end of a wedge."

While this response was confusing to Dr. Salenger, Bion was a sincere man. It was not his intention to confuse, but only to explore as best as one can do the issues that were involved. It took quite awhile for Dr. Salenger to formulate a new perspective regarding the concerns he felt he would have to be involved with. They were "What do you say to a patient, what do you say to your audience, who are you writing the paper for, who are you doing analysis for, and for what reason, and to whom?" Bion's comment forced him to confront these fundamental issues.

Because human beings feel a need to orient themselves through things such as class, time, money, objects, degrees, knowledge, Bion examined the relationship between these things. For example, Dr. Salenger said Bion would state that the analytic setting is an environment in which to explore the experience of two people in space. These two people create something between them; something in the space that alters both people forever. And the experience of the analysis is the analysis of the experience of that space and what goes on between analyst and patient in that space. So then Bion was also interested in a space between things, in the relationship of things in space as they related to the experience between analyst and patient.

Bion felt when people are frightened by the experience of a space, or as Bion would say, by a gap, they may or may not be able to listen and they have to take in what they hear on whatever level they are able to integrate. While Bion worked on multiple levels of experience patients would often distort and change the experience to fit their past experience, or to something that gave the illusion of safety. Multiple levels of experience refers to different levels of organization of the same phenomena. For example, the transference, the "here and now" interactional level, the intuition level, the personal level, the group level, and a fine-tuned degree of sensory perception level are among the multiple levels of experience with which Bion would deal. Bion would struggle with a patient so that his work would be experienced on all these levels simultaneously. However, patients would struggle to stay in the particular levels in which they felt most secure.

Bion felt that patients attempt to fill the space by presenting something through ignorance because they cannot tolerate empty space. Bion felt that patients had a dislike of frustration, a dislike of ignorance, and a dislike of having space which is not filled. The totality of these frustrations can stimulate a premature desire to fill the space.

In summary, I feel that this human dilemma leaves the psychoanalyst with a dilemma. The psychoanalyst has to decide if he or she has come to terms with how to deal with space, whether he or she is promulgating theory, space filler, or is actually doing the kind of analysis that would help patients deal more effectively with the space between two human beings in relationship to the here and now experience that takes place between psychoanalyst and patient. For it is only with such a separateness between analyst and patient that they may contact each other in ways whereby meaningful experience, or existential moments, are likely to occur.

On a more personal note it is only when I feel that I am dealing appropriately with space that I feel a clear sense of separateness and actually feel that I can breathe easier. My lungs take in more air and my body feels bigger. My sense of presence expands. When I become more physically myself at this "here and now" level, I am then able to think much more clearly as well as deal with my feelings and experiences in a fuller way. But to be able to do this I have to be able to withstand what is clearly a very separate feeling from the other person or other people. In addition, I have to pay particular attention to what are my own thoughts and feelings as opposed to being so concerned with their thoughts and feelings that I just become a reactor to them instead of someone who is living my life as richly as I can. And Bion's ideas about space are at the core of what I feel are the crucial elements in facilitating these richer and more expanded levels of being; dealing with the complexity of human life in very simple ways while taking into consideration multiple levels of experience.

Bion: Impact and the Supervision of the Practical Analysis of Being There, with Wilfred R. Bion, M.R.C.S. and Stephen E. Salenger, M.D.

> When it comes to the question of psychoanalysis, you do get a chance *if the chap will turn up.* I say a chance. It's a minimum requirement. Not the maximum, but the minimum. After that point, you could start, you see. You could even say, "Look, I can see you tomorrow or I suggest that you come five times a week and we can now fix up the times because I have to ask you to keep certain hours and to try to conform to my vacation times and to pay for the time whether you use it or not." It's about all you can say. The minimum requirements. After that, is where it starts.

This is a direct quote (as will be much of this section except for my commentary and organization of the issues and ideas) excerpted from a cassette audio tape recording of a supervision session by Wilfred R. Bion of Dr. Stephen E. Salenger. Dr. Salenger was kind enough to make six tapes, totaling twelve hours of supervision, available to me. Further, Dr. Salenger was very courageous in permitting me to write about Bion's supervision of him, particularly as he was a very young analyst at the time of the supervision.

Notes were not used in the supervision hours. Bion felt that it was important to let the experience of the patient filter through and whatever the training analyst remembered, just like an analytic hour, the associations of a dream, etc., would be the hour. Bion would then analyze by making some comment that had to do with the primitive misperceptions or conceptions of what was going on. However, I am sure that Bion would strongly urge that these interpretations not be used as the ideal way to respond, but only be used to stimulate freer and more truthful thinking and responding on the part of analysts and therapists.

The first segment of supervision on "impact" has much of the dialogue uninterrupted. This is intended to give a flavor of how Bion responded in the course of a supervision session. However, the confrontations in response to Dr. Salenger's responses are included more sparsely throughout. The focus moves to what Bion had to say about critical issues in doing psychoanalysis, which as I see it, relate to the practice of all psychotherapy.

The kind of interventions that Bion discussed are particularly useful when patients throw the responsibility back to the therapist, particularly when the therapist assumes a false sense of guilt, a false sense of power, and a false sense of responsibility.

When I heard these tapes I was fascinated. Bion concerned himself with supervising around the issues of whether the patient was *there, not there*, the minimum conditions of psychoanalysis, money, and several other issues that are rarely talked about. Further, the issues around which Bion supervised are those in which therapists often feel that they become *impotent* with patients. In a sense Bion was supervising on a simple, basic existential level of two people in a room, and the basic truths of the condition that exists between them. The level of *integrity* Bion suggests of the psychoanalyst would certainly create an environment where interpersonal existential moments were likely to occur.

When referring to the kind of issues that Bion discussed he said, "This is where the trouble arises, in that *practical analysis*, instead of some goddam business that one writes in a book and so forth."

From this point on I will use 'B' to refer to Bion and 'S' to refer to Dr. Salenger in the dialogue excerpts.

The Impact of the Analyst/Therapist

S — The problem I have with him is that I feel like when he presents the stuff and I understand what's going on, he just destroys, attacks or shits on my interpretations. I am *not able to have any impact on him*, at least that I can see.

B — You might be doing a pretty good job with him, but it doesn't mean that it has the slightest use. I don't see why you bother with what he's really saying.

S — It doesn't seem to have any effect on him. He doesn't seem to listen to it.

B That's right. It raises a question, you see. What good does he suppose it does, coming to you? If you behave like that?

Bion puts this in such a way that the responsibility for coming is thrust right back upon the patient, thereby restoring the potency and impact to the therapist. Also, Bion's intonation fully suggests that the patient may not want to continue coming. At this time Dr. Salenger was a young analyst beginning practice. To put out straight this issue, when one has more open time than one would like, is certainly most difficult. However, while there are risks of the patient leaving, to not deal with the issue leaves the analyst/therapist in a position of impotence due to fear of losing the patient.

S I have asked him that question.

B What does he answer?

S He says, I don't know.

B Well, who is to know? On what grounds are you supposed to make another appointment?

Bion's methods become even more ruthless in that he is suggesting that the tables be turned and the patient be threatened with loss of the relationship if the patient cannot come up with the responsible involvement necessary to convince the analyst that the patient really desires the relationship, and for substantive reasons.

S I've told him that if he was not able to take in what I was giving him, and if he didn't feel it was of any use, he is wasting his time.

B It seems to me to beg the question. You see, if that is the case. But according to him, it is the case. According to him the facts are as he stated them. The only problem about it is what's he doing there, that morning or afternoon, when he was coming to you! And what does he suppose you are to do about it! Are you supposed to make another appointment or what are you supposed to do? And if so, why?

Bion again forced the assumption of responsibility upon the patient. Some patients have unrealized fantasies about their reasons for wanting relationships with therapists, as well as infantile fantasies about how therapists will magically make them well. Bion's comment will force the patient to delve into those fantasies, if that patient, does choose to continue. Bion's work is quite existential in that it confronts responsible involvement. It either forces such involvement on the part of patients, or forces them out of treatment.

S   What he tells me is he feels he is getting a lot out of treatment. He doesn't know why.

B   He has told you what he's getting out of it. He's told you that he's getting this very bad treatment from you and you behave in this very bad way. Well, so what? What is the point of his telling you that, if it's untrue? And if it is true, what's he doing again? Is he expecting you to make another appointment or what are you supposing to do?

Bion refuses to let Dr. Salenger off the hook. His attention is continually focused on the area in which therapeutic potency has been diluted. Bion calls for *action-oriented interpretation* to the patient to restore therapeutic impact.

S   I felt that one of the things he gets out of the session is a kind of triumphant feeling that he really wants me to come, and to work hard, and to feel impotent.

B   You see, that may be your opinion, but that's not what he has said. Why shouldn't you respect what he says? Why shouldn't you assume that he isn't a liar?

S   I don't assume that he is a liar.

B   Very well then. The answer is simple. These are the facts. Now what does he expect you to do about it? (All of Bion's comments are stated emphatically, in a challenging way)

S   I point that out to him and he says I'm hopeless. Nothing can be done about it.

B   Are you supposed to make another appointment with him or not? (a return to the action that would restore therapeutic potency). After all, he must know that you purport to be a psychoanalyst. You have office hours and all that kind of thing. Is he expecting you to make these hours or sort of thing that you are doing available to him? If so, why? You see, it seems to me it's a free country. I don't see why he isn't entitled to say or think about anything he damn well pleases. Well, if that's what he thinks, that's fine. But what are you supposed to do?

S   I have pointed that out over and over. It doesn't do a damn bit of good.

B   Right. That's fine. There is nothing good you can do for him. Now do you want an appointment for tomorrow or don't you? (Bion role plays Dr. Salenger talking to patient) And why do you expect me, you see, to give you an appointment tomorrow in view of the information in which you have given me? See from my point of view I can say about this, not that I would (he leaves room for choice open to Dr. Salenger), but that it's just too bad. Clearly my ideas about such psychoanalysis as I can do are completely erroneous. Either that or you are a liar who misinforms me, but what is the point? Why should I fix up with you to get some more misinformation? (Bion stops the role playing and makes his comments directly to Dr. Salenger) Now I'm not you and I can't very well tell you what to do about it, but I can ask you, and I can discuss the matter with you, and I can say, what are you proposing to do about it? It seems to me that you are proposing to give more interpretations, or more analysis. But it begs the question altogether as to whether analysis is of the slightest use. Such analysis as you can do, or in my case, such analysis as I can do. You see, for all I know you may be in a position to be able to afford to see him again. You have the time or the money or whatever it costs to see this fellow. I can't tell you anything about that. But it does seem to me, you see, that you can say to him, "Well, you tell me that these are the effects. I suppose you are really purporting to speak the truth to me, and I don't doubt it at all. I can't see what you suppose to see in point of continuing this association." However, whether you'd be wise to say that or not, I do not know, because I am not there. But you are.

S   I have some anxiety that he would leave treatment altogether, even though he feels he needs it.

B   What of it?

S   I just have enough of a practice to keep going.

At this point Bion has hit the bottom line in the supervision.

B   It doesn't matter, you know. This is the snag about it. You may be in a helluva jam and so forth in the same way as I may, but then, that does not really answer the problem which I've got–"Am I supposed to make another appointment or what?"

S   I suppose that would really be a much better interpretation because he would be bound to listen to it.

B   It is an administrative job. All that you can do as I gather from your account is to give him another session and to tell him things which he's been told a hundred times. They're no damn good to him anyway, so there doesn't seem to be any point in telling him 101 times. I can perfectly well see that if you were a better analyst and all that kind of thing or did something else, it might get a better result but that's not the problem. The problem is you being you and he being him.

Bion, while being rather severe in his supervision, reassures the younger colleague by empathizing with him. These are equalizing statements said in a respectful way, while still maintaining the authority necessary for supervision.

The Minimum Conditions

This situation involved a patient who will only come for psychoanalysis three times per week.

B   You can tell him that you don't know what to do if you aren't allowed to do psychoanalysis if it happens erroneously or whatever, that you think you want to see him five times a week and you aren't allowed to do it, what the hell are you going to do? . . . You can draw his attention to the fact that while in his opinion he can afford to do this (come three times per week instead of five), he leaves out of account whether you are able to spend your professional time on analysis or not. Now if he cannot afford the time or the money it's just too bad. The minimum conditions don't exist.

S When I drew his attention to the minimum conditions he said he was of two minds. He said there was one part of him that needed to come and that missed me when he didn't come, and that felt that he got something valuable. But there was another part of him that just didn't give a damn. It was too much of a commitment for him to give his time. Money was not a problem.

B He is either there or he isn't. All that he is saying may be true, but the plain effect is, he is either in the office or he isn't.

Bion's focus on the facts cuts right through interpretations that lose power because of adverse facts on the part of the patient to the minimum conditions, and/or the lack of action on the analyst's part to confront the issue.

S He went back to saying, "I'm not sure what I'm getting out of it and I feel like three days is sufficient."

B You could say, "As far as you're concerned it's sufficient. I don't know anything about these different parts of you. But for you it is sufficient. For me it isn't. I've told you what is the minimum that I want, not the maximum, the minimum." If he can't afford to give you the minimum of your requirements there is nothing more that you can do about it. You can't analyze him.

S But there is nothing I feel like I can do about it. I can point it out to him again. But the question is will he see that as my trying to get rid of him, or telling him that even three times a week is not worth it?

B For all you know you might be in a position of having no patients at all, but that isn't the point.

> The point is that you feel that the probability is that you wouldn't have him.

S

> That's so.

B

> He's not doing anything to you. Not if you're analyzing him. He is either coming or he isn't. . . . You see, your habit of mind is such now that you are really not bothering with what I am saying to you. You are bothering with what the interpretation is of what I'm saying to you. I'm trying to draw attention to a situation in which you are not allowed to have the conditions in which to analyze him. You may for some reason or another believe that you can indulge him or even that he can indulge you if you have to have rest or breaks. But these breaks aren't analysis. It's conceivable that if there are two people who are proposed to cooperate on this that those things can be swept into the analysis. But they aren't analysis.

Here again Bion focuses on the integrity of the analyst maintaining certain boundaries that are consistent with this particular analyst's view of what it takes to be effective. This sense of separateness, or space, is important to the practice of analysis. It forces the patient to come to terms with the issue of abandonment.

B

> As far as I'm concerned, included in these minimum conditions is all the psychoanalysis one is ever likely to know.

B

> You hardly need a model to see how absolutely up against it you and the most cooperative patient you are ever likely to get are up against it. Now if he or you either are under the impression that this analysis can be done with even fewer conditions still for doing it, it is a very serious matter.

The Demanding Patient Who Is Never Satisfied

B

Why not draw his attention to the fact that he, who presumably knows the facts in a way which you cannot possibly know, except whatever he is pleased to pass on to you, is in fact telling you that there isn't the faintest chance of his paying even the slightest attention ever to what he knows already. Now since that is the case, what does he expect a mere stranger like yourself would do, or what notice does he expect that he would ever pay to a mere stranger like yourself? How is it you are coming here again this morning? What do you expect me to do by coming to see me?

Patient Who Came at the Wrong Time

B

But of course the whole trouble with analysis is how to do it. You called him, as if it mattered to you when he should come, or to make available to him a time to come. This is something you see, which you do know about (Dr. Salenger's prior comment was that he didn't know). Nobody can know better than you what your feelings and so forth were, and why you acted as you did. . . . Now that may be a step toward knowing why he thinks he knows what you did. The question is then, how did he react to what he thought you did?

S

I have a feeling that what you have hit upon may really be the crux of the matter. I am concerned that he come, and I think that is evident to him. And it's evident to him on a number of bases. I called him about his appointment. I made up for him this time. I offered him more time than he was coming in for.

B   You could say something like, "I think you must have been impressed by the fact that I called you," or you could say, "What is all this about? How did you come to discover that I need you?" Now this becomes a matter of expertise, if you could get to what would be the correct approach there. As to whether to say to him "I think this is your reaction to my having called you," or whether to get some sort of further evidence which is convincing.

S   He came at the wrong time yesterday.

B   The point is this, that he did come at the wrong time and he knew damn well, somewhere, probably, that you knew this. Now the question is this: This patient can tell something from what you do. Now you're giving his interpretation, his conclusions, if you like, from what you did do. Now if you hadn't done that, that would also be interpretable. After all, your behavior is peculiar to you. Therefore, it is not unlikely that if he knew what you would do, he could make a sort of guess at who you are. He could analyze you. (Pause) What is also quite clear is that it doesn't matter a damn what you do about this. If you move to give *her* (Bion's use of "her" with a male patient was an unconscious reaction) no reply at all that surely would tell *him* something as well. Just to debate the possibility he could argue, well, obviously, you don't give a damn. If you don't mind whether he keeps the appointment or not, if you don't give a damn about his having engagements or work to do, but behave in this offhand way, well, that tells him something about what sort of person you are. So I think that the question arises what should this patient be told? What interpretation should one give? Bearing in mind of course that one would like, if possible, to give the correct interpretation, but God knows what a correct interpretation is.

Bion posed the question from both sides and left Dr. Salenger in a position to search for his own solution. Bion further challenged him to provide the correct interpretation, implying that in a way it didn't make any difference, because no matter what he did, he would have his hands full.

The Stingy Patient Who Strings You Along

B

Some people that you meet will be masters at having you in that situation. When you show signs of terminating the analysis, they give you a little bit more to keep you going. So you are left in the position of teaching in the state of the barest possible minimum in so far as the patient knows what the barest possible minimum is.

S

He's sure doing that to me.

B

What are you to say to this man next session?

S

I pointed out to him that it is not enough to come to get help just enough so that he could maintain some contact.

B

Yes, but who does he think you are? Does he think, for example, shall we take a few extremes, that you are a young psychoanalyst who's got no damn patients anyway, or if you have got patients they are patients that can't pay, or what? What is his game? Let me suggest another sort of a visual image about this. A sort of game of *last across the freeway without getting run over*. How far are you going to carry that? (challenging) Now it isn't quite the same thing, but, how far can I go with my psychoanalyst which is to give him the absolute minimum and at the same time not get him to chuck up the game.

S   Precisely.

B   Now, the question is then, have you reached a point at which it is possible to give him that interpretation, or have you not?

S   This is a real problem because I don't enjoy having a patient like this insofar as there is a great deal more pressure than I might ordinarily have.

B   See, you are then more in a position of the person playing the game, because your problem is not, "How late can I leave running across the road," you see, or "How close can I get to telling him the truth which is now available to me." (Pause) Because you can still feel that it would be helpful for the analyzing to go on, and not just to terminate then and there, because you couldn't stand it. So the analyst in a sense is also involved in this problem, this dangerous game. How far can you go in the way of telling the truth? (Pause) Thinking all the time, what is the alternative, anyway? *(a comment that focuses on the strain of holding back the truth of what exists between them)*. And how far can you go if you are going to commit yourself to having to say something which isn't correct? There may be limits indeed, to the amount of analysis in inverted commas that you can stand.

Fear of Losing the Patient

S   Well, I see it either as saying I can not work with you, and/or I'm not willing to work with you under these conditions, at which time I would have no patient. I also see him as a patient I desire to keep in as much as I feel that I have learned an extraordinary amount from him.

B   Well, there are all these conditions you see which are possible to debate here and not possible to debate in the office. The snag is you see that in the office then and there you are supposed to make a reply. Suppose you make no reply. That is a reply.

S   It doesn't make much difference what I do with this guy. He knows something from whatever I do.

B   That doesn't matter. What does matter is what he thinks he knows. That is where you come up against your cutting edge, you see. You might know quite a lot about him. You might know quite a lot about the interpretation. The question which arises is "Are you going to give that interpretation, or not?" And if you are not going to give that interpretation, how long are you going to stand being able to do analysis in these conditions?

S   I don't know.

B   But then I'm not suggesting you do know. All that you can say about that is it takes time to answer. Not only with one patient, but with the whole boiling lot. (This kind of comment again would give Dr. Salenger the feeling that these issues are not unique to him, nor that the question of how honest the therapist can be are unique to him, but the entire profession of psychoanalysis including Bion, himself have to face "the whole boiling lot.")

The Patient Who Either Wants to Terminate For Lack of Money and/or Chastises the Therapist for Making Money

S	The patient is saying that he recognizes this need for him to continue analysis, but he wants to keep busy and make money and use those as substitutes.
B	Who wants to make money? (challenging)
S	The patient. That's what he says, and–
B	(Even more challenging) Who is it who wants to make money?
S	Well, I pointed out to him that he had this feeling that all I was concerned about was the money, and that–
B	Be careful about what you see, because you can draw attention, why not say, "Since you feel that you need money I think this makes you remember the possibility that I do." (Pause) "Now, I don't think you like the feeling that I also might want to make money. It is much nicer to feel that if I do want to make money you can do without me." Now I am not putting this forward as being the ideal interpretation because I think this is just damn nonsense. I do think you see that it is important that you should yourself have some kind of formulation or some sort of idea of what it is you ought to say to him. But what you are to say to him can't be determined unless he comes to see you and you see him. It can't be determined by me.

The Patient Who Diagnoses Himself as Insane

S   . . . I asked him and he said it has to do with his not being able to be functional; his not being able to be in relationships with other people. And he has not been more specific about that.

B   Well, you can point out to him then, that in his opinion, that if somebody can't function you feel that the correct diagnosis is insane. To make the point a bit clearer by making it all that ridiculous would be, you would hardly argue about a baby, or would you? Would you say that when a person is a baby that can be the diagnosis but when he is forty, or fifty, or sixty, some other diagnosis is required. (Long pause) If he could feel that he was a baby, then he could always feel at some time or another he'd grow up and all would be well. (Bion giving Dr. Salenger a possible response to the patient) But what I want to draw attention to you the patient is that "You are not telling me this. You are actually using a sort of psychiatric formulation. You're talking about your mental health. And the explanation can't be that you're only an infant or only a child."

The Uninvolved Patient

S   He's half here and half not, and the result is that whatever point he feels is half enough. He is not getting a proper analysis.

B   Well, you can point out to him, "Look, you don't even have to get off this couch. Thanks to being able to think you can absent yourself even while you're here."

Ending the Session

B   "We are ready at time, now." (In a firm voice that doesn't permit hanging on)

The Patient Who Terminates over the Telephone

S   He called and said, "I called to tell you that the check I sent you bounced, and to redeposit it in the bank. I also wanted to tell you that I have decided that I no longer need your services, nor can I afford them, and so as of this coming Monday, please cancel all of my appointments." And he said "Thank you," in a manicky way, and hung up. He was really having the feeling I needed him for the analysis.

B   Now, look at it a different way. Supposing you had called him, what about? You made a perfectly definite statement to me, which is that he isn't about to come to you for analysis or anybody else. He may not be able to afford the time or the money which it costs. Now he says he can't, alright, that's fine. Now what have you got to that? What is the alternative if there is one? What excuse would you have of calling up, and so on? Now I'm raising this question because it's going to happen over and over again.

S   I don't know. If a patient misses an hour or something I can call to see what happened. But this particular patient, the only thing that I was left to do was to make an interpretation on the telephone.

B   Not analytically. Not in my opinion. Anyway, on the face of it you can, but dammit all, just consider whether you can give an interpretation when the fellow hasn't come to the office.

B   Superficially you could answer it on the telephone, in fact, it is true. This is a matter where nobody can judge the answer except yourself.

The Lying Patient

B   The only point here is to be sure that you consider the various possibilities, including the possibility of what the hell you would be saying if you aren't going to accept what he says. This possibility crops up when you have a patient come to you who you know perfectly well is just lying, or at least shall we say is not telling you the truth. You may feel that it is very important to be correctly informed, but if the patient is not in a position to keep you correctly informed, well, the conditions can be as far as you are concerned, lacking.

Can you afford to see the patient? If a patient is allowed to tell you any lies that he chooses he may be in a position to afford analysis from his point of view. The question then arises, are you in a position to afford to to see him? You can say, "Yes, I will see you at so many dollars a session and so many lies a week," to make it rather ridiculous. But the real question is whether in fact the conditions exist for analysis. As far as you're concerned, the fundamental question is whether you can afford to associate with him, and not only whether he can afford to come to you. Now fundamentally this encompasses the whole of analytic practice. The kind of people that you're dealing with and associating with and relying upon are the people who almost by definition are unreliable. So the point is that it isn't altogether surprising that analysis is no bloody good or has a bad reputation, because analysts are dealing with people who are pretty sure to get analysis and the analyst a bad reputation. Either that, or they are not patients. Now as far as you are concerned, the point is, where do you draw the line?

Patient Threatening Suicide

Dr. Salenger is worried that he may say or do something that would trigger the patient to commit suicide.

B *(Discussing suicide)* The point is not whether he will kill himself or he won't. The point is, what does he expect you to do?

Such a response is more than likely to trigger off anger in the patient as opposed to suicidal, depressed feelings.

B The point is to draw his attention to the fact that there is no use, no point whatever, in his coming to you who are a stranger and at the same time expect you to collude with him and to behave exactly as if there was some point in his coming to you.

B In a sense it is true that it can be said that a patient's feelings of *envy* and *rivalry* triggered a suicide because they were so powerfully aroused with the patient that the patient was even prepared to commit murder to see that you don't have a success. Therefore, you are certainly vulnerable. It can certainly be said that you pressed the trigger. But as you can see, it isn't in fact, not from an analytic point of view, quite true, because there is a long history. But the point again is, what does the patient expect you to do about it?

The Patient Who Continually Complains about How Bad You Are

Dr. Salenger presented a woman who was referred by a friend who was in analysis. The referring source said that Dr. Salenger was a good analyst but now the woman is complaining about him. Dr. Salenger does not know what to say.

B So to this point all she has to go on is hearsay.

S   Yes, but she has come for one and a half years.

B   So that must be pretty surprising, too, although by this time she ought to know how bad it is or how bad you are, or something like that.

S   She knows.

B   And yet she comes.

S   So indeed one of the problems could be, "How does she manage it? How, in spite of this experience with you, she still turns up?"

Bion's way of forcing people to deal with why they are coming to therapy is paradoxical, for it continually goes with the resistance, instead of against it. Patients cannot just take hold and begin to fight against the analyst. In fact, they must fight the other way in order to stay. Or they may find out that it is really not in them to stay and pay the price that analysis or psychotherapy involves.

S   This question has puzzled me.

B   Has it puzzled her?

S   No.

B   So in this respect, you see, there can be known to you a puzzle which is not in fact known to her. The question isn't so much that she has this sort of difficulty, but in spite of all that how she has turned up again. However, it's not really quite the point in a sense, because that is your puzzle as it were, and that may be something that is known to you but hasn't come over the horizon to her.

S   She says she comes because she now sees what she has been doing and is horrified by it.

B It doesn't explain why she should come.

S No it doesn't.

B You see, because to discover the horror of herself and her doings and so on does not sound like a particularly agreeable experience. In fact, it deepens the mystery.

Why Am I Not Better after All the Time I Have Been Coming?

S He said, I've been here a year. Why am I not better already? And he gets enraged with me when I point out to him that the minimum conditions are that he come, and that all I can do at best are give him interpretations; that I am not with him to tell him what to do and to show him what to do. Even if I could, it probably wouldn't be of any use. And that I've got to have someone help me take care of him (Bion), he doesn't want to recognize. It enrages him even more.

B This is the snag–that he can then say upon your own admission, "It's got nothing to do with you." So this improvement, you see, can't be done to him. It can't be done to you. Anyway he hasn't talked about improvement. He has talked about changes. Whether they are good, bad or indifferent, he hasn't said.

S The feeling is that I am a purveyor of shit, and I just don't give him anything good, and he expects me to do all sorts of things for him which I haven't done yet, and I'm just no damn good, which I accept, and I point out to him if he's got these expectations of me, I wonder where he's gotten them from?

B   If this is the case, you must point out to him that there is an unresolved problem. Why has he turned up again? Either this cannot be true in his estimation, or there is a question as to whether so much time and money is taken up in an association that's no damn good.

S   He will say, there has been improvement, but there just hasn't been enough for him.

B   Well, you can point out that this is again still another story.

While much has been presented about Bion and his individual approach to psychoanalysis and supervision, little has been said about Bion's work in the development of a psychoanalytic method that also dealt with group dynamics. I experienced his approach with Dr. Lars Lofgren and Dr. Marion Solomon in a group experience referred to as a Tavistock group. Bion's view of this process is explored in depth in his book *Experience in Groups*.

A TAVISTOCK GROUP EXPERIENCE, WITH LARS LOFGREN, M.D., AND MARION SOLOMON, PH.D.

Dr. Lofgren is a Psychiatrist, Residency Education Service, Brentwood V. A. Hospital; Associate Professor in Psychiatry, UCLA Medical School, Los Angeles; Fellow, A.K. Rice Institute; and in the private practice of psychiatry and psychoanalysis.

Dr. Solomon is a Program Consultant, Mental Health Professional Training Series, UCLA Extension; and is a Clinical Social Worker in the private practice of individual and group psychotherapy.

The Tavistock method of analysis of group experience was developed by Bion. His work provided a basis for synthesizing the approach of classical psychoanalysis with group dynamics and the nature of unconscious processes in groups. Tavistock is also based on the open systems concepts of organizational life developed under the leadership of A. K. Rice at the Tavistock Institute of Human Relations in London.

I was curious about Tavistock. A psychiatrist friend had told me that he had gone to a weekend Tavistock group with Drs. Lofgren and Solomon, and the experience made his hairs stand right up on his head. He described experiences and issues that are nearly always thought about by both men and women in group situations, but never commented upon.

He said that different people at times lost so much contact with reality that they appeared psychotic. One group member was described as saying, "I have a fantasy that people here are walking to the gas chamber in Auschwitz." Later the group members had a joint fantasy humorously expounded upon of breaking Dr. Lofgren's head open and stomping on the contents. It was only later that the reality of what was being said was taken seriously.

My friend said that the group dealt with the way men and women made objects of each other and with the anger and resentment that this caused. The competition between men was overt but covert competition amongst women, often ignored in other groups, came to the surface quickly, as did the fierce competitiveness between men and women for which sex would have the power in the group. From what was said and from repeated role switches, it appeared at times as though women had penises and men had vaginas.

The group repeatedly asked how men and women could work together productively without competing. They seemed bewildered, as though this was an impossible task. They could never figure out how Drs. Lofgren and Solomon worked together, so the group denied that it was happening.

My friend went on to say that he learned much about working with women rather than his usual experience of competing with them or "killing them off" emotionally.

The other groups I had experienced in the past were quite different in that the kind of opinions my friend was discussing did not come up for discussion among the group members. The issues struck me as quite unusual in that they usually go on at a very subliminal level of awareness, but are never dealt with among people–as it is not socially courteous to do so.

As I was particularly interested in Bion and his work, in addition to my friend's description of the experience, I decided to sign up for the weekend group given at the UCLA Extension. While I feel that what I learned is directly applicable to doing group therapy of all kinds, it must be noted that the course was an educational endeavor, and was not meant to be group therapy. Its purpose was to explore and study group processes.

As Dr. Lofgren and Dr. Solomon have different themes for different Tavistock groups, they have given me permission to quote from two information sheets so that a more adequate description may be given.

The Self in a Small Group: An Experiential Event

Background

The formulations in Bion's *Experiences in Groups* formed a landmark for the understanding of covert group processes.

(As a result of Bion's work) it now became possible to understand why persons coming together in order to perform a particular kind of work instead behaved as if the basic assumption for their endeavor was entirely different. Instead of doing work they seemed content to give up their competence and rely on an idealized leader (Basic Assumption Dependency). Or, they flew collectively into a rage, trying mercilessly to destroy the work, or at least flee from it (Basic Assumption Fight-Flight). Sometimes they resorted to sexually tinged fantasies about two of the members getting together in order to produce a messianic solution for the future (Basic Assumption Pairing). Bion showed that these basic assumptions competed with the Work mode. Only one Basic Assumption was present at a time, permeating the life of the group.

Bion's explanation is that the group collectively is trying to act out fantasies about the internal parts of the early oedipal mother. His argument is not easy to follow and the experiential correlates are hard to isolate. It may be somewhat easier to compare the Basic Assumptions to the Freudian partial drives. Dependency then appears to have prominent oral characteristics, fight-flight seems related to the anal stage with its spiteful rages at a time when progress of locomotion increases the ability to escape, and the pairing may have a lot to do with the oedipal fantasies of creating an offspring in an incestuous coupling. The question still remains, however, why these drive manifestations appear in a small (leaderless face to face) group. The Psychology of the Self as formulated by Kohut has important contributions to make to this situation. Kohut states that frustration in susceptible persons leads not only to a drop in self-esteem but a return to archaic narcissistic positions; the phase of the grandiose self and the phase of the idealized parent imago. Kohut further states that the movement of the cohesive self in the direction of threatening fragmentation may cause the appearance of isolated raw drive derivatives. These tenets contribute effectively to the understanding of the phenomena as first described by Bion. The leaderless group represents a taxing and frustrating experience for the members. The Basic Assumption Dependency corresponds to a creation of a charismatic, idealized leader on whom members can depend without exerting any competence and/or authority except in functional union with the leader. The Basic Assumption Fight-Flight corresponds to the narcissistic rage that is caused by an intense frustration. The oedipal qualities of the Basic Assumption Pairing can be seen as an attempt collectively to create stimulation for the endangered selves in the group in order to prevent further fragmentation. It is not yet clearly known what group phenomenon corresponds most closely to the grandiose self.

Principles

For persons involved in group work or organizational life, a theoretical knowledge of the formulations described above is not wholly satisfactory. A direct experiential and emotional experience of the group situation and one's own contribution to it creates a much more workable knowledge. Thus the main principle in offering these events is a didactic-educational one. Many participants report, however, experiences that they describe as definitely therapeutic. The reason for this may be related to Kohut's thesis that the work around the temporary regressions of the self constitutes the main therapeutic agent in dealing with the disturbances of the self. There is thus at least a theoretical possibility that participation in the offered event may lead to a state of more stable cohesiveness of the individual self.

Methods

Up to 14 members meet with the two consultants for 10, one and one-half hour experiential sessions. The stated task of the group is to examine its own behavior in the here-and-now. The consultants try to avoid nurturing attitudes, believing that these are at best condescending and at worst degrading. Instead the consultants try to explain group processes, especially unconscious ones, in simple everyday language.

The last and eleventh session of the event is a one and one-half hour discussion in seminar form with participation of members and consultants. Persons in frail health are not recommended to participate in these groups.[15] The theme of the particular Tavistock group that I experienced was "Authority, Leadership and Responsibility in a Small Group" and in their paper Lofgren and Solomon explain:

Aims and Principles

This small group event is designed to provide opportunities for members to enlarge their understanding of interpersonal and group relations through learning by direct experience. Experience has shown that problems of authority and leadership are essential in determining the development of events and the fate of the individual in groups. The ability to maintain authority in a small group is probably closely related to the problem of maintaining a cohesive self. At times there is a clear investment of authority in one or several members, but there are also times when forces of conscious and unconscious nature seem to make it impossible for a person to maintain authority (and a cohesive self). This leads to difficulties in pursuing the task of the group and realistically appraising the events that are taking place. The method of study is entirely experiential, and there is no attempt to prescribe what anybody should learn. The attempt is to provide an opportunity for increased intellectual and emotional awareness of the relevant issues. It should be stressed that the purpose of the small group event is increased understanding. There is no attempt to provide leadership training or to make more efficient group members.[16]**My Experience with Tavistock**

Drs. Lofgren and Solomon referred to themselves as the consultants. The initial focus of the group was the exploration and analysis of group processes by the group members in relation to each other and the consultants. Yet there were other important ramifications of the group. While most groups I experienced focused on either an individual working through intrapsychic conflicts in front of the group, or group members relating to each other creatively and authentically, I had never before experienced what I consider a crash course in the unconscious ways that group members relate to each other. The unconscious awareness was brought to consciousness and explained many of the previously unresolved difficulties in my social relationships. For this reason I think Bion's Tavistock method of group experience deserves further exposure. Once the unconscious issues are clear it becomes more possible for me, the self, to pursue an inner direction. This is different than the rehearsal of skills in that action flows naturally from being in tune with the unconscious self, other members of the group, and the group as an entity. If an individual is unaccustomed to dealing with the unconscious processes as they unfold in the group situation, that group may very well swallow up its members as a separate entity. Perhaps with awareness of the unconscious processes action is based on courage and authenticity. These points of insight combined with action may spark the freedom and contact of an existential moment.

I came about five minutes late to the group. It started at *exactly* six p.m. on Friday evening. I was told that the consultants had stated the purposes of the group, and left the members to discuss those purposes and get acquainted until six-thirty. I vaguely wondered about the consultants starting at exactly six p.m. and then leaving after five minutes. They returned exactly one-half hour later, walking at about the same pace. They gave me the feeling they knew what they were doing, although I wasn't quite sure what that was. Neither was the group. So we began the process of exploration. We had no instructions on how to begin. But we were told that the task was to examine the group process as it was occurring.

We introduced ourselves. Each of us said what we did for a living, and some went a bit further about themselves personally. But whenever the focus became talking to each other personally, or on a one-to-one basis, the consultants intervened and brought the talk back to the exploration of the group process. At one point, for example, Dr. Solomon said, "The group has chosen to talk about this subject at this time." Or, "I wonder for what purpose the group seems to have chosen to have these people talk about this subject right now."

The group felt frustrated with the leadership. We didn't quite know what to do with the consultants. They had a baffling way of establishing and maintaining an authoritative control that we felt kept us to the task of exploring authority and leadership in the group and the group processes.

Shortly after about an hour of exploration, the first shocking event took place. Dr. Lofgren said to the group, "Well, it looks like John is going to make himself the resident crazy in the group." I had never seen a group therapist, consultant, or leader come right out and say it! Of course, it was understood that we put on other people parts of ourselves. So Dr. Lofgren's comment was a group comment indicating that it wasn't that the one member of the group was crazy, but that the group was putting all its feelings of craziness on that one member, and he was choosing to take on the group craziness and act it out in the group. This certainly gave the group members food for thought. Were we contributing to John's craziness? Were we making him a scapegoat? Was he leading us into his game plan, that of being the group crazy?

At the break both consultants got up simultaneously and left the room. Members of the group asked them questions and tried to make contact as the consultants were leaving, but they did not respond. There were a variety of reactions among the group members to this behavior. I felt distant and cool because I couldn't pursue my need to be treated as special. Some were angry. Some said, Well who the hell do they think they are? Yet this simple, responsible behavior–starting and leaving on time–had the same effect on us as an analyst doing individual psychoanalysis might have on a patient, by being a blank screen that would leave the patient free to explore his or her own countertransference.

After leaving the group that evening a psychiatrist and I decided to go for a drink. John was walking along with us, and although I had mixed feelings about him joining us, I could tell he was hurting so I asked him if he wanted to come. Indeed, he spent most of the time talking about how terrible the group was and that he wouldn't return. He also asked us not to disclose his feelings to the group. I agreed, thinking it was no big thing he requested. However, the events that followed taught me that I should pay more *attention* to the nuances and implications of social communication–just as I would do if I were doing therapy.

When the group members assembled again, the consultants kept John's chair in the group. They said they were not informed that he was leaving so they would proceed on the basis of his still being a group member. During a break the psychiatrist that went for a drink with John and me asked me to share with the group our Friday evening experience. I refused, saying that I gave my word to John. Yet there was much discussion in the group about the missing chair, and what would now be done with the craziness in the group, now that John would no longer be there to absorb it.

There was quite a struggle for leadership, and against leadership. Some wanted it. Some didn't want it. None of the group members could agree on the agenda of any leader. While we couldn't agree on anything for any length of time, we did agree to kill off the consultants, to make John crazy, and at times, to work on the task of the group.

Perhaps the term *killing off* is a bit puzzling. This was the term used when through extended silence, one or a number of group members, appeared not to be present in the group. Men might be attempting to talk to Dr. Lofgren, or challenge him as the male authority figure. Women were not included, which "killed them off." The women might talk to each other or attempt to talk to Dr. Solomon while excluding the men. The subtle and powerful ways in which this was accomplished were startling.

By Saturday afternoon I became fascinated in the way we were struggling for our own individuality and integrity. There was a fear throughout the group of getting sucked into a whirlpool of problems. Many group issues came up. The competition among the men was overt, among the women, covert in that the women were not openly willing to confront the unspoken hierarchy of who were the most attractive women. Some of the men withdrew from competition with the consultants and from participation in the group. Others challenged the male or female consultant.

At one point Dr. Lofgren said that the group had effectively killed off Dr. Solomon and were now deciding what to do with him. He felt that the group was ambivalent about whether he should be killed off because the group members were so divided about authority and leadership. Dr. Solomon commented that the group had relegated her to a role of either being attractive competition among the women for Dr. Lofgren, the father, or killed off, having existed only as an object attached to Dr. Lofgren. She further commented that the women in this group seemed to have all the power, and the men were working hard to have more say and more power in the group. Dr. Solomon stated that the women seemed to have decided that they must choose between competing for men or destroying the potency of men, taking over the power for themselves. At this point, the men in the group were feeling either overpowered by the women (who outnumbered the men), or childishly dependent on them, while resenting the women for this dependency, even to the point of rage. The men tended to kill the women off by barely acknowledging their existence.

As time went on, the men became more reluctant to challenge each other. There was a feeling that as there weren't many of us, we had better stick together. The competition became covert.

I noticed that I'd like to kill one of the men but felt like I was much too gentlemanly to do anything like that. Fantasies emerged to the surface about rage, murderousness, pairing, male and female, power, fight-flight. These fantasies were running rampant throughout the group. Staying with these feelings felt intolerable to me at times. It was difficult to just sit there and experience the pain of just feeling. There was a lot of anxiety. There were many ways to try and contain the anxiety, by challenging the leaders, dependency, wanting somebody to take charge, wanting mother-father Dr. Lofgren to take over. We kept asking, What do we do now? Yet, no one would say, I feel helpless and dependent and I feel frightened and I'm going crazy. Dr. Solomon at one point commented that "some people in the group are opposed to feelings and punish those who are willing to tolerate feelings." At one time I tried to stop the feelings of craziness by offering to lead a structured experience because nobody was taking charge. My offer was rejected. By Sunday the group was more able to tolerate anxiety and other feelings and proceeded with the group's task, that of understanding the group process. But thinking and feeling were more difficult to put together at the depths with which the group was dealing. After Dr. Lofgren smiled once, noting that the group paid a great deal of attention to his smiling in their quest for nurturance, said, "It's more important that people smile than that people think."

It was becoming clear what was different about Tavistock. While most therapists have had experience getting in touch with the neurotic parts of themselves, a Tavistock group gets to some very primitive feelings, even psychotic parts that have been long split off. This is unusual because with the customary good manners of a group one does not usually talk about these kinds of things. People act as if they believe there are no such things as murderous rage and believe there are not infants within us that are demanding and greedy.

If a therapist and a group can allow the craziness of the group and of its members in the group, then the crazy part of its members are allowed. This process permits integration of the psychotic parts of the personality that are usually kept out of awareness. It was now clear why the consultants were specific that if people were trying to solve personal problems they should not come to this group, because people have to be pretty well integrated before they can delve into these deeper psychotic levels and come out of it all right in a one-weekend course.

The group had a need to have one male challenge Dr. Lofgren's authority, and set this man up to destroy him. It was during this time that I was feeling bored. The male member that was taking over leadership of the men certainly wasn't leaving much space for me. I sublimated my own aggression, felt bored, and came out in a quiet way. I didn't allow myself to have my own rage in competition with the other male, and yet I wasn't getting what I wanted and what I needed. I had too much invested in being fair. I began to wonder what it was I needed when I felt dependent–to get to the happy baby underneath.

When I felt "killed off," I felt that I was wearing handcuffs. It was hard to figure out how to get back into the group. There were long periods of time when I said nothing. I was thinking to myself, "Dammit, there must be some way I can take control of this group, so that my needs will be satisfied."

While I often felt the same handcuffs, until Tavistock I never really understood the *basic issues at the unconscious level.* The primal awareness I experienced in the group process that I have been describing led me to understand that is how people might behave, and that perhaps I should not be offended, become hurt and angry, and then withdraw and pout when people are doing what people naturally do according to their unconscious motivations. Until this time I saw much of what happened among people as being tantamount to jungle warfare, and had a feeling that it was easier not to participate. But the Tavistock group gave me a good sense of the primal motivations that were going on and the aggressions I needed to become a part of the jungle, and even turn the jungle into a well-orchestrated symphony. In other words, the awareness of group phenomena at the unconscious level helped me to become a more social person and move out of my basic "loner" position in life. While I didn't want to be a loner, I was never quite sure why I made that choice, nor was I sure of what to do about it.

About six-thirty Saturday evening the group had another thirty-minute break. During all the breaks, contact among us was quite enjoyable; the people were relatively warm and friendly. As soon as the group started the meeting again it was as if we didn't know anyone else in the group. We responded entirely differently. We were taken over by the group process. But during this particular break I discussed revolution–a coup! While none of us agreed on what would be done overtly, unconsciously we must have agreed it was time for Dr. Lofgren and Dr. Solomon to be effectively neutralized at the same time.

When I came back into the group I had decided to move John's chair out of the group circle and faced it toward the wall. It was Dr. Lofgren's responsibility to keep track of the time for starting and stopping, and Dr. Solomon's job to shut the door after the breaks when group began. Dr. Solomon had closed the door but was sitting with her back to the door. One of the group members came in late and left the door open. Thus a second challenge had been presented. The open door represented the breaking of the consultant's rigidly constructed boundaries. For the next hour and a half the rebellious spirit in the group pervaded. Dr. Lofgren was silent during this time. Dr. Solomon did talk about the chair that was taken out of the group. The group, however, was working toward making both consultants avoid hearing anything significant they said. During this time I was having an unusually playful time considering the task of the group (to focus on leadership and authority and its ramifications in terms of group process). Dr. Lofgren got wiped out around the chair and Dr. Solomon got killed off around the door.

Finally, after a long period of non-functioning in that we had killed off the leaders (authority) in the group, Dr. Lofgren acknowledged that the chair had been removed from the group, and that the door had been left open. He said he was quite surprised that the group unconsciously had set both incidents up simultaneously to kill off the consultants. He was angry and said that group members must surely be questioning the competence of the consultants, and rightly so. I was quite surprised at the level of therapeutic responsibility assumed by the consultants. Who cared whether the door was open or closed? After all, no one else was in the building anyway. I probably would have thought of closing the door only so the group experience would be private. I must admit I did have a feeling of satisfaction that the leaders both got a taste of what it was like to be effectively killed off for awhile, but I was glad to see them back. I think there was a fear in the group that the group might become quite vicious if it were left to its own ways without the consultants. There certainly were a lot of mixed feelings about whether Drs. Lofgren and Solomon should be welcomed back or not.

That was the last breath of rebellious fresh air that the consultants were unaware of. Sunday was a continuation of the exploration of group processes at what I experienced as a deprivation of individual personal contact. It certainly was hard for me to run my self-indulgence number in this group.

One issue stood out for me on Sunday. The psychiatrist who had gone for the drink with John and me blew the whistle on John's conversation and my insistence on confidentiality. Some people thought the psychiatrist acted irresponsibly toward John and some thought I acted irresponsibly toward the group. No matter how I reflected on the incident, I realized that by inviting John for a drink against my better, instinctual judgment, I had a price to pay! I have since become more assertive in saying what I want, and don't want, and in choosing who I want to be with and who I don't want to be with. Further, I learned to discriminate more sharply between a felt compassion and a compassion mixed with a rescuing quality that was actually disrespectful toward a person.

In terms of personal tyle of interpretation when leading a Tavistock group, I thought Dr. Lofgren had an unusual way of commenting on group phenomena that would often throw group members into chaos who were in search of meaning in the group process.

Dr. Lofgren feels there are times when the consultants have to be drastic to get the attention of a regressed group. I was particularly taken with the way he would intervene in some of these situations. "A bunch of porcupines trying to get together for warmth and that's dangerous when you are a porcupine. We are all covered with custard." Another of his comments was "Mirror mirror on the wall, shut up."

As a result of this Tavistock experience, in other social situations I was able to prevent myself from being killed off for the most part. Or, when I did get killed off, I understood what was happening and began to use my own fire power, my own aggressive and assertive participation. I found that before this experience I had not been quick enough to assess the primal group dynamics at both the conscious and unconscious levels and then respond at those levels as fully as was required of the situation. For example, the natural, overt or covert competition among men and women in social settings, the aggression and hostility that also accompanies love and tenderness, in relations, the exclusions by those on power trips, and how to aggressively deal with some of those issues so I would enjoy myself instead of being defensive. Before, if someone were not coming from a place of good heart *all* the time, I would write them off. My expectations were humanly unreal. In any case, my social life has been much fuller since this very brief experience. This suggests that while a Tavistock experience may be brief, it can be powerful.

While Bion's way of doing psychoanalysis and group analysis were representative of one segment of psychoanalytic thought, the work of Dr. Martin Grotjahn may help the reader understand how group analysis might be practiced from a more Freudian point of view, with a focus on the individual within the group.

ANALYTIC GROUP THERAPY–AN APPROACH TO NARCISSISM, WITH MARTIN GROTJAHN, M.D.

This section focuses on Dr. Martin Grotjahn, past president of the Society for Psychoanalytic Medicine of Southern California, former director of the training school of the Institute for Psychoanalytic Medicine, and formerly chairman of its educational committee. He has written several books, among them: *The Art and Technique of Analytic Group Therapy* and *Beyond Laughter: Humor and the Subconscious*. Dr. Grotjahn worked with Franz Alexander in Chicago, and was influenced by him. He was trained at the Berlin Institute before 1933.

Although I grew up in a middle-class environment, after getting my doctorate I began practicing with an entirely different kind of patient population. They were affluent, bright, and had a sophistication with which I was a bit uncomfortable.

These people were used to being treated as *special*. They had money, physical attractiveness, positions of excitement and power, whereby people would either treat them as special to get near them or to jump on the bandwagon and milk them. But from their point I found when I treated them as I treated other patients–setting firm limits–they would not comply and felt outraged that I would not treat them as exceptions. The problem–narcissism. However, I recognized part of the difficulty with working with them was that narcissism was alive and well on both sides of the couch.

These "special" people have a particularly difficult time receiving effective psychotherapeutic as well as medical care. They either antagonize their psychotherapist or physician until they are unable to continue in a working relationship or are given limits by the psychotherapist or physician and choose to leave of their own accord, all the while continuing to treat their helpers as of less consequence than themselves.

While most therapists have a frustrating time dealing with narcissistic patients on an individual basis, I had heard that an old and well-known analyst, Martin Grotjahn, actually worked with them in analytic group therapy. I went to a presentation of Dr. Grotjahn's and saw a charming, sophisticated man who was both brilliant and quite responsive.

During the coffee break I asked Dr. Grotjahn if he would send me a paper he had written about working with famous people. After asking me where I practiced and finding out we were next door neighbors, he invited me to lunch. I felt flattered at the way he put it, "It must have been at least ten years since I have invited a young doctor to lunch." He was telling me that he was both interested and sensed something "special" about me. I replied, "Well, I did come to meet you," thereby appealing to my narcissistic qualities. I thought, Grotjahn is much more soothing than me in terms of getting the ball rolling. This was my first existential moment with Dr. Grotjahn. It was important in that it both appealed to my narcissistic need to feel special while Dr. Grotjahn was quite sincere and open about his interest.

I was expecting to go out for lunch. To my surprise and delight Dr. Grotjahn (or Martin, as we were on a first-name basis) had fixed lunch for me. He had a little lunch tray with fruit, a variety of sandwiches, some nuts, and coffee. With his European accent and mannerism, I felt that I was having lunch in an outdoor cafe in Vienna. I fantasized that's how it must have been when the psychoanalysts got together in Freud's day.

Martin was not slow in getting to know me. He asked very pointed and extremely personal questions. He zeroed in very quickly. I had a feeling that he must have seen so many people in his life he knew right where to go!

He gave me one of the books he wrote, and I bought another. He told me I could take any of the articles he had published, so I took one of each–and there were many.

I began to tell him about the book I was writing and he offered to give his response to the chapter on Dr. Erickson. I received a telephone call in a week. Martin invited me to lunch and gave me a word-by-word review of the chapter. I noticed the difficulty I had with more subtle, sophisticated people was tied into what he was saying about my writing. I wouldn't *pay attention in choosing the most correct choice of words* or phrases to say to people. I didn't want to think that hard and gave way to low frustration tolerance. This left me a bit too abrasive when working with narcissistic people until I learned to make the effort to polish my shoes, so to speak. Martin would spend a great deal of time on each word that was of interest in his critique–telling me how important the choice of just the right word could be when writing. HE LIKED THE CHAPTER, SAYING THAT I CAME TO LIFE WHEN TALKING ABOUT THE INTERACTIONS BETWEEN MYSELF AND DR. ERICKSON, AND HE FELT THAT I HAD WRITTEN A BOOK FOR PROFESSIONALS IN A WAY THAT THE LAY PUBLIC WOULD BE INTERESTED.

I told him I was working on a psychoanalytic chapter and asked if he would like to see it. He said that he would. However, his response to this chapter, particularly the part about Freud, was quite harsh. He felt I did not make my points with enough zest, and that my writing was somewhat banal. He then proceeded to tell me what needed to be included to bring the chapter to life. The word banal hit me. My struggle was to reach the existential moments, to not be banal but impactful. I noticed that Martin was opinionated but still open-minded and quite outspoken. Certainly, he was not banal in any sense of the word. I had a second existential moment of insight when I realized I needed to start speaking my mind and give up my fear of offending people. His frank expression of opinions help make him an interesting character. As I later saw in his groups, he had no qualms about rendering an outrageous opinion. He told one woman that she should go out and have a passionate affair, so she would know "how it felt to be a woman." He said it with an almost fascist authoritarian sense of conviction. He and I and everyone in the group knew the woman would not do it, but his comment set the stage for lively, opinionated interaction.

Upon first entering the group I felt quite frustrated. All the members were like one big happy family involved in what appeared to be little more than social chit-chat. Each had a great deal of difficulty acknowledging their problems; most of the group members were having troubled relationships. When they did this there was an energy drop among group members, and the speaking member would appear to get more hyper–getting carried away with his or her own tale of "how wonderful my life is today," or "how awful things are" without feeling any real sense of what they are saying or doing. That is, without feeling an acknowledgment of the tragedy of the self encapsulated person. The loneliness. The despair. They were suffering from narcissistic encapsulation.

I felt frustrated that I had little to say. One man said that he made an enormous sum of money that day. I silently thought, that is a lot of therapy hours. Another stated that he was living six months in Europe and six months in California. Each had fascinating careers. I thought, what could I possibly share that would interest them? I began to see three problems. I was a loner in life and my position was clear from the start in the group. I was outside looking in. I was ambivalent about whether I wanted to make the effort to break into a group that was doing something I didn't particularly enjoy, or just quit. The second problem was lack of empathy; I had difficulty fully appreciating the pain of their existence because it is so well-masked by charming personalities and quick wits. The third problem was not having developed myself to the degree of worldliness in the group. I was used to straightforward, simple communication. There was a large part of me that would have felt a lot more comfortable eating pizza, having a few beers, playing cards with the neighborhood gang and betting on the football game of the week. I found myself feeling a cultural gap in terms of the arts, the extent of travel, and of a wider experience of the world in general.

A type of existential moment came about quickly in the first group session. Martin did not ignore the fact that I was a psychotherapist just because I was a group member to protect his own ego and position of power. He encouraged me to respond to people as a member of the group and as a person who had therapeutic skills. I found his active encouragement refreshing. He neither needed nor wanted protection. In fact, he openly challenged and even insulted me on a few occasions. When I came back at him he looked delighted. It was a situation of a proud father who encouraged his son's competitiveness and aggressiveness, fully appreciating that I was among the generation that would succeed him. Each time I felt this kind of encouragement, I felt freer. These were existential moments.

While Martin can be very direct, on occasions he says things that sound a bit like psychobabble. He uses this as a method of distraction to get to the unconscious. I did have unconscious reactions to what he said, but had the obsessive need to double-check. Once I had my boots off and was sitting on the couch with my legs folded in a yoga position. Martin said in a forceful tone, "Why do you wear those boots?" I said, "Because I like them." He screamed, "That's precisely what I mean! How could you like them!" My unconscious thought was that he was criticizing my lack of sophistication. However, I came after him to check out what he meant. He gave me an answer that sounded like psychobabble. Then one of the men in the group began to speak for Martin. He told me of Martin's brilliant ability to reach the unconscious. I said, "Why don't you let Martin speak for himself? Why does he need you to talk for him?" Out of the corner of my eye I saw that Martin was delighted that I was challenging him. I told Martin, "Explain yourself!" He gave me a bit more mumbo jumbo. I looked him right in the eye and replied, "What did you say!" in a tone that implied his words were preposterous. He came back with a sophisticated insult. I did not respond. I felt a bit frozen. A woman in the group tried to rescue me. Martin said, well, he insulted me. But he was evidently enjoying the lively interaction. He then became a bit more serious and made it clear where I was having difficulty making contact. He described me as having the kind of narcissistic qualities that would make me internalize as compared to his narcissistic qualities, which were more exhibitionistic.

Martin knew himself well. When I said I was fascinated by him, he said "Good." I then realized that his use of narcissism was partly why he dealt so successfully with narcissistic people. They all saw Martin as an absolute genius, perhaps one of the most brilliant men of his time. Thus, he was a man who was as important as they were. They were fascinated with his style and mannerisms as well as with his ability to make accurate responses that pinpoint the issues. He hooked people on his exhibitionistic narcissism as a way to draw them out to make contact and to sustain an interest in group therapy.

Nevertheless, this did not intrude upon the caring aspects of his personality; he invited me to lunch in front of the other group members, because he was genuinely interested in doing so.

Martin's interventions are high in vicarious introspection. That is, he has an uncanny ability to demonstrate empathic recognition of the patient's experience. For example, as one group session came to a close he introduced me to a group member for the first time, "And here is Len, who has yet to talk to the group. (Then directly to me) Len, are you feeling that this group is so different from any other group you have ever been in and so different from how you work that you want to leave the group?" (This was not only a question, but an accurate assessment.) He encouraged me to call him during the week, assuring me we were colleagues and could talk about what he was doing in the group if I had reservations. The following group session he approached me immediately and asked me to tell the group what I felt was wrong and why I did not want to stay. In other words, whatever real or imagined disappointments I had with him, the group members, the way he worked, and so forth, were up for grabs. He needed no protection.

I told him that I wasn't sure if the group would not only fail to be of help to me, but that I might even get worse. I revealed that I felt the group members were talking to themselves in front of people, the basic problem of narcissistic people who have difficulty overcoming their egotistical side to make contact. I felt that my more direct methods of contact were more useful, or at least more comforting. But as I was saying it, I knew at a deeper level that I needed to develop my capacities to become a more interesting person. The group welcomed me as a member, showing genuine interest in my challenge. As I began to relate more to the group, I found my ability to empathically put myself in the shoes of the narcissistic person increasing. I thought, my narcissism must be decreasing a bit or at least, I am using it better. Martin felt that narcissism was not something to overcome, but something to make friends with.

Narcissistic patients were used to talking about themselves, and an empathic interest in them could heal their narcissistic wounds without the more confrontive measures which their injured egos would or could not tolerate. So it was in the way of empathic understanding, of putting himself into the patient's shoes—as opposed to having them deal with the object of the analyst as a primary mode of intervention—that Martin was able to reach people who would have otherwise run away from therapy. In addition, he used his own exhibitionistic narcissism and his reputation as an important and interesting person to keep the narcissist in therapy while Martin slowly cultured a healing environment. The feeling of being understood so well that it is almost beyond belief was an existential moment for me. I had often felt misunderstood in my life, never realizing that feeling misunderstood and the ensuing disappointment was a problem of narcissism.

Martin's use of empathic understanding and vicarious introspection, his analytic technique in a group, aided by his enchanting personality, helped people reach a type of existential moment. When I really felt understood to that degree a more natural empathy came from within me for other people. It was not something that I had to tell myself to do. The existential moments provided by his analytic technique felt as if soothing medication were being placed on the narcissistic wounds.

Grotjahn said that the "aim of treatment is to learn how to trust, to disclose, to develop intimacy without fear and guilt, and to express one's self courageously, and to respond honestly and freely to others. Together with the strength to accept one's feeling of intimacy goes the strength to express one's hostility or aggression and to master it."[17] Such a viewpoint is existential in nature and facilitates an environment in which existential moments occur.

ENDNOTES

[1] Lawrence Friedman, Psy'-cho-a-nal'-y-sis. Paul S. Eriksson, Publisher, Battell Building, Middlebury, Vt. 05753, 1968, p. 133.

[2] Ibid., p. 134.

[3] Ibid., p. 134.

[4] Ibid., p. 135.

[5] HD Hilda Doolittle, Tribute to Freud. Pin Farm, Carcanet Press, (Oxford: 1971), p. 6.

[6] Ibid., p. 23.

[7] Ibid.

[8] Ibid., p. 7.

[9] Ibid., p. 24.

[10] Ibid., p. 57.

[11] Leon Grinberg, Dario Sor; and Elizabeth Tabak de Bianchedi, Introduction To The Work of Bion. (New York: Jason Aronson, Inc., 1977), p. xvi.

[12] Ibid.

[13] Ibid., xvii.

[14] Friedman, Psy'-cho-a-nal'-y-sis, p. 143.

[15] Lars Lofgren and Marion Solomon, "The Self in a Small Group: An Experiential Event," mimeographed, 1980.

16 Lars Lofgren and Marion Solomon, "Authority, Leadership & Responsibility in a Small Group," mimeographed, 1979.

17 Martin Grotjahn, The Art and Technique of Analytic Group Therapy. (New York: Jason Aronson, Inc., 1977), pp. 6-7.

REFERENCES

Friedman, Lawrence. *Psy'-cho-a-nal'-y-sis.* Paul S. Eriksson, Battel Building, Middlebury, Vt. 05753, 1968.

Grinberg, Leon; Sor, Dario; and Tabak de Bianchedi, Elizabeth. *Introduction To The Work Of Bion.* New York: Jason Aronson, Inc., 1977.

Grotjahn, Martin. *The Art and Technique of Analytic Group Therapy.* New York: Jason Aronson, Inc., 1977.

HD (Doolittle, Hilda). *Tribute to Freud.* Carcanet Press, Pin Farm, Oxford, 1971.

Lofgren, Lars, and Solomon, Marion. "The Self in a Small Group: An Experiential Event," 1980.

Lofgren, Lars and Solomon, Marion. "Authority, Leadership & Responsibility in a Small Group," 1979.

AS MANY OF BION'S BOOKS ARE DIFFICULT TO PURCHASE IN THE UNITED STATES, INTERESTED READERS MAY WRITE TO H. KARNAC (BOOKS) LTD., 56-58 GLOUCESTER RD., LONDON, SW7 4 QY FOR THEIR CATALOG. THEY STOCK NEARLY EVERYTHING HE HAS PUBLISHED AND A FEW WORKS THAT HIS WIDOW, FRANCESCA BION, IS CURRENTLY EDITING. BION'S BOOKS ARE DIFFICULT TREADING, BUT THOSE WHO ARE WILLING TO DEVELOP THAT LEVEL OF ATTENTION IN THEMSELVES MAY BE SURPRISED AT THE DEPTHS OF PRIMAL EXPERIENCE INTO WHICH BION DELVES. THE BOOKS ARE A RARE EDUCATIONAL OPPORTUNITY TO VISIT THE FAR CORNERS OF THE UNCONSCIOUS. IT IS RECOMMENDED THAT THE READER BEGIN WITH *SECOND THOUGHTS*, AND THEN MOVE INTO THE *SEVEN SERVANTS* IN THE FOLLOWING ORDER OF ITS PARTS: "LEARNING FROM EXPERIENCE"; "ELEMENTS OF PSYCHOANALYSIS"; "TRANSFORMATIONS"; AND "ATTENTION AND INTERPRETATION." THEN ANYTHING YOU WISH.

When sharing my problem with retention of some of the work of Bion, Francesca Bion wrote to me, "I don't believe that your 'problem of retention' is anything to worry about; in fact it might not be a good idea to 'remedy it.' Others have experienced this flash of understanding and then have been unable to recount it in words. Nevertheless I'm sure that once it has been 'felt' it can then be used–and that is much more important than the verbal repetition which so often is nothing more than parrot talk." Her comments affirmed my feeling that Bion is one of those few who has himself reached such an extraordinary level of experience, that his work merits study throughout the course of a lifetime.

Bion, Wilfred. *Second Thoughts:* London, William Heinemann Medical
    Books, Ltd., 1967.

Bion, Wilfred. *Seven Servants:* New York: Jason Aronson, Inc., 1977.

Bion, Wilfred. *Experience in Groups.* Tavistock Publications, London,
    1961 and reprinted in 1977.

Bion, Wilfred. *Bion's Brazilian Lectures 1.* Imago Editora Ltda., Rio de Janeiro, Brazil, 1974.

Bion, Wilfred. *Bion's Brazilian Lectures 2.* Imago Editora Ltda., Rio de Janeiro, Brazil, 1975.

Bion, Wilfred. *A Memoir of the Future, Book One, the Dream.* Imago Editora Ltda., Rio de Janeiro, Brazil, 1975.

Bion, Wilfred. *A Memoir of the Future, Book Two, The Past Presented.* Imago Editora Ltda., Rio de Janeiro, Brazil, 1977.

Bion, Wilfred. *Bion in New York and Sao Paulo.* (ed. Francesca Bion), Clunie Press, Perthshire, Scotland, 1980.

Bion, Wilfred. *Four Discussions with W. R. Bion.* Clunie Press, Perthshire, Scotland, 1978.

Bion, Wilfred. *The Dawn of Oblivion. Book Three of a Memoir of the Future.* Perthshire, Scotland: Clunie Press, 1979.

Bion, Wilfred. *Two Papers: The Grid and Caesura.* Rio de Janeiro, Brazil: Imago Editora Ltda., 1977.

A Case Against Self-Assisted Suicide

– Len Bergantino

One of my skills as a clinical psychologist is to get deeper quicker and get to the rock bottom heart of the matter while doing so.

SOMEWHERE BETWEEN 1993 AND 1999 I consulted at a nursing home with the elderly who were disabled enough that they weren't coming back to any degree of normalcy.

My job was to knock on the room door and introduce myself and do one hour of psychotherapy per week with them, albeit I only stayed two weeks.

On the first week, I knocked on an African-American woman's door and opened the door while saying, "I am Dr. Bergantino. I am your new psychologist." Immediately, as she had had a stroke, with a dislocated tongue, she said, very, very slowly and with great difficulty, "I want to kill myself!" I said, "Let me try this one more time," and I went outside the room and knocked again on the door and while entering said "I am Dr. Bergantino, your new psychologist." Again, she said in exactly the same manner, "I want to kill myself!"

I sat down beside her on the bed and said, "Lady, if you to kill yourself, you have come to the right guy! Jack Kevorkian is a personal friend of mine. All I have to do is spin twenty cents in that telephone and you are dead. (This was prior to Kevorkian's incarceration.) She said, "What's your hurry?"

The thing is, a less-skilled clinician might have felt she really wanted to kill herself, and yet when I pushed her to the wall (even with no apparent reason to me as an outsider why someone in her condition would want to live) there it was at the deep levels after her first two demands of me were to help her kill herself––when I pressed her to the limit, she wanted to live!

Further, a medical doctor not trained by such people as I was (Milton Erickson, Carl Whitaker, or Jim Simkin) with somewhat unusual and bizarre responses, might have felt they had made a "good faith effort" and think the woman actually wanted to commit suicide. Therefore, this small sample statistic of one on its face justifies the law being rather safe than sorry, as even the best clinicians cannot say for certain that they know a person wants out.

LEN BERANTINO, PH.D, ED.D., ABPP, was in the private practice of clinical psychology specializing in telephone psychotherapy or supervision. He is a diplomate of the American Board of Professional Psychology and a licensed psychologist in the states of Arizona, California, and Hawaii, and he can work with those who call from one of those three states or internationally (1)310-207-9397. He resides in West Los Angeles, California. In addition to being trained by Milton Erickson, M.D., and Carl Whitaker, M.D., and other world-renowned therapists, he has authored 80 publications and the book **Psychotherapy Insight and Style: The Existential Moment**, *1981, Allyn & Bacon, Boston.*

From Beverly Hills Psychologist-Psychoanalyst
TO PSYCHOLOGIST ACTIVIST
IN A STATE PRISON

By Len Bergantino, Ed.D., ABPP
Los Angeles, CA

I practiced psychoanalysis in Beverly Hills from 1979 through 1999 and found the work very interesting and personally rewarding. I retired fairly well off but lost 40% of the value of my annuities, so I found work as an independent contractor in a state prison. As much as I enjoyed my private practice, I never really got to use certain skills that I brought to my work with the prison inmates. I had trained with Milton Erickson and Carl Whitaker, two pioneers who helped me create a style of work that I referred to as "existential shift," where I had a chance to make a difference in a person's life each and every time I saw him, no matter how short the session.

I have always held the existential viewpoint that one's decisions in the world should be in good faith and that ethical decisions need to take into account a) oneself; b) significant others; and c) all other people in the world. My training analysis, with an analyst who was himself trained by Bion, gave me the strength to be "a solid rock of truth" in a system that hardly ever treats inmates in a humane way.

Bion once said that the entire psychoanalytic library was good for about the first hour and a half of an analysis, and that after that you needed to know what to say to the patient. It was like that, working in the prison.

I had about 100 inmates in my caseload in the Administrative Segregation section of the prison ("the hole"), which was reserved for "lifers," mostly men who were in for one or multiple murders. The state had decreed that 70% of the inmate population needed to be seen one time per week for a five minute session of psychotherapy or the prison would be closed down. Inmates did not want to be seen for five minutes of psychotherapy because they felt there was nothing in it for them. Further, they had to be brought from their cells in hand and leg chains and put in a cage (like Hannibal Lechter in the movie: The Silence of the Lambs) by two correctional officers. The inmates hated the chains and the cages.

My treatment approach was simple. I was straight with the inmates. I did not lie to them, because they could smell it a mile away. I was asked to do cell-to-cell canvassing to recruit inmates to attend sessions. One inmate asked me, "Why should I come out to see you for five minutes, to be dragged down in chains and put in a cage?" I was straight with him. I said, "Because I need a favor. If I don't get 70% of you guys to come out every week, they are going to fire me!" He shocked me when he replied, "You are a holy man! You can make a difference around here!"

My job was to keep inmates' spirits up and stop them from committing suicide, an understandable temptation when you are 30 years old and have two life sentences plus eighty years ahead of you. I used the psychoanalytic principle of maintaining a non-judgmental attitude of fairness toward the inmates, regardless of the crime they were in for. I treated them as tabula rasa, as if I knew nothing of their histories, nor did I really care; it had little to do with what I was hired to do.

A few clinical vignettes

A senior correction officer, one of the "good guys," said, "You'd better see Mr. Smith in Cell X; he tried to kill himself last night. They brought the man to the cage and he was drooling saliva, his head downcast; he looked totally dispirited. He had tattoos all over his body and rings coming out of his nose, bellybutton, ears, etc. He was a big, bulky tough guy you would not want pissed off at you. His projective identification, as received via my countertransference, showed me how to intervene. Looking at him in the most scolding way I could, I said, "What the fuck are you still doing here?" That pulled him out of his stupor, as what I said to him had been totally unexpected. "What do you mean? he asked. I responded, "I thought you would have escaped by now!" He beamed from ear to ear, having heard me tell him I had enough confidence in him that I believed he could escape from an impossible situation. All I needed was five minutes. One comment was the psychotherapy that day, and I reached him at a very deep level.

The administration never knew what I said to inmates in their sessions but in general they did not trust me as one of their own.

For group psychotherapy, six cages, one for each inmate, were arranged in a semicircle. Guys dressed like Darth Vader sporting black machine guns were on hand to monitor the session. Sometimes I found myself wondering, since all the inmates were locked up in cages, who were they planning to shoot? One little fellow seemed to have little contact with reality that day and shouted wildly at me, "What are you, one of those correction officers?" I had been taking notes throughout the session (mandatory in prison psychotherapy), and told him "I'll get to you next." Finishing my notes, I shouted at him, "What the fuck makes you think I am one of them?!" The inmate looked up at the guards and said to me, "I don't trust them." I leaned over and whispered to him through the cage, "I don't trust the sons of bitches myself." He trusted me implicitly after that session, and that one sentence laid the groundwork for the therapy that followed.

PUBLISHED IN SOUTHERN CALIFORNIA PSYCHIATRIST

VOL. 46 NO. 4, DECEMBER, 1997

<u>Guest Book Review</u>
by: Scott Carder, M.D.

Making an Impact in Therapy:
How Master Clinicians Intervene

by: Len Bergantino, Ed.D., Ph.D., ABPP. *The first soft cover edition was published in 1993 by Jason Aronson*

The book is a new release of a 1981 edition that was originally entitled, <u>Psychotherapy, Insight, and Style: The Existential Moment</u>. As a psychoanalyst I usually read and review almost exclusively psychoanalytic psychotherapy material. I was surprised to find my positive reaction to reading this "moveable feast" where Dr. Bergantino very openly and artistically describes his experiences with some of the top psychotherapists of different theoretical schools. The reader is first prepared to understand Dr. Bergantino's approach and purpose, and then accompanies him as he and sometimes his wife, My wife at the time, participate in a wide range of psychotherapy techniques. As an eclectic psychoanalyst, it was refreshing to read about the good learning experiences of Dr. Bergantino in other than psychoanalytic therapeutic modalities. My psychoanalytic work, especially my application of object relations theory, has been constructively enhanced by reading this text.

There are two sections to this book: the first relates the author's view of how he developed an existential perspective of psychotherapy and how he found the pursuit of emotionally impacting events which he calls "existential moments" as a foundation to effective process oriented psychotherapy. Part two is a detailed discussion of his exploration and understanding of different therapeutic experiences. It begins with his psychoanalytic exposure and continues through a wide range of transactional, gestalt, behavioral, somatic, hypnotic, confrontational, and family therapy experiences.

Only recently has the field of psychoanalysis discussed theoretical ideas concerning the intersubjective aspects of our work. This study of intersubjectivity more openly focuses on the influence of the psychoanalyst's beliefs and style on the treatment process. Over fifteen years ago, Dr. Bergantino made the attention to the therapist's style or his unique treatment enhancing qualities, the subject of this book. The author attempts to define and demonstrate existential moments that impact both patient and therapist. He also focuses on the liberation of the therapist: his effort to free himself to use the full range of his personality to constructively influence the patient.

The author's clear writing style makes it easy to understand the different therapeutic modalities and to experience the many clinical examples as if we were actual participants. The self-disclosure in the process of relating his efforts to become a more liberated therapist gives the book a real human feeling.

Of course from a psychoanalytic view, the best of the book is his fourth chapter, "Psychoanalysis and the Existential Moment" in which he describes his and other people's experiences with Wilfred Bion. It did appear to me that Dr. Bergantino, himself, had an unconscious idealizing transference to Dr. Bion since after only minimal personal contact he speaks in somewhat grand terms of the influence of Bion's personal presence. However, Dr. Bergantino was able to very clearly present a number of Bion's ideas such as the importance of language, of a clear mind, of a state of discovery, and of the ability to tolerate pain. In the subsequent pages, Dr. Bergantino marvelously edits material from several analysts who had intimate contact with Bion in Los Angeles. It was a special treat to read how psychoanalysts such as Richard Edeleman, James Grotstein, Lars Lofgren and Michael Paul experienced personal psychoanalysis and supervision from Bion.

Dr. Bergantino skillfully clarifies Bion's understanding of Melanie Klein's contributions. Using Dr. Grotstein's thinking on Bion and Klein, the author clarifies many good ideas that were Bion's particular focus as an extension of Klein's ideas. For instance: he explains Bion's "selected fact" concept; his use of deprivation and interpretation of projective identification in analysis to help the patient experience their own human richness; and Bion's emphasis on <u>attention</u> in the here and now of the analysis. I was especially appreciative of Dr. Bergantino's clarity in explaining many concepts of Bion's.

After this review of Bion's ideas, the reader is given a unique opportunity to experience the process of Bion's supervision of Stephen Salenger, M.D., who was at that time a clinical associate from the Los Angeles Psychoanalytic Institute. <u>It is the only published process material of Bion doing supervision</u>.

The remaining one third of this book has many refreshing comments as Dr. Bergantino relates his experiences with the styles of therapy of such non-analytic greats as: Albert Ellis on behavior modification, Milton Erickson on hypnotherapy, and Carl Whitaker on family interviewing. Dr. Bergantino looks for and underscores the existential moments as he saw and experienced them in his work with transactional analysis, analytic group therapy, Tavistock group experiences, Gestalt treatment, somatic therapy and direct confrontation of seriously disturbed psychotics. The book has many enlightening clinical examples, many of which are very personal as Dr. Bergantino and his wife My wife at the time traverse this therapeutic terrain.

I can heartily recommend this book as a learning experience to all psychotherapy clinicans and especially to psychoanalysts who would like a clear view of Wilfred Bion and his application of some of Melanie Klein's concepts.

5

Transactional Analysis and Existentialism with Bob Goulding, M.D. and Mary Goulding, M.S.W.

D R. ROBERT GOULDING, M.D., and Mary Goulding, M.S.W., are co-directors of the Western Institute for Group and Family Therapy in Mt. Madonna, Watsonville, CA. They teach members of the International Transactional Analysis Association and give workshops throughout the United States and in other parts of the world. They have authored two books: *The Power Is in the Patient* and *Changing Lives: The Power of Redecision Therapy.*

She was a gorgeous looking woman of five feet six inches, 130 pounds, with long blonde hair and a shape that would attract every man from New York to California. Her way of relating was as seductive as a kitten. But she had the venom of a sidewinder–particularly toward men. There were many affairs in her, a desperate search for meaning in life. And yet all she could muster up were hysterical tears which came like the turning on of a fire hose, even for insignificant reasons. I tried the two-chair technique of gestalt therapy, having her be the seductive little girl talking to her latest boyfriend. She would only break out in more tears. The difficulty was that she couldn't tell when she was being an adult and when she was being a seductive little girl–she mixed both into the same process without knowing it. Furthermore, any awareness I facilitated was only internalized by her, which made her feel worse.

I told her I felt the best way to approach the problem was transactional analysis, and in particular, work that would help her separate ego states. That is, her parent, adult, and child parts of her personality. Each of these conceptualizations called ego states had a particular set of thoughts and feelings that accompany them.

I asked her to use three chairs instead of two. I asked her to sit in one chair each time she was ending parent messages. A second chair was for her adult ego state, which I described to her as giving straight information. A third chair was for when she was feeling like a child.

She was in tears and sat in the child chair. I said that if she was crying she must be telling the child something that would make her feel bad. I asked her to sit in the parent chair. She then told the child, "You are inadequate. You are not measuring up to . . ." I asked her to switch chairs back to the child. She began to cry hysterically. I asked her why she was crying. She said because the parent was correct; she was inadequate. I said, "So you are going to buy that bullshit so easily?" She insisted it was true. I asked her if it was her mom or her dad that was saying that to her. She said it was her mom. I had a hunch that the injunction she was giving herself was "don't grow up." She said, from the child chair, that it was true. She got into the parent chair and said, "I don't want you to grow up. I need you to be inadequate so I will have a purpose in life." The child responded by saying "Yes. You're right" (in a sickeningly compliant sugar sweet voice). The child again gave no fight at all and was in full agreement with the parental message. I asked her if she could remember feeling that way when she was very young, perhaps five years old. She said that she could never remember feeling any other way, and described an early scene where her mother gave her the message that she was inadequate and she crumbled to tears within a moment. She remembered deciding that she had no choice but to live her life that way, because she also needed her mother's love and protection. The five-year old child did the only thing she could do to survive. The question now became, "Do you think this decision still fits for you today?" The answer was an emphatic no. I told her to get into the child chair and to tell her mother what she was going to do in the present. My question was ambiguous enough so that she switched into her adult ego state and gave a response that she was going to decide to grow up and to live her life as a woman. However, I did not feel any conviction in her words. I asked, "What's in it for you? What's in it for the happy child in you?" Then she began to get in touch with the desire to live that she had buried deep inside of her. She told her mother, "No, I'm not going to go along with this bullshit anymore. I'm tired of protecting you. I feel bad that you don't have a reason to live. But, I'm going to live as a woman. I am adequate. In fact, I am the most adequate person among the group that I belong to." As she went on she felt more and more confident about herself, and her feelings, and she was no longer breaking into crying jags. I knew she felt the redecision in her guts, that she made the decision to grow up and disobey the parental injunction, feeling the full desire of the opportunities that she could have from making such a choice. Romance in her life. Children. Love. Affection. Meaningful sex. She realized her feeling of competency, which she had previously refused to acknowledge or utilize. I then asked her to get into the adult chair and give me a computer readout on what had just happened. She was very clear. She did not return to a contaminated little-girl voice while thinking she was an adult. She experienced a feeling of potency in being able to control her responses in the adult chair while feeling the joy of life in the child chair, and when the session ended she felt like dynamite! These moments were existential moments that I could not have reached without the following background and working knowledge of transactional analysis.

Before training in transactional analysis I had several years experience with a humanistic existential approach to psychotherapy that included one and a half years of gestalt therapy training. While both the existential and gestalt approaches were relatively free-floating and almost theory-less in terms of practice, the transactional analysis approach is very heavy in theory and foundation. Learning this modality was somewhat difficult for me because my natural inclinations were to respond moment to moment and not be too concerned about theory. However, I believe that the existential approach and gestalt therapy can be bolstered by the solid theory of transactional analysis as it is applied to the practice of psychotherapy. For that reason I studied transactional analysis and became a clinical member in the International Transactional Analysis Association. While this chapter certainly is not meant to be a comprehensive presentation of Transactional Analysis theory as applied to an existential framework of psychotherapy, its purpose is to show how Transactional Analysis theory does fit into an open-ended, existential way of doing therapy and can be quite useful in helping therapists to become well-balanced, so they know *what* they are doing, besides being able to do it. Otherwise, existential therapists may be stuck with learning the art of intuition without a solid theoretical base from which this intuitive response takes place. TA provides the map that accompanies the territory.

While reading the TA journals, bulletins, and books, I had the impression that Eric Berne had taken his psychoanalytic background and put it into manageable terms. He was both rejected and inspired in his development of transactional analysis by his psychoanalytic peers who looked upon him with disdain for his breach with the "true faith." Yet a psychoanalytic and objective rational foundation is quite obvious throughout transactional analysis literature. While attending a one-week workshop with Dr. Bob Goulding and Mary Goulding, I saw how they integrated transactional analysis with gestalt therapy and came out with a lively, responsive, and enjoyable therapy that certainly was existential in focus because of its here-and-now orientation. (While they are excellent psychotherapists who could supervise people in many therapeutic modalities, the Gouldings are primarily known as transactional analysts.) In addition, many existential moments occurred in their transactional analysis therapy.

When Eric Berne wrote of existential and transactional analysis he said, "Insofar as actual living in the world is concerned, transactional analysis shares with existential analysis a high esteem for, and a keen interest in, the personal qualities of honesty, integrity, autonomy, and authenticity, and their most poignant social manifestations in encounter and intimacy."[1] The addition of transactional analysis to the existential camp meant that therapists, and especially young therapists who are learning their trade, could have a better grasp of the overall picture, and could have a consistent direction to which the moment-to-moment existential responses might flow. Otherwise, existential therapies may certainly provide healing moments and authentic relationships, but may not help patients achieve meaningful goals, at least those patients who could not initially withstand the existential anxiety of open-ended therapy.

Transactional Analysis has diagnosis, a treatment plan, and a clear direction as part of its process. There is a focus on contracts. While gestalt therapists also use contracts in that they ask people what they want for themselves, they are nowhere near as specific as TA therapists in providing a contract that may cover the scope of the entire therapy. While the existentialist-gestaltist may be quite content to go with what develops and to amplify what develops in an experiential sense, TA therapists provide a concrete framework from which unsophisticated patients find it much easier to begin therapy. For example, patients may be expected to assume responsibility for themselves in the form of the following kind of contract.

1. What do you want to change about yourself?
2. What will you do to bring about the change you want in yourself?
3. What behaviors do you now engage in that might prevent you from bringing about the change you want in yourself?
4. In behavioral-measurable terms, how will other people know you have changed?

Two kinds of contracts are possible, social control contracts and autonomy contracts. Dr. Bill Holloway, a transactional-analysis therapist, describes social control contracts as

> those that have as an end point some change in behavior, attitude or feeling, whereby the patient makes a more effective social adaptation to his world. For example, "To stop being angry at my wife," "to stop drinking," etc. All of these may represent significant change for the individual and in that sense are meaningful and valid goals in treatment.[2] Holloway commented that the types of therapeutic intervention in social control contracts were interventions whereby the therapist gave the client permission "to stop drinking," or "to stop being angry at

his wife." He differentiates the limits of the permission intervention when compared to autonomy.

In talking in terms of cure through TA, the cure being the completion of a contract, we must also look at the other type of contract, the autonomy contract. Holloway defines autonomy as

> the ultimate individuation and implies that the person is capable of the full use of options in attaining strokes from multitudinous others and that specifically excluded is the option of a single fixed dependent relationship (including a fantasied dependency). Dependency is considered antagonistic to autonomy, since ongoing dependency, especially beyond childhood, is only granted in exchange for obligation. Obligation is accompanied by resentment and resentment prevents intimacy. Autonomous functioning, therefore, is the condition which permits of intimacy while ongoing dependency precludes intimacy between adults.[3]More specifically, Bob Goulding says he asks the

> patient what he wants to achieve now, or today, or this week, or in the next eight weeks. Then we look for the Injunction, the script or first act, the early decision, the games, and the rackets–in short, we look for all the ways in which the patient denies his autonomy.[4]So the therapeutic work then becomes providing an environment for redecision whereby the patient can "feel the change in his guts, feel the flood of relief of having made a real decision to grow, or play, or live."[5]While existential therapies such as gestalt and humanistic existential therapy are not concerned with diagnosis or a medical model framework, Transactional Analysis is concerned with diagnosis. However, there is a clear distinction between TA diagnosis and the traditional diagnostic classifications in the *Diagnostic and Statistical Manual of Mental Disorders of the American Psychiatric Association.* Bill Holloway puts it well when he says,

. . . Berne's model is a decisional one–not a disease model. In this sense, it has the appeal of the whole humanistic approach, i.e., it is based in, appeals to, and builds on the health, strength, or inherent worth of the individual and does not seek to find what is 'wrong' with him. Additionally, the patient rather soon senses the self-mastery which is available.[6]In this context treatment becomes a decisional process. Based upon what patients are willing to do, the contract is made, providing a clear direction or treatment plan for therapists. Cure is thought to be the completion of the contract. There is a responsibility for both therapists and patients living up to their part of the contracts. New contracts can be renegotiated upon the completion of social control contracts once patients have removed themselves from crisis situations and are interested in pursuing autonomy contracts.

Before describing TA any further, I must tackle one of the initially awesome problems with TA–the definitions. While the general public usually gets a superficial exposure to TA definitions that at times have a cute and catchy ring to them, don't let this be misleading. I at one time was dismissing TA as something I couldn't take seriously because it had so aggressively marketed itself. About all I knew was the TA book, *I'm OK, You're OK*, and the terms "Parent-Adult-Child" ego states, and that supposedly the entire therapy was built on three circles. What I was to later find out was that TA had an awesome amount of terms and the scope of the therapy was comprehensive. However, for purposes of this chapter I am only going to present a few definitions.

Strokes are units of recognition and can be either positive or negative. For example, "I like you" is a positive stroke.

Injunctions are parental prohibitions or negative commands that a person has accepted. Bob and Mary Goulding list the specific injunctions as, "Don't be: Don't be you (the sex you are); Don't be a child; Don't grow; Don't succeed; Don't be important; Don't be close; Don't belong; Don't be well (or sane); Don't think (don't think about X–forbidden subject); Don't think what you think, think what I think; Don't feel (don't feel X–mad, sad, glad, etc.); Don't feel what you feel, feel what I feel."[7] These injunctions were given to people when they were children, at which time they made decisions about how they were going to live their lives based on the injunction or injunctions. When a therapist provides an environment for redecision the patient has an opportunity to see what fits in terms of current reality, and decides both at a cognitive and emotional level to choose options that are now in the patient's best interests.

Script is "a life plan based on a decision made in childhood, reinforced by parents, justified by subsequent events, and culminating in a chosen alternative; the script determines the person's ultimate outcome; a decision made by the child between his own autonomous needs and the expectation of his parents and the injunctions he encounters in his primary family group."[8] Thus the analysis of script becomes the analysis of these life dramas that people unconsciously play out.

Adapted Child Ego State is composed of (a) Child-feelings that are rebellious to authority and parental ego state. The feeling is freedom, although the rebellious child does not realize rebellion is only another form of adaptation; an archaic ego state. (b) Compliant child-this archaic ego state is also under the influence of the Parent ego state. It elicits responses that are most likely to draw the best responses from others. (c) "The Little Professor," or intuition, figures things out.

Free Child Ego State (Natural Child) is the part of each person that is childlike, in spontaneity, joy, and abandonment.

Nurturing Parent Ego State is the part of the Parent ego state that gives strokes for being oneself. It is protective.

Critical Parent Ego State is the part of the Parent ego state that is controlling, prohibitive, and may have non-rational attitudes.

Adult Ego State is "an ego state adapted to current reality and not affected by parental prejudices or archaic attitudes left over from childhood structure; an aspect of the personality which is primarily engaged in objective data processing and computing probabilities."[9] *Life Positions* is a "basic existential position arrived at by age seven; the four life positions are: I'm OK–You're OK; I'm OK–You're Not OK; I'm Not OK–You're OK; I'm Not OK–You're Not OK."[10] Corresponding to these positions are slogans regarding relationships. I'm OK, You're OK leads to people developing fruitful relationships. I'm OK, You're Not OK leads to relationships in which one person is 'getting rid of,' as in divorcing, the other and is usually accompanied by anger. I'm Not OK, You Are OK leads to relationships in which one person is 'withdrawing from' the other and is usually accompanied by a depression. I'm Not OK, You're Not OK describes a relationship position that is going nowhere.

Transactional Analysis is a theory of personality and social action; a clinical method of psychotherapy based on the analysis of all possible transactions between two or more people, on the basis of specifically defined ego states."[11] *Structural Analysis* is the analysis of the ego states of a patient (Parent, Adult, Child) and their relationships to each other along with the analysis of the properties that compose the ego states.

Passivity is "the syndrome manifested by the four behaviors Doing Nothing, Over-adaptation, Agitation, and Violence"[12] or incapacitation. These behaviors are in opposition to the active behaviors of thinking, feeling, and acting autonomously.

Game theory (Schiff) is the "theory that all games develop out of unresolved symbiotic relationships with discounting as the mechanism and grandiosity as the justification. There are four possible ways to discount: (1) discount the problem; (2) discount the significance of the problem; (3) discount the solvability of the problem; (4) discount the person."[13] When patients are confronted with their discounts, they begin to establish goals, make a plan for how to reach these goals, think about their actions, and then *do* what they need to *do*.

Contamination is "the intrusion of the Parent and/or the Child ego state in the boundary of the Adult ego state."[14] *Decontamination* is ". . . realignment of ego states."[15] *Exclusion* is ". . . rigidity in one ego state."[16] *Counterscript Drivers* are the five behaviors that people manifest in a driven and compulsive way to accommodate others, e.g., "Try Hard," "Be Perfect," "Hurry Up," "Please Me," and "Be Strong."[17] *Ego States* are "coherent systems of thought and feeling manifested by corresponding patterns of behavior."[18] *Discounting* is "the functional manifestation of either a contamination or an exclusion. The person who discounts believes, or acts as though he believes, that his feelings about what someone else has said, done, or felt, are more significant than what that person actually said, did or felt. He does not use information relevant to a situation."[19] Schiff and Schiff "bypass analyzing games by confronting the discount, which is identifiable as the initial unstraight transaction and is the point at which the patient's Adult ceases to be aware of what is happening. Recathecting the Adult in this transaction effectively stops the game at a time when the patient is in touch with the feeling motivating the behavior."[20] To recathect the Adult means to intervene in a way that facilitates the patient's use of the Adult ego state.

Game is "a series of transactions that ends in at least one player feeling badly or being injured in some way. The game begins with an ostensibly straight stimulus. However, this stimulus also includes a secret or covert message. This secret message is responded to in an overt fashion. At the end of the game, the player experiences a payoff–he is unhappy or hurt. The entire series of transactions is not within his Adult awareness."[21]

Racket is an inauthentic feeling that is repetitively used to cover an authentic feeling. For example, a patient who is repetitively angry, and drives others away with this anger, also uses the anger to cover sadness.

The First Act Experience, as defined by Bob Goulding: "To review, then, the individual gets an Injunction from his parent, which is implanted by strokes (which may be positive or negative, conditional or unconditional), makes a Decision around the Injunction, and then develops a script to support the Injunction. Sometimes, however, the child has some kind of first act experience, in the course of which he develops some bad feelings from the strokes he gets and the things that happen to him, but also gets some satisfaction from the strokes, and often, when young, some kind of reward for his bad feelings. . . . When it occurs, it is this first act experience which sets the pattern for the feelings and modes of behavior that the child retains until (and if) he decides to change)."[22]

While the TA definitions are tedious, they are a base from which therapists may begin to think about patients. While existential therapies are concerned with the territory of *being* and *staying*, and gestaltists are concerned with the amplification of human experience, TA theory provides a framework for the exploration of the territory. Perhaps the best way to begin to provide an overall picture is to discuss what was required in preparing for the clinical exam.

When preparing for the clinical examination (1976 standards) of the International Transactional Analysis Association, the examiners concerned themselves with several issues that fall under two basic categories:

1. *Competence:* Examinees will demonstrate their ability to integrate theory into clinical practice.
    A. Does the examinee have a theory (primary TA) explaining what he/she is doing? Does the examinee understand how theoretical concepts (structural analysis, transactional analysis, game and racket analysis, script analysis, etc.) are manifested in the client's life?
    B. Does the examinee have a direction in therapy, i.e., how to arrive at goals and contract of the treatment?
    C. Does the examinee have awareness of the various approaches in and branches of TA: significance, methods and options?
    D. Does the examinee have awareness of discounts and response to them; uncovering and confronting incongruities; does the examinee support scripty issues and pathology?
    E. Does the examinee demonstrate that he/she is crisp and clear in assessing and managing clinical work?

II *Judgment*

    A. Does the examinee show a lack of significant harmful interventions?
    B. Does the examinee demonstrate significant helpful interventions?
    C. Does the examinee demonstrate significant potency?
    D. Does the examinee demonstrate intuition (an awareness of what's going on in the client) and creativity?
    E. Does the examinee demonstrate a firm ethical foundation?[23]

This examination was the culmination of about two thousand hours of preparation in terms of classwork as well as TA therapy, workshops, and clinical supervision from TA therapists. Having previously been trained in existential therapy and gestalt therapy I found there were a few areas that gave me particular difficulty.

First, TA therapy was comprehensive in scope. I had never been trained to look at a patient in such a comprehensive way–and in fact, had been trained that such comprehensive objectification of a patient was counterproductive to the subject-to-subject healing that is at the heart of existential therapy. Second, while I would intuitively and/or by moment to moment observation pick up what patients were doing and how they were doing it, I saw no particular value to having these patterns of behavior at my disposal from the beginning of therapy; I dealt with them when they came up. Third, except for session-to-session gestalt contract work, I had no particular interest in therapeutic outcome other than the responsible involvement of patient and therapist in the pursuit of an authentic relationship. Fourth, this meant that I had never concerned myself with an overall direction in therapy other than the pursuit of purer states of being, and therefore a treatment plan had been meaningless. Any goals and contracts of therapy had always come up session by session at the patient's request. In this sense all of the existential therapies of which I am writing lacked a continuity, which in my belief could make a significant impact with certain patients getting what they want for themselves over the course of therapy. The issues mentioned in preparation for the TA clinical examination write the probability of successful therapy right into the contract–and in a sense therapists need to have far less skill before they can begin to effect meaningful change in the lives of patients than existential therapists who depend more fully on the art of intuitive responding. This is not to say that TA therapists do not have to be skillful therapists, but that the structure provided by TA theory and its application to clinical practice makes the transition of becoming a competent therapist more likely since the map is drawn. Beginning therapists can be successful by filling in the blanks until they become more experienced. TA structure also makes it easier to work with a wide variety of patients who might find the demands of other existentially-oriented therapies a bit too open-ended. TA structure is relatively non-threatening since patients make contracts based upon their goals, and a nurturing parent ego state is written right into the contract from the start. That is, in patients are getting well when their Adult, Nurturing Parent and Free Child ego states become strong enough to counterbalance the heavy Critical

Parent tapes that leave patients responding as either Compliant or Rebellious Children, not really knowing the meaning of autonomy or freedom. The heavy confrontation due to assumption of responsibility did not seem as harsh in TA therapy as it did in my prior existential and gestalt training. The focus on Nurturing Parent, Free Child, and Adult ego states made therapy seem relatively safe for those patients who felt weak to begin with.

This did not mean there was a lack of focus, however. With a contract, there was a focus on movement in the therapy, movement in the direction of the contract. The focus on movement was often pursued by a focus on discounts of patients and therapeutic response to the discounts. (Discounts are ways that patients discount themselves, the problem, others, the seriousness of the problem and the solvability of the problem.) There is more of a focus on a problem than in existential therapies where the generic problem is the authenticity of the patient. Yet I found that existentially I would more naturally concern myself with the way patients interpersonally discounted. In this way TA and existentialism are congruent in terms of the pursuit of an authentic relationship. A keen focus on discounts made the therapy work crisper. That is, there is a sense of solid movement, direction, and clarity.

There was a step-by-step movement. Each discount was confronted. During tape supervision the movement, and the increasing crispness of the work became more apparent. TA theory was useful in my learning to refuse to support scripty issues because patterns, games, and rackets were imbedded in my head from my initial diagnostic procedure. Thus, I had both my experience and my cognitive knowledge to draw upon when doing therapy. It's OK to be experiential. It's OK to be cognitive. It's OK to pursue therapy with a balanced approach that gives therapists options to accomplish tasks. The crisper the work became, the more potent I felt as a therapist, which increased patients' confidence. Intuition and creativity were a natural part of my working style and just complimented the cognitive, structured aspects of TA.

Perhaps the case of Joan (recorded on an audio tape presentation similar to that required by the International Transactional Analysis Association at a clinical examination) would be helpful in demonstrating how an overall picture of a patient may look in TA terms.

CASE OF JOAN

Joan was a thirty-year old divorced woman who was a clinical social worker in a large metropolitan hospital. She was very conscientious about her work, to the exclusion of much else that might have been her life. Although she was intelligent, her eyes were dull. Life appeared to be a drag for her. She dressed shabbily, and from her appearance, sex would be the last thing on her mind. She was depressed much of the time.

Her overall contract in therapy was an autonomy contract–to feel good about herself and to learn to be happy. This meant that part of her therapy would be to learn how to choose options that would let her experience joy instead of her chronic bad feeling which perpetuated script behavior. She maintained a life position of I'm NOT OK, You're OK, and generally had a desire to withdraw from people. Her life position and withdrawing behavior also needed to be dealt with as part of her contract.

Her contract for this particular session was to learn how to handle her feelings regarding a patient with whom she was working. The short-range treatment plan was to help Joan deal with her depression by staying in the present. She laughed when I snapped my fingers each time she drifted away. This was a playful way of creating an existential moment between us that helped Joan leave her obsessional and depressive thinking and enjoy living.

A second direction of the session came in the area of structural analysis. I was dealing with a contamination that existed between Joan's Parent ego state and her Adult ego state. Joan thought she was giving clear information but did not realize she had both a critical tone and choice of words that were contaminating her information. When turned inwards, this is one way a Critical Parent ego state is used for self-torture. Ego state separation was accomplished by having Joan use a Parent chair and talk to the adult chair, switching back and forth until she was able to take control over the contamination. Such control gives a patient the freedom to choose new options in responding. (Sometimes such ego state separation can be done with five chairs–Critical Parent, Nurturing Parent, Adult, Rebellious Child and Compliant Child.) The object of the treatment was accomplished because Joan acknowledged that she had control over producing depressed feelings or good feelings, and that she was able to separate her Adult ego state from her Critical

Parent ego state–thereby freeing herself to allow her more opportunities for her Free Child ego state to experience joy.

Looking at Joan's long-range treatment plan–that of providing an environment whereby Joan would have the opportunity to make a new decision to live autonomously–several factors must be considered.

Joan's pattern of behavior was depressing herself over and over (script pattern). When observing her moment-to-moment behavior she tried hard, geared her responses to please others, and although she attempted to have fun for awhile, was saddled with the feeling that she should not have too much fun! Joan reported that she decided on this life course when she was three years old. She said she was riding along with her father in the car. She wanted to kiss him. For reasons only known to him at that time, he said no. She decided that she was not OK, that she had to try hard, to please others, and that it was not all right to have fun, and that she would live her life that way. This early scene, whether it was the actual decision point or not, provided the basis for redecision work so Joan could live her life based on present-day reality. She did not have to live forever with the life position she was maintaining–I'm Not OK, You ARE OK.

The parental injunctions that were most prevalent–"Don't be a child" and "Don't make it" explained Joan's fear about having fun and about being successful in her work. Success can oftentimes be alarming to the Parent ego state of the professional. The program that Joan kept responding to was "keep thinking about all the bad things that will keep you depressed." Her basic game was, "I'm Only Trying to Help You," in which she switched from rescuer to victim while working with her patient. The thesis of her game was that her patient wasn't doing what she told him to do and the aim of her game was the alleviation of her own guilt. Thus, while Joan was trying to prove how adequate she was, the Child ego state of her patient responded by saying, "I will make you feel inadequate." The dynamics of Joan's game are masochistic, since she suffers feelings of inadequacy. Joan's existential position was that all people were ungrateful. She certainly experienced her patient as ungrateful, and yet, another advantage of her game was to avoid dealing with her own inadequacies. The antithesis to Joan's game was for her to learn to get loving strokes, while avoiding the game. While "I'm Only Trying to Help You" is one of the games described by Eric Berne,[24] I find it easier to pick up a game by thinking of whether a patient is engaging in rescuing, persecuting, or victim behavior. Any of those behaviors can be switched, by the patient, as switched from rescuer to victim. This idea was originated by Dr. Stephen Karpman and is referred to as "The Drama Triangle."[25]

When viewing Joan in terms of her passive behavior, we see she was engaging in over-adaption, trying hard to further the symbiosis between herself and the patient. Behaviorally she was discounting or minimizing the solvability of the problem as well as her own ability of solving the problem. Functionally, her role was that of caretaker, in that she was playing "I'm only trying to help you" whether the patient needed it or not. Structurally she pursued a symbiotic relationship in which she discounted her Child ego state needs and feelings. Her symbiosis left her dependent in relationships. Her games were an attempt to get back to the original symbiosis. She chose passivity instead of solving problems. This was done by discounting the solvability of the problem and Joan's ability to solve it. Grandiosity was her justification. With her "please me" driver she responded to her interpretation of others expectations. She redefined by discounting, grandiosity, and overdetailing. Her racket feeling was depression.

I have presented you only a part of the TA comprehensive system—enough to give you an idea of how Transactional Analysis provides a map for therapists to explore the *territory* with patients, either through TA or other therapies. This map is very important in helping therapists reach existential moments with patients because it provides a preface to experience. Therapists' creativity and intuition will always be a part of the therapeutic process, but having a structure can certainly help therapists confront patients in ways that will lead to ever-increasing responsibility, authenticity, autonomy, and the existential moments that are at the heart of healing relationships.

Two of the finest TA-oriented therapists that I have experienced have been Bob and Mary Goulding, in a one-week workshop. I am going to include some work they did with me so I can show how and where existential moments made a difference in their work.

Me	What I want to do is claim the passive part of myself. I understand it intellectually, but emotionally I can't experience myself that way.

Bob   Describe yourself as passive.

Me   Stubborn, resistant, refusing to move where I could make my life a lot more interesting if I did.

Mary   That's not what most think is passive. Resistant rather than passive.

Me   OK. I'm not sure I see the difference.

Mary   What you are describing involves a lot of activity.

Me   I was thinking about a particular kind of patient that I have trouble working with. A kind of person who won't do anything. However, I can sense that it's not all them and I am not sure about what part of me gets in the way.

Mary   What is your contract? What are you going to change about yourself so you won't be in danger of anyone thinking you're that kind of patient! (Entire group laughs)

Mary confronted my behavior by being playful and somewhat provocative, but with a warm look on her face that let me know I was among friends. I felt touched by her at the same time I was being confronted. This was an existential moment that I remembered, and one of the moments that made a difference in the work–its impact made a lasting impression.

Me   (somewhat embarrassed) I'm really resistant to change.

Mary   God knows, you're not one of those patients! (Playfully)

Me   I really want to sit here and give you a bad time. That's where I stop. There's nothing else I want to do.

Bob   Say that to your father what you just said to Mary.

Bob's comment takes the work back to an early scene. I could visualize being in the backyard with the lawnmower.

Me   Dad, I really want to give you a bad time. You're such a pain in the ass. You're always hounding me. Do this. Do that. When I mow the lawn you say I missed a spot. You're a haunt. Just leave me alone.

(It became clear to me that this struggle was going on with me, both the haunter and the haunted.)

Mary   I think you really did a nice job getting your doctorate and your TA clinical membership and the other things you have done in spite of that tape going on in your head. You did it.

(Mary's comment helped me acknowledge my power; I had succeeded, despite the resistant tapes.)

Me   I did it. It was murder.

Bob   Nobody got killed by it. You said it was murder. Tell your father that you did it. (Between Bob and Mary hardly a discount goes by unnoticed.)

Me   I had all this shit going on and I did it. I did what I needed to do in spite of your baloney and I did it my way. I'm feeling powerful.

Bob   Good.

Me   I'm only passive when it doesn't hurt me. I can be pretty tricky in how I want to be passive. (I am now owning my power in taking responsibility for when I am passive instead of playing the victim of my passivity–a step toward autonomous behavior.)

Mary   *My guess is the reason you have problems with passive/ aggressive patients is that your Parent ego state wants to get on their case the same way your father got on yours.*

While I had owned my power in the previous comment, I was also being tricky by sidestepping the primary issue I wanted to work on–my passivity in relation to resistant patients.

Bob   You started off by saying what you want to do is find your passivity.

Mary   You claim that you are very picky with your passivity and can hurt yourself.

Me   Yeah. Like if I say no and I'm tricky about how I do it and can really keep you two working.

Mary   No you can't.

Me   When you said what you said before that, my head went blank. I blanked everything I had experienced. Now that I just said that, I don't know if I'm being tricky or if the trick gets played on me, because I don't remember.

What I had just done with Mary and Bob could have discounted the entire piece of work and removed it from my experience, or I could have profited from the work while somehow discounting them, putting them down, and making the work less powerful so I would still remain in control–as evidenced by my statement that I could still keep them working. Mary's next comment was an absolute stroke of genius, for she completed the work and I got the message. We felt an existential moment occurring, and there was a mutual respect between us.

Mary	I think you remember. I think you remember what you did in the last few minutes. And besides that you brought a tape recorder so it doesn't matter whether you remember or not. You can hear it again.

Although I hate to admit this I had been at my most stubborn worst to work with as a patient and I had been effectively therapized in a playful and loving way where I had experienced an early scene, owned my power, made a redecision about using my power as a result of this work, and had fun while doing it. This is TA therapy at its best.

I can't ever remember feeling as if my entire body was on a dime. I was frustrated, dumbfounded. I didn't know what to say. The entire group laughed again. I let go of the control–as if I had a choice at this point!

Me	(Tipping a cap I was wearing during the session) You're trickier than I am!

The last interchange between Mary and myself was an existential moment that captured the reality of two people being with each other in a real, loving, warm, and playful way. Bob, Mary, and myself were master duellers, and I could only say touché! at being taken on my own terms.

A few other things stick in my memory from the week I spent with the Gouldings. Script issues did not pass without being confronted. When the workshop first began people were introducing themselves. I said my name in a low voice. People repeated what they thought I had said: Lon, Lan, Glenn, etc. I said, "It looks like I can get a lot of attention by mumbling around here." Mary rebutted, "If that's how you want to spend your time!" I felt like I had been hit with a sledgehammer. There were a few more instances like this, but by the end of the week I knew the difference between real belly laughter and gallows humor that sucked others into reinforcing my self-destructive behavior. Also Bob's comment during the work, "Nobody was killed by it. You said it was murder." I can't even recall how many times Bob stunned me by cutting into overdramatized scripty comments such as, "It was murder!"

Bob and Mary usually worked between ten to twenty minutes with a person. They confronted the discounts. The work was crisp. People made redecisions and felt good in their guts while also being able to redecide cognitively. The work was powerful. Throughout the work, existential moments were abundant!

TA MARITAL THERAPY WITH BOB AND MARY

Some three years after my initial work with the Gouldings my wife and I went to a three-day weekend workshop. While marital therapy has always been one of my primary therapeutic interests, I had primarily viewed it from an interactional perspective. What I found to be unique was the focus Bob and Mary took when doing marital therapy. Essentially, they would do a brief check with each partner to see what they wanted for themselves, and then from each other. The focus was then on individual therapy in front of the spouse and in front of a group. Each spouse would have an opportunity to work through his or her own difficulties that might have previously been inappropriately laid at the door-step of the other spouse. The spouse watching would feel a sense of freedom and relief to know what belonged to whom. It became very clear what steps needed to be taken to break the game that existed between partners. The new behavior would usually be worked out using the empty chair, or by other individual therapy methods, before the couple would interact at the end of the work as a final check to see if all were well. Some of the following dialogue will demonstrate TA marital therapy done by the Gouldings, with my wife at the time, and myself. The statements in italics are what I experienced as bullseye remarks that left us more liberated.

Mary asked me what I wanted for myself. I said I wanted to have more fun.

Mary   Test out, "How do I get in the way of my having fun?"

Me   I worry a lot. I worry about the future, and I think about what didn't go right in the past.

Bob began dealing with the split in me. One side wanted to put out more instead of laying back and waiting. The other side was cautious, feeling that the first side was a person who would leap off into anything, and that needed to be watched. The first side responded to the second by saying, "I feel that way because you keep such tight wraps on me. I feel like I want to leap out of my skin. Like I want to explode." The second side then cautioned, "You better be careful. You'll get in trouble like that." Bob asked if any of that sounded familiar to me. It did. I remember messages from my father that were telling me to be cautious.

Mary then brought it between my wife at the time and me by saying, "So what do you two do for fun?"

Me	I have the most fun with you, when you break up my obsessions with your humor; when you spoof this trip I go on.
My wife at the time	You think your boredom with stuff falls into that also?
Bob (To my wife at the time)	You think so?
My wife at the time	We went to a concert last weekend and left in the middle. Len was bored and I didn't want him to sit in the car by himself, so I left.
Mary (To my wife at the time)	*I'm hoping the contract for you is that you can do what you want no matter how bored he is.*
Mary (To me)	What's the kind of fun you want?
Me	A freedom or happiness in responding to life in a here-and-now way.
Bob (To me)	Get an image.
Me	I'm talking to people and I'm just really loose and saying some hot things.

Mary (To me)	How's your breathing? (Mary knew that I was adept at monitoring my tension through awareness of my breathing.)
Me	Feels a little looser right now. I'm breathing easy and my body feels much, much looser. I feel freer to move and less constrained.

Later in the work Mary said she was wondering aloud *"How you'll do with a wife who isn't guilty and who's willing to stay through a conflict, a concert, while you sulk in the car."*

As something was bothering me about my wife at the time, I turned and said to her, "I wonder where you're at with your 'don't grow up' situation."

Mary (To me)	*Oh, goodness gracious. Why don't you tell her what it is you want or don't want and not psyche it.*
Me (To my wife at the time)	I want you to relate to me as an adult more often. I have a lot of fun relating to you as a little kid but I would like to experience you in other ways, too.
Mary (To me)	Could you give her a for instance? Is that okay with you, to hear a for instance?
My wife at the time	Yes.
Me (To my wifeat the time)	You will say something to me where I feel that what you want to do is get my approval or impress me. Then I feel like I'm in the role of big daddy and I want to go away at those times.
Mary	That's not an example because the something isn't clear, but do you want to respond anyway? (to my wife at the time)
My wife at the time	I need approval sometimes, and I like to get approval from you.

Bob (To my wife at the time)	*You want to say, "I want approval rather than I need it?" You really don't need it, maybe you want it.*
My wife at the time	I want approval. I'd like to hear someone else say, yes, you're great. I don't need it all the time but I like to hear it sometimes.
Me	Most of the time it occurs to me that you're great when–
My wife at the time	When I don't need it.
Me	When that kind of situation doesn't happen.
Mary	Could you give an example, one of you?
Me	My wife's driving the car. My wife is telling me some story. I can't remember what–about, teaching, teaching her class a certain way in school. While in the content of the story she does a nice job with the teaching or how she reaches the kids, there is a message that comes across to me–"Oh, look what an important person I am and look how foolish these other people are." Then I feel, uggh. I feel almost frozen and am not quite sure what the hell to do.
Bob	*You want to stop feeling frozen when she brags. This is your side of the contract, not hers.*
Me	She's not bragging about it. (Denial by switching the issue)
Mary	Or whatever the hell it is that she's doing, you want to stop freezing yourself.

Me   I want to not hook into certain behaviors or things she does.

Mary   Stay at this scene. There she is telling you a story that proves she did a good job with the kids. What are you saying inside your head to get you to freeze up?

Me   She needs to feel good about herself right now and by telling me this story, she is feeling better about herself.

Mary   And what do you say in your head to freeze up?

Me   On the other hand she is coming from an adapted child position. I don't know quite what to say or do. I just feel quite uncomfortable. So I think the best thing for me to do is nothing; then I space out.

Bob   *You freeze up and she misses her stroke.*

Mary   *And when you were six years old,* (referring to the early scene that I have been reliving with her) *how did you space out when you didn't know exactly how to please your mother?*

Me   I felt obligated with her. I'm supposed to make her happy.

Mary   Would you tell her (mother) what you mean while she is living her life and you are six years old?

Me   You are living your life depending on me for all your happiness.

Mary   So at 3, 4, or 5 you were working on making her happy and it wasn't working. Can you feel your stomach crunch?

Me   Yes.

Mary   If you didn't freeze up and be silent what would you do?

Me   Either way I'm caught. I'm either going around being pissed at you or freezing up. I would just as soon not do either, but be able to stay in a good space myself no matter what you're doing (to mother in empty chair).

Mary   So you freeze up and you're pissed. So there she is doing her scene . . . and how could she be happy?

Me   I can ignore you.

Mary   That's sort of like freezing up. But that's one way.

Me   I could go in my room and play with whatever toys I have by myself.

Mary   You do that, don't you?

Me   Yes.

Mary   *It's called "give up." Would you get in touch with what would be wrong about saying to her, "Yes, you're wonderful, Ma." Look and see what would be wrong with that.*

Me   It feels like I would be feeding her bullshit when she is pulling the strings on me.

Mary   *SO THE MORE, "YES, YOU'RE WONDERFUL," YOU SAID, THE MORE WHAT WOULD SHE DO?*

Me   She would probably lay off.

Mary   And then?

Me   AHH–THEN I CAN BREATHE MORE.

Mary   (Laughing) Would you say it to your wife?

Me   (Chuckling to my wife at the time) Yeah, you're wonderful, my wife at the time.

Mary   How is your breathing?

Me   I feel air coming in. I don't feel a need to be tight and defensive.

Mary   Okay, there's some significant differences between your wife and your mother, aren't there?

Me   Yes. (And I tell some differences) (Mary pointed the focus to where they were the same and where I was painting my mother's face on my wife).

Mary   (To my wife at the time) I have a cue for you, just for fun. When you want a stroke for some of the things you have done, would you say to him I want a target stroke? And tell him what you want it for? That will set him off on target.

At another point she is saying that she wants to go to concerts, but resents that I won't commit myself to going. She then procrastinates so we both end up with poor seats. Then I want to leave the concert because I can't see very well at such long range and she feels guilty.

Bob   So he's got the choice of buying his own crummy seats.

Mary   That wouldn't be any fun.

Bob   Stop the game, probably.

From there her work was her feelings of guilt, but when Bob and Mary went back to track an early scene they did not find significant guilt in her past. She also talked about her desire to pull a fast one on people, and how much she enjoyed that.

Bob (Later in the dialogue)   What's wrong with a little guilt?

My wife at the time   If I didn't get a headache it would be fine.

Bob   *Guilt is great if it reminds you to check out something and you decide to do or not to do something and you absolve the guilt. I don't hear you doing that. I hear you just feeling guilty and letting it sit there. Is there anything you can do about it? The answer is yes. Either buy the tickets or tell Len to buy them.*

Mary   *Instead of deciding to take action, you go to headaches.*

My wife at
the time
(Turns to me)   I don't want to go to the Flamenco concert. I will buy you a ticket if you want to go. Or you can buy the ticket.

Me   Buy me a ticket.

Mary (To my
wife at the time)   Is that satisfactory to you?

My wife at
the time   Yes.

Mary   That seems less painful than a headache.

So Bob and Mary got to several significant issues in each of our personality structures, and left us with steps we could take for positive action. They started with us together, then moved to us as individuals while having us talk to each other every now and then and then brought us back to an interpersonal interaction that was relatively free of hidden agendas at the end of the work. This left my wife at the time and me with a clean, fresh feeling when we interacted.

ENDNOTES

[1]   Eric Berne, Principles of Group Treatment (New York: Oxford University Press, 1966), p. 305.

[2]   William Holloway, "Beyond Permission," Monograph III, The Monograph Series, No. I-X (Medina, Ohio: Midwest Institute for Human Understanding), p. 12.

[3]   Ibid.

[4]   Robert Goulding, New Directions in Transactional Analysis: Creating an Environment for Redecision and Change," in Progress in Group and Family Therapy, ed. Clifford Sager and Helen Singer Kaplan (Brunner/Mazel, 1973), p. 122.

[5]   Ibid., p. 123.

[6]   William Holloway, "Decision for Change: Facilitation Through Group Psychotherapy," Monograph I, The Monograph Series, No. I-X, (Medina, Ohio: Midwest Institute for Human Understanding, 1973), p. 5.

[7]   Robert Goulding and Mary Goulding, "Injunctions, Decisions and Re-Decisions," Transactional Analysis Journal 6 (January 1976), pp. 41-42.

8   June Ellis, "TA Talk: Terms and References in Transactional Analysis," Child and Family Consultants, Inc., 512 S. 16th St., Fort Smith, Arkansas, 72901, 1974, p. 81.

9   Ibid., p. 3.

10   Ibid., p. 56.

11   Ibid., p. 92.

12   Ibid., p. 70.

13   Ibid., p. 41.

14   Ibid., p. 20.

15   Ibid., p. 25.

16   Ibid., p. 34.

17   Taibi Kahler and Hedges Capers, "The Miniscript," Transactional Analysis Journal 4 (January 1974), p. 32.

18   Eric Berne, What Do You Say After You Say Hello? (New York: Bantam Books, 1974), p. 11.

19   Aaron Schiff and Jacqui Schiff, "Passivity," Transactional Analysis Journal 1 (January 1971), p. 73.

20   Ibid.

21   Mary Goulding, and Robert Goulding, Changing Lives Through Redecision Therapy (New York: Brunner/Mazel, 1979), p. 30.

22   Robert and Mary Goulding, "New Directions in Transactional Analysis," p. 115.

23   International Transactional Analysis Association Guidelines for Clinical Examination (1976 clinical standards).

24   Eric Berne, Games People Play (New York: Grove Press, Inc., 1964), pp. 146-147.

25   Stephen Karpman, "Fairy Tales and Script Drama Analysis," Transactional Analysis Bulletin 7 (April 1968), p. 39.

REFERENCES

Berne, Eric. *Games People Play.* New York: Grove Press, Inc., 1964.

Berne, Eric. *Principles of Group Treatment.* New York: Oxford University Press, 1966.

Berne, Eric. *What Do You Say After You Say Hello?* New York: Bantam Books, 1974.

Ellis, June. "TA Talk: Terms and References in Transactional Analysis." Child and Family Consultants, Inc., 541 S. 16 St., Fort Smith, Arkansas.

Goulding, Mary, and Goulding, Robert. *Changing Lives Through Redecision Therapy.* New York: Brunner/Mazel, 1979.

Goulding, Robert, and Goulding, Mary. *The Power Is in the Patient,* San Francisco, TA Press, distributed by Transactional Publications, 1772 Vallejo St., San Francisco, CA 94123.

Goulding, Robert. New Directions in Transactional Analysis: Creating an Environment for Redecision and Change. In *Progress in Group and Family Therapy*. Edited by Clifford Sager and Helen Singer Kaplan. New York: Brunner/ /Mazel, 1973.

Goulding, Robert and Goulding, Mary. "Injunctions, decisions and redecisions." *Transactional Analysis Journal* 6 (January 1976).

Holloway, William. "Beyond Permission." Monograph III, The Monograph Series, No. I-X. Medina, Ohio: Midwest Institute for Human Understanding, 4004 Huffman Road, 44256, 1974.

Holloway, William. "Decision for Change: Facilitation Through Group Psychotherapy." Monograph I, The Monograph Series, No. I-X. Medina, Ohio: Midwest Institute for Human Understanding, 44256, 1974.

Kahler, Taibi, and Capers, Hedges. "The Miniscript." *Transactional Analysis Journal* 4 (January 1974).

Karpman, Stephen. "Fairy Tales and Script Drama Analysis." *Transactional Analysis Bulletin* 7 (April 1968).

Schiff, Aaron, and Schiff, Jacqui. "Passivity." *Transactional Analysis Journal* 1 (January 1971).

6

Gestalt Therapy and the Existential Moment

WALTER KEMPLER, M.D., is the founder and clinical director of The Kempler Institute, an organization for the development of family therapists, and author of *Principles of Gestalt Family Therapy.* Presently, Dr. Kempler divides his time teaching throughout the United States and Europe.

Dr. Kempler views the relationship of the couple as the target center of family therapy, and the children as essential participants when they are the symptomatic signals; thus, I have commented on his work as it relates more directly to marital therapy and the existential moment.

Robert L. Martin, D.S.W., is a gestalt therapist and trainer in private practice in Portland, Oregon. His special interests are creative expression and work with sensory perception. I was frequently surprised by his range of freedom in expressing the unusual.

Dr. Erving Polster is a trainer of gestalt therapists. He has contributed to a number of volumes, including *Gestalt Therapy Now; Recognitions in Gestalt Therapy; Encounter;* and *Twelve Therapists.* He founded the postgraduate training program of the Gestalt Institute of Cleveland.

DR. MIRIAM POLSTER has taught psychology at Case Western Reserve and Cleveland State Universities and at the Cleveland Institute of Art. Her gestalt training includes work with Fritz Perls, Laura Perls, Paul Goodman, and Isadore From. TRAINED ALSO AS A MUSICIAN, SHE HAS LED WORKSHOPS IN WHICH MUSIC SERVED AS A POINT OF DEPARTURE FOR EXPLORING PERSONAL EXPERIENCE.

The Polsters were now in private practice in San Diego where they were continuing to develop training programs in gestalt therapy. They were co-directors of the Gestalt Training Center of San Diego and have co-authored *Gestalt Therapy Integrated.*

Dr. James S. Simkin was a gestalt therapy trainer who resided in Big Sur, California. Dr. Simkin has authored *Gestalt Therapy Mini-Lectures.* He was a student, friend, and colleague of Fritz Perls and often co-led professional workshops with him. Dr. Simkin is a Diplomat of the American Board of Examiners in Professional Psychology and director, Simkin Training Center for Gestalt Therapy.

STYLISTIC FOCUS ON "THOU VS. I," WITH MIRIAM POLSTER, PH.D., ERVING POLSTER, PH.D., AND JIM SIMKIN, PH.D.

It is only with the basic premise that each moment of existence is important that one can appreciate the focus on what I refer to as an existential moment.

While each moment of existence is important, there are certain moments that have more impact upon patients than others. So within a gestalt framework I am referring to existential moments as those in which an accentuated contact takes place: (1) between patient and therapist, I-Thou; (2) between alienated parts of a patient suffering from inner conflict; and (3) between patient and environment.

In terms of style, some gestaltists work more with *I-Thou, interpersonal contact.* Others work more with gestalt experiment as a way to approach *intrapsychic conflict.* In other words, they suggest experiments that become obvious to them as they are working with patients, and these experiments help patients to integrate both sides of an inner conflict.

While I am exaggerating for purposes of making style more explicit, I certainly do not mean to stereotype one approach as being exclusive of the other, because most gestaltists would certainly use all working with patients, both at the interpersonal and intrapsychic levels. I am making the distinctions so that therapists may have a clearer focus while pursuing a balance to make the greatest impact when working with patients.

The therapist engaged with a patient in gestalt experiment who is following the patient one step at a time, while still being very in tune with his or her (the therapist's) own experience, may facilitate a different type of impactful experience. When doing this type of work the therapist finds each moment of existence to be of equal importance, but facilitates the experiment so there will be a gradual crescendo of experience of the quality of contact the patient makes with self, others, and the environment. Such a crescendo can often lead to a therapeutic breakthrough, as will be shown later.

Impact, which results from a *crescendo of experience* into an almost euphoric state, builds one moment upon the other. The accumulated impact of a series of such natural moments begins to help patients become more interested in being as alive as they dare instead of partaking in old, deadening ways.

Accentuation of moments when making I-Thou contact (interpersonal existential moments) can help therapists stir patients at the primal level, thereby affording those patients the opportunity to make changes in their lives that might otherwise leave them as tragic figures. These types of moments can be either direct, such as my telling a woman I experienced her as precious when I felt some anguish about sharing that with her; or indirect, such as the following: A thirty-eight-year old man who was the son of a very rich woman came to see me. He was quite sensitive to any direct comments. He had lived all over the world and would come back when he went broke, basically promising his mother that he would reform. He was very bright and capable, but took more pleasure in proving he could once again fool his mother than he did in making his life work. I told him, "I think the problem is that you are willing to settle for crumbs. Your mother is willing to make you the head of a large corporation, but what is that? I would demand a Rolls Royce and a large mansion to immediately accompany the position. Further, I can't really understand what you are complaining about. You are living out fantasies that most people have. In fact, I would appreciate your asking your mother if she would like to adopt me as a second son, because I would really enjoy the opportunity to do what you are doing." This cut into the man's apologetic behavior for his actions quickly. He laughed at his own process, but got the message, while we had an enjoyable contact between us.

Sometimes unpleasant things emerge from me in response to a patient. At these times, it may be important for me to be as fully absorbed as I dare in making an impact. I may be authoritarian. I may be intimidating. I may do it with such force that the message rings in the patient's head in a way he or she will never forget. This type of impact also provides the patient with the opportunity to change a self-destructive and tragic behavior pattern.

Perhaps gestalt therapy, of all the therapies, comes closest to having the concept of the existential moment in its theoretical framework. Gestaltists have been primarily concerned with contact as a basic function of gestalt therapy. The contact boundary may also be referred to as the point at which each of us meets with that which is not ourselves, that is, others or the environment. A third way of thinking about contact is contact as those alienated parts of the self that need to be restored to each patient. These parts are not ourselves because they have been disowned. When each type of contact is effected, an existential moment occurs. Now let us look at some of the issues involved in reaching those accentuated and impactful existential moments.

While gestalt theory has the contact issue written into its theory, there may be some problems making contact and reaching peaks. Again I want to emphasize that I am exaggerating to make stylistic differences clear, and that things are not as clear-cut with individual therapists. However, I believe that problems arise due to a lack of balance in the style and personality of the therapist. For example, one type of gestalt therapist may be quite good at making contact in an I-Thou encounter. Yet that therapist may have more difficulty following the ongoing process of patients one step at a time in ways that will help patients amplify their ongoing experience; or in reaching contact moments through intra-personal awareness. (By intra-personal awareness I mean the working through of the patient's inner conflicts.) These type of gestaltists tend to be more "I" oriented than "Thou" oriented. On the other hand, the "Thou" oriented gestalt therapist may be quite good at facilitating the ongoing process of experience until patients come to a closing of the gestalt–a contact between two alienated parts of themselves. This type of therapist may make an error by tending to leave him or herself out of the relationship. Yet, the very fact that gestalt therapy considers the *contact issue as primary* makes it potent. Those who practice it well can reach and change people at the primal level. Erv Polster, in describing Fritz Perls, wrote of this primal quality when he said,

> He was counterintellectual and, as I now realize, he moved fast into primal familiarity. He described the nature of good contact and exercised it, stripped of amenities and professionalism. He showed how good contact joined with techniques for heightened awareness could provide new leverage into developing profound emotional experiences. The resulting emotionality was a rarity in those days. Even to cry in public, among fifteen people that is, was remarkable then and, in fact, quite suspect for the rest of the community who saw his methods as dangerous and irresponsible.[1]

Polster went on to say that

> The basic novelty to me was the accentuated possibility for entering into the experience of therapy rather than trying to understand the therapy. . . . I gave up being merely professional and permitted myself to become as deeply absorbed as is necessary for the sense of primal familiarity. I moved from the periphery of people's lives, which was a tease away from the personal absorption I wanted. I moved out from behind my desk and began to allow myself authentic centrality.[2]

In such a potentially powerful therapy as gestalt, there is one particular concern that must be raised: facilitating awareness so that it leads to amplified existential moments in patients who have weak Nurturing Parent ego states. The problem can become magnified if both therapist and patient have a tendency to look for what is missing as opposed to what is plus or neutral–even if it's only five percent.

Patients who cannot look at things in perspective (underdeveloped Adult ego states) run the risk of becoming overly critical of themselves while feeling helpless to break out of the vicious cycle. This is particularly true when these patients also lack a substantive ability to nurture themselves. In these cases their behavior becomes either rebellious or compliant–adapted, instead of autonomous. *When patients use awareness against themselves they may set up a project of self-reform which only takes them away from the moment-to-moment unfolding of experience that is at the very heart of gestalt therapy.* Such patients may close up, regardless of the fact they are becoming more aware. They are astute enough in their own critical process and scared child feelings to pick up even *the awareness that they use their awareness against themselves as an awareness that they can use against themselves* (a very complex process).

When working with these types of patients, therapists who tend to view the glass as half empty as opposed to half full need to pay particular attention to being as nurturing and compassionate as possible. Once I was strong enough to deal with those who look at what was missing, after working with the more nurturing therapists first, they were effective and necessary to my personal growth. I experienced them as supportive at very primary levels in that I knew they would help me get to the core of the rotten feeling I had in my guts.

Those therapists who tend to work more from the nurturing parts of their personalities are more likely to be successful with very self critical and scared patients by focusing on whatever is alive about those patients, rather than on what those patients are avoiding or missing. Scared and very self-critical patients must be taken on a faith in the phenomenology of what is happening each moment. Their contact doesn't have to be a true delineating of their nature at the beginning stages of therapy. Wherever these patients get beyond neutral they are to be believed. They do not have to be congruent with their being. If 95 percent is phony, go for the five percent that is not phony. By responding in this manner, therapists can become more interested in providing the kind of environment that will help these patients unfold into their natural selves. Therapists can provide a different kind of experience for patients–one that shows them through experience that the world isn't as bad as they had perceived it to be. In this type of work it is not of primary importance that therapists comment on everything they see, but that they keep a facilitative type of environment in mind. It is a full appreciation of each moment of patients' current experiences, whether they are commented upon or not, that may eventually lead to the accentuated existential moment. But the existential moment is not to be sought as an end in itself–else patients and therapists will be little more than dogs chasing their tails! Each moment of existence must be appreciated for itself before heightening of experience may take place. And these moments build from the emerging needs of patients as opposed to the projected demands of therapists. (Of course, this is not necessarily true for stronger patients who may value the opportunity to deal with both the therapists' demands and projected demands, as long as that therapist is also able to pick up on which demands are projected). In this way patients will not feel as if they are in a battle for control or power because what is building is flowing from their own needs. Unless this approach is taken, patients who are dealing with problems of power and control may even view the slightest suggestion to experiment with new behavior as a power play on the part of therapists. Such patients may even view it as strange that other patients in a gestalt group would be willing to experiment when therapists make a suggestion. They tend to view the process as one whereby therapists are in control of patients, and feel they must not comment on this awareness in order to gain other kinds of awareness in working with therapists. With these kinds of patients, gestalt therapists would be best to avoid beginning their comments with the word "You." For example, "You are toxic and you are a gameplayer" or "You haven't done anything for yourself" are the type of comments that make such patients more defensive and more controlled. They just tighten and close up. The ultimate tendency is to rebel or comply. Thus, the opportunity for free choice and autonomous behavior will have been missed.

When working with defensive and controlled patients it is important for therapists to be secure enough in themselves to deal with attacks that may be forthcoming. Therapists must have a good grasp on what they are doing with patients and be willing to share themselves as well as what they are doing if this is what is needed to make these patients feel more secure. It is when therapists do not know what they are doing, and do not own their behavior when called to account by patients, that these patients tend to escalate rebellious or compliant behavior.

Erv and Miriam Polster, when speaking of therapy without resistance, say,

> The psychotherapist must exercise considerable connoisseurship in distinguishing between what is happening in the present moment and what is distractingly preoccupying. The distinction is a subtle one; rules about what is a present experience will only clutter up one's good sense. The very act which appears to be a preoccupation, when focused on, may turn into present occupation. For example, the woman who looks around the room when talking seems preoccupied rather than presently engaged. When the therapist suggests that she notice how her eyes wander and that she say what she sees (rather than telling her she is resisting), what may be revealed is inordinate curiosity, which, when acknowledged and accepted, results in lively visual experience. So, although the original inclination of the therapist may be to consider looking around the room as irrelevant to the current process, a mere deflection, the fact may well be that looking around the room is basic and talking to the therapist would have been a deflection. The basic propellant to change is the acceptance, even accentuation, of existing experience, believing that such full acknowledgment will in itself propel the individual into an unpredictable progression of experience.[3]

When therapists do not assume that patients are behaving wrongly they are more likely to be able to stay with the unfolding of fresh drama. A faith that all will turn out well, even when the current moment is filled with suffering or a problem, makes acceptance of the ongoing experience much easier. Erv and Miriam say that behavior change is related to the heightening of present experience, which, at its apex, can be defined as an existential moment. They say,

> Always, the return to experience, to the acceptance and reengagement with what is, leads to a new orientation

for behavioral change. Animating these principles is the move beyond the concept of resistance into the view of the individual as a population of ideas, wishes, aims, reactions, feelings, which vie for full expression.[4]

The more expression given to the existence of each moment, the likelier one is to experience an existential moment.

While participating in Erv and Miriam Polster's three year training program in gestalt therapy I saw many magnificent things happen. One such experience took place when a couple who were naive about therapy and had had little or no exposure to gestalt concepts accepted an invitation by one of the trainees in our group to participate in a demonstration so the group could see how the Polsters worked with couples. The man readily admitted that he was a closed book, and that he didn't believe in sharing. He had that defensive look about him that let everybody know if he wasn't treated very gently he would remain exactly where he was–well-defended and non-trusting. But there was also the feeling that he would remain there in any case. This couple was the kind that might come into any therapist's office and provoke a feeling that a fifty-minute hour was going to be a long time to spend together. The session began and I found it to be boring for about fifteen or twenty minutes. However, Erv and Miriam were interested in the couple from the very beginning. At first they made some comments that didn't seem to go anywhere. However, Miriam discovered that she was being "spattered with words" and said, "I'm beginning to feel how important it is for you (to the husband) to explain yourself–to be understood." Then the intensity began to build. An unfolding of experience began to crescendo, heightened by intensity. The man began to talk about his need to be understood and progressively became more open about it. Miriam *found a basic need that had so long gone unfulfilled.* Soon both the man and his wife were crying and sharing the tragedy of both of their brothers being killed, one recently, and one five years earlier. It was the anniversary of his brother's death. This was such a moving experience that it sent chills up and down our spines. When the session was about to end Erv asked the man to tell him the moral of the story. While I do not remember the man's exact words, they were something to the effect that he was quite surprised that he had been able to share himself that deeply in front of a group of strangers. He and his wife were both quite moved when he spoke.

This story interests me for several reasons. It relates directly to the Polsters' article on "Therapy Without Resistance", from which I quoted. As I mentioned, these were people that came in off the street without any gestalt training or psychological sophistication and would have presented a challenge to most any therapist (most group members talked later about the point at which they would have given up). There was relatively no use of "I" in the I-Thou way of working. Erv and Miriam's emphasis was on staying with the couple, while simultaneously probing gently until finding the "five percent liveliness." On top of the experience turning into one both surprising and extremely moving, the man's realization of his ability to share was absolutely incredible in one session–considering the place from which he started. Although the work started out in a very boring way both Erv and Miriam had faith that all would turn out well–and it did; they paid attention and valued each moment of experience, and the valuing of each moment led to the building up of an intense experience that capitulated in an existential moment.

Miriam said she experienced the couple as being authentic. They were authentically cautious, holding in their shared sorrow, supportive of each other in awkward but clearly loving ways. They were suddenly in front of fifteen or so strange people and expected to talk about intimate things. This is not easy for inexperienced people. Miriam went on to say, "I did not (I think Erv didn't either) find them boring so the faith that all would turn out well was just a process of staying engaged and in contact with them *and* aware of my own experience."[5]

Miriam was a warm, touching, and loving woman who was genuinely moved and moving in much of her work with people. Her sense of caring, quick eye, and sense of creative imagination often helped people turn corners that were ever so slight and subtle. In fact, I often think of her as a subtle soloist. I, as her patient, suddenly felt I wasn't stuck anymore–but had broken through to a much richer place in my life. Her low-keyed style of working made the breakthroughs all the more surprising and delightful. A few of these existential moments follow.

I talked of a recent trip to Las Vegas. Miriam asked me if I could imagine myself as a card dealer. I said that I could. She suggested that

I deal myself a hand. One by one I dealt each of the cards out. I had dealt myself a royal flush, which I was quite pleased with. However, the last card was a joker. My reaction was amazement. I had a conscious disdain for anxiety that accrues from not knowing. While much of my conscious life was spent trying to reduce this anxiety, my unconscious mind was keeping the surprise in life for me. It dealt me a joker. I never forgot this piece of work because it put my entire life–past, present and future–in perspective.

I was telling the group how much disdain I had for having to sell myself to build up a private practice. I was not only blocked in doing so, but quite stubborn about it. Miriam asked if I was willing to sell the ottoman in front of me to the group. I began to describe "a beautiful blue-covered ottoman, and when you touched it there was a feel as soft and enticing as velvet. This ottoman would let you feel warmth throughout your body, just being near it." I went on for about ten minutes. When I finished each member of the group said there was no question that they would have bought the ottoman from me. I was astonished that I had that capacity within me, and never forgot it! A few years later I was talking with Bob Goulding. He said that of all the thousands of people they had worked with over the years, they knew the name Len Bergantino. I asked him why this was so. He laughed and said that I was a good PR man. I thought of Miriam's work with me immediately, and was tickled that it stuck. Of course, one of the values of existential moments such as those I have described throughout the book, is that they do stick! They can be used over and over so people can continue to put to use the lessons they have learned in therapy.

When thinking about existential moments Miriam provided what I might, for lack of a better term, refer to as a non-specific existential moment. That is, when I think about her I am enriched by the legacy of a warm, tender, caring human being and am further inspired to develop my humanity.

What first attracted me to working with Erv Polster was seeing him reach closure (a resolution) in twenty-minute sessions with three different patients in a demonstration before two hundred people. It was at that point that I contacted him about becoming a trainee in the three-year training program given by him and Miriam. During that first year I taped a segment of my work as a patient with Erv as the therapist. I find the work interesting because it involves my particular request to get better at reaching closures with my own patients. I use the experience below to show how one moment builds upon another until I become absorbed enough in what I am doing to attain the closure I was seeking.

Me   I'd like to work on something that ties in with the piece of work I did yesterday, when you were supervising me. There were a couple of places you made comments about where I didn't stay with the issue and where I didn't confront when the patient didn't answer my question. I became lazy and didn't pay attention. I do it right before a closure takes place most of the time I make that kind of mistake. I wonder if you've had any more thoughts about what you pointed out yesterday.

Erv   Would you believe that since yesterday I never really thought of it. (Erv, in a playful way, is picking up on my grandiosity.)

Me   Well, let me see if I can get out of my grandiosity for a minute.

Erv   That was a very humble statement. (still being playful)

Me   (Feeling there was enough of this playful stuff, and I wanted to get down to business–or at least how I perceived the business) I would like to avoid missing closure and I want you to help me get to a place where I can do that.

Erv   My guess is that from now on you will be alert to whether somebody has given you the answer to your question or not.

Me   I get more alert and then I feel like coasting. I seem to repeat the pattern. (I laugh)

Erv	What are you laughing at?
Me	I was laughing at your facilitative qualities.
Erv	(teasing me, to the group) I like him for saying something like that–positive reinforcement. (group laughs) Ah, what was that sarcastic thing you had on your mind?
Me	I have the feeling when I start to work with you that I don't know if I'm finished right after I start.
Erv	You mustn't be compulsive. (Which I usually was; Erv kept me loose and present.)
Me	(With a laugh) You seem to take great delight in seeing me work on stuff?
Erv	I take great delight on seeing you work on stuff?
Me	Yeah, like most of the time I get into saying something, you laugh a lot more than anything else.
Erv	More than anything else are the key words.
Woman in the Group	You're so good at working hard.
Erv	I do find that I'm either laughing uproariously or I'm very serious about something that I don't quite understand the seriousness of. Like the kind of thing you're talking about. You talk as though one of these days you're not going to miss anything. So you put it in a very serious way but it really is so funny put in perspective. I don't want to discourage you from your research or enlightment but I don't want to take that perfection trip. I would like to take a trip with you though.

Me   Well, what kind of trip?

Erv   Wherever we go is OK with me but you must know
            I can't seriously try to help you never miss anything.
            (I laugh) You get so enlightened when you laugh.

Me   That's because I'm so heavy when I don't.

Erv   See if you can set up a dialogue between your light
            side and your heavy side.

Me   Basically I just really enjoy having a good time
            bullshitting. OK, for my heavy side. How are you
            ever gonna make it to the top if you don't work
            hard and if you don't pay attention to what the hell
            is going on? Your trip is to take a twenty-four-hour
            holiday every day. My light side says––you're right.
            That's what I want to do. But I'm clever and how
            I am going to pull it off is to play when I work. If I
            work hard playing I can satisfy your demands while
            I am satisfying my own. How does that grab you?
            My heavy side says–it's kind of distasteful.

Erv   Kind of distasteful?

Me   There is a feeling that nobody should have that
            good a time.

Erv   Who do you sound like when you say that?

Me   I sound like my Dad. He was always working.
            He had a day job and was a musician by night.
            When he wasn't playing a gig he was practicing.
            But being a musician was what he really loved.
            He was playing while he was working. It had an
            unusual effect on him. He is in his seventies and
            he still plays gigs with the kids. He plays jobs with
            guys thirty, thirty-five, forty-years old and he stays

vital doing that. That was the message I got, how to stay vital by playing while you work. But there was a non-accepting overtone to it–as if there were something wrong with doing it.

Erv   (Moving toward increased absorption, but I didn't know it at the time). How did you feel about his being gone so much?

Me   Pretty good. He was a pain in the ass a lot of the time he was around. He was always trying to work me. Trying to get me to work.

Erv   Would you talk to him?

Me   (Talking to my Dad using empty chair)   You're always bugging me to work. Mow the lawn. Do the dishes. Practice your mandolin. You wanted me to work while you were out having a good time. I wasn't going to do that. I'm not going to do that.

Erv   Now be your father.

Me   (playing my Dad) I'm really going to put the squeeze on you. I'm really going to pressure you. I feel kind of shitty about the fact that I'm playing all the time and your mother misses me. So I can't train you to be an irresponsible guy like me who looks responsible. Yeah, oh, that was something that I never thought about–how to look responsible while being irresponsible.

Erv   (following one step at a time–breaks from the two chair dialogue) So you're Len thinking that, right?

Me   Yes.

Erv So go over there and be Len so that we can get the distinction.

Me When that came out I was surprised. I really needed to know that. I don't know what to say to my Dad anymore.

Erv So you're not talking to him?

Me He is in the background and you (Erv) are in the foreground. I'm feeling like a little kid.

Erv So what does that little kid in you say to me?

Me I need a lot of acceptance and nurturance until I can do that for myself, until I will do that for myself. That's why I'm here. I was aware of waiting for you to give that to me. You were a little slow. I'm feeling solid. I'm willing to stop now.

Erv I'm somewhat confused about who you are now, whether you're your dad or your own man. Sounds like you're Len, but I didn't get the transition. What I'm missing is something between you and your father, something more substantive. I feel like you slipped out of your dialogue and aren't taking your relationship with your father seriously.

Me I'm puzzled now. I don't know how to have a real relationship with an empty space. What I was doing was exploring different parts of me. I don't have an appreciation of what I would need to do for you to have a sense of completion.

Erv Is it important that I have a sense of completion?

Me Insofar as that I assume I would have one too.

Erv — You don't have one, is that it?

Me — Well, I felt one earlier. I felt one and not quite. Yeah, but not quite.

Erv — You said you felt solid. Is that the moment you are talking about?

Me — Yes.

Erv — I'd like to know if there's anything that you want to say to your father that you didn't say.

Me — (I hesitate. I'm not used to talking about loving and warm feelings in front of a large group. It's easier for me to play tough guy.) I feel a resistance. It's hard to say–

Erv — Would you tell your Dad what you feel?

Me (Talking to Dad in empty chair) — (My Dad was in the hospital with a heart condition for two weeks prior to this session, and only recently had gotten out.) I mainly love you and I'm really concerned about your heart problem. I really want you to live forever and the thought of you dying makes me nervous and teary and I don't know how to fight off telling it that way. That's why I tell you to keep swinging.

Erv — Can you see him now that you're talking?

Me — I start to and then I saw the shoes of people in the group.

Erv — Close your eyes and see if that helps you to see him.

Me — You know, you're a cute old man. I used to think you were a pain in the ass when I was a kid but I think that you're a really cute old man now. Just about the time I began to see you that way I moved away so I've never been able to know you. Three thousand miles away. I see you once a year and I talk to you on the telephone on Sundays for five minutes. I'd like you to move to California. I know you'd be kind of scared and you think you are too old to start over again with your music.

Erv　　Can you walk toward him?

Me　　I want to go the other way. I want to trick him into walking towards me.

Erv　　Oh, you want to trick him into walking towards you?

Me　　Right! He's as tricky as I am. (to Dad) You're as tricky as I am so you're not moving either.

Erv　　What's in it for you to trick him into coming to you?

Me　　I was always on your turf. You used to tell me I had to do it your way until I moved out. I want to balance things out. I really want to be with you, but I'm not like I used to be with you. I'm more. It seems that you hold your ground and I hold my ground and there is no give.

Erv　　Is that the way you want it?

Me　　No. That's not the way I want it.

Erv　　But you're not ready to move towards him right now. Are you ready to call out to him?

Me　　Call out to him?

Erv　　Dad, come over here. I'm coming, whatever feels routine.

Me	Dad, come on over here. You've got all this sunshine out here. I've got you some neat possibilities for studio work with your music. Come on over here. I got more to offer than you've got back there.
Erv	What happened?
Me (Playing Dad)	Nothin! Cause you're my son, I love you, I care about you, I appreciate you had the strength to get as good at what you're doing as I do at what I'm doing. I respect you a lot. I'm an old man. My dreams are over. I feel safe back in Connecticut. I grew up back here. I lived my entire life here. I enjoy rapping with you but I ain't comin'. If I come out to visit you in the summer or if you come back for a week, that's how it's gonna be. (speaking as Len) It doesn't feel like enough–it seems like it's not enough.
Erv	What do you feel bad about? Do you feel sad, for example, or do you feel rejected?
Me	I don't feel rejected. I feel sad and a little teary.
Erv	You're skipping over your teariness and sadness (noticing that I had turned toward the tape recorder)

Just about this time my tape recorder had run out and I stopped to change the tape. For sure, this was obsessive on my part, but then again maybe my unconscious mind knew how important it was for me to have this particular session on tape. It exemplifies all that I wanted to learn.

Erv	I feel like you could have had a good experience untaped and now you may not have any experience taped. That's sad. (long pause)
Me	It's hard to get back to where I was. I resent your interrupting.

Erv   You resent me interrupting?

Me   Yeah! I felt when I changed the tape I could still maintain what I needed to do to get through that piece of work and I wasn't counting on your interruption.

Erv   That's what happens sometimes. Some things happen that you don't count on. I couldn't get back into it myself. I had to say what I had to say and you resented it. (noticing what I was doing) You point your finger at me and you tell me.

Me   It's hard for me to point my finger at you, but I'm doing it, so it couldn't be that hard.

Erv   You're not exactly pointing the finger. (My finger was curved.)

Me   I'm not exactly pointing my finger at you because on the one hand I know what you did and I appreciate what you did and on the other hand you were a pain in the ass. So I understand you and resent you doing what you did at the same time.

Erv   What can we do about that?

Me   So what we can do about it is shift right back to where I was.

Erv   It's almost like interchangeable parts. It's something we might find in a bargain store. (Recognizes with gentle sarcasm my mechanical quality.)

Me   (pissed) Do you want something more?

Erv   I want to feel that it's more than a game. Because I don't think you're going to get anything out of your father anymore. That's a human being there. I'm a human being here. You're a human being there. This is more than psychotherapy.

Me   Sometimes I'm really fond of you and sometimes I have a lot of fun with you and sometimes I love you and sometimes I feel really competitive with you and sometimes I feel like I can do things you can't do and I'm better at them than you are and I like that feeling. Sometimes I'm gaming with you and I'm pissed off when you don't bite. I care a lot about you and I want the same back. I get some of what I want back but not enough. When I don't get enough back is when I get into gaming. I feel fully equal and mutual and I dig relating to you in that way, except you have this craft that you are an expert at–and while I am learning your craft there is certainly an inequality between us. I feel that and when I do it's hard being with you. Then I get gamey.

Erv   Is that happening now?

Me   Not now.

Erv   There's some anger in you.

Me   Where in the fuck are you at?

Erv   Deprived.

Me   For?

Erv   Something, just fullness!

Me   I just gave you one helluva statement. Are you disappointed?

Erv   No. I'm not disappointed. I'm not going to settle for this shit. (Still feeling my internal distraction)

Me   What will you settle for?

Erv   *Full absorption.* See what happens if you raise your voice.

Me   (Louder) I feel OK about raising my voice. (Louder) I feel OK about raising my voice. How do you feel about it?

Erv   I feel good. I like hearing your voice like that.

Me   I never knew that. You have the most self-accepting group and with such self-acceptance being your trip I just felt awkward about raising my voice. It feels counterculture in here. I'm gonna raise it! So how's that grab ya?

Erv   How's it for you?

Me   Super.

Erv   Do you know what I mean about absorption? When you raised your voice, did you feel any difference in your absorption?

Me   Yes. I felt really engaged and involved with you, not just on your terms but on my terms and your terms.

Erv   Alright, try it again. Raise your voice, then I'm going to ask you a question.

Me   (Loud) I feel fantastic raising my voice!

Erv   Can you imagine yourself changing a tape in the middle of that sentence?

Me   (Screaming) No!!

By following the flow of what was happening one step at a time it can be seen how Erv was able to facilitate my moving toward a fuller experience each step of the way–until I reached a *full absorption–an* existential moment. Basically this was therapy without resistance–with one exception. I changed the tape and Erv experienced that as so intrusive to the flow of things that he switched to an "I" frame of reference as opposed to staying with me in terms of where I was flowing. Although I initially chose to work with Erv because of his ability to stay with patients, as I felt this would provide the balance I needed in my style and personality, I was angry when he switched to an "I" frame of reference as opposed to focusing on "Thou." Yet, my natural way of working focuses more on the "I" experience. Interesting that a dose of my own medicine annoys me the most. However, Erv had the balance and range to not only stay with me step by step, but to be tough and confrontive when it was necessary. On several occasions he interjected himself into the work. Thus, the pursuit of a balance between "I" and "Thou," or being and staying becomes one of the tasks of the therapist.

While I was involved in Erv and Miriam Polsters' three-year training program, and was learning how to work in a gentle and often playful way, I had a feeling that I was neglecting the authoritarian parts of my personality. This may very well have been a result of my stereotyping the Polsters to be more on this side of the coin than what I felt myself to be–an authoritarian policeman with super quick awareness, who did his best not to let any bullshit slip by helping patients get to a lively energetic place as soon as possible–both for their own good as well as my own! The Polsters were more inclined to not be as concerned about crispness, but be more concerned with the unfolding of the patient's experience into a fullness of being. While both the easy flowing and authoritarian approaches lead to a fuller unfolding of experience, I felt I needed a bit more experience being authoritarian. Again, I do not mean to stereotype anyone as being authoritarian or non-authoritarian, but there was a part of me that wasn't using all my power. The part of me that felt unsatisfied, the authoritarian part, was keeping itself in check and telling itself that for me to be more authoritarian I needed to work with someone who appeared to me to work more from that style. Of course this was my own way of reducing my potency. Nevertheless, that is how I saw it.

I had heard tales of a man who didn't let very much slide. Although I had a great deal of ambivalence, and it took me several years to get the courage to finish some unfinished business with myself, I finally made it up to Big Sur, California, to spend a week with Dr. Jim Simkin.

While Erv and Jim both can work well in either an "I" or a "Thou" mode, there are distinct differences in styles of making an impact on patients. Both have helped me to become a fuller human being in addition to benefiting as a therapist.

A gestalt therapist in the early 1970's sent me a note saying that I was too slippery for him and that my avoidance maneuvers were so sophisticated that I should take time to go to Big Sur to work with Jim Simkin. His words stayed buried in my unconscious for several years, but I never forgot what he said. I heard that Jim had an extraordinary ability to focus on nuances of expression in movement, voice, and demeanor, and helped patients explore the personal meaning in these subtle expressions. From all that I had heard about Jim I knew I would be called on each discount–he would be a super policeman. In many respects this style was more similar to my own than that of the Polsters. That made my ambivalence even greater about working with Jim. I sensed it would be a rough week, and I made sure I had a couple of years under my belt with Erv and Miriam Polster, and a week-long workshop with Bob and Mary Goulding, all of whom were very nurturing in working with me. This nurturance helped me to feel good enough about myself to risk engaging Jim at the level of truth he demanded.

Jim didn't do any private practice. There were two options to work with him. I could either go as a trainee for one month or as a patient model for one week. However, this format posed a problem for me. I only wanted to go for a week. As a patient model I would have the opportunity to work as a patient in a large group setting with Jim and as a patient with the therapists who committed themselves for a month. The therapists who went for a month would have the opportunity to be therapists with patient models who went for a week in addition to being supervised by Jim on video tape. I wanted to have the option to be a patient, a therapist, and be supervised by Jim while I only went for one week. I called him six months ahead of time to work out the details. The conversation went as follows:

Me   Jim, I have had several years experience and training in gestalt therapy. I want to come for a week but I want you to make an exception and permit me to work as a therapist in addition to being supervised by you.

Jim   No. (Long pause–maybe a minute)

Me   (Feeling anxiety, not quite knowing what to say, wanting to work with Jim, and not liking this experience). Isn't there any way you would be willing to reconsider?

Jim   No. (Long pause–about another minute)

Me   (My anxiety continuing to rise as I had never been dealt with so firmly). Alright, I'll come for a week.

Jim   Just a minute. My wife will give you the details. (No wasted energy here).

Anne   Len, I'll send you the application for a week program.

Me   Anne, why don't you send me the application for both the week and the month-long program.

Anne   Len, I'll send you whatever Jim wants me to send you.

Me   (Frustrated) All right.

I had the distinct impression after this short conversation that Jim was not to be taken lightly. Not only did Jim refuse to engage in courtesy or social amenities, but the entire group was responding in the same way. Each discount was called. I couldn't make up my mind if it was going to be a long week or a short week. The feeling was similar to having my appendix removed. I knew I needed it out. I felt better when it was over. But the process of removing the appendix was painful. All the people at the workshop were highly committed to pursuing this level of truth within themselves and with each other. I was going to get the strongest taste of relationship–and existential moments via the I-Thou encounter as I had ever experienced. Then again, I had a habit of letting direct confrontations run right off my back unless they were written with indelible ink.

To give you an example of a few of the people, there was a psychiatrist from Germany who was spending his third month and third summer with Jim. There was also a gestalt therapist from Italy and one from Holland doing the same. In one instance while I was talking to about four people after dinner, they all got up and left. I hadn't realized that I wasn't making contact with them. This was the kind of impact I was not likely to forget. With this introduction let's take a look at the "I-Thou" gestalt oriented approach of Jim Simkin working with me. Again, I mention that both Jim and the Polsters are very well balanced in both "I" and "Thou" modes of working, so what I intend to demonstrate is a matter of personal style and emphasis. (Dr. Simkin requested I delete any sentence that cannot be reproduced exactly due to inaudibility on the tape.)

Me   I'm a little anxious. The transactions are really moving quick and I feel like I'm in fast company.

Jim   How's that feel?

Me   A little threatening.

Jim   (Being playful) I'm going to slow my transactions down.

Me   (Being playful) I don't feel any less threatened.

Jim   So how are you threatening yourself? (Switching into a very serious mood. There was never time to get set with a particular mood of Jim's because he shifted so fast–terrible for an obsessive to deal with.)

Me   I was telling myself, maybe you're not quite as fast as the other people here.

Jim   Say that as a statement . . . I'm not fast . . .

Me   I'm not as fast as the other people here.

Jim   How's that sound?

Me   It sounds solid. Which is another part of me saying, well, you should be–

Jim   (Shifting quickly into an I-Thou mode and taking me by surprise while speaking very quickly) Len? Len? Who were you talking to just then?

Me   I don't know.

Jim   Did you experience any contact?

Me   Yes, when you asked me the question I started thinking about it. I sort of went into my head and was out of contact with you.

Jim   Did you know that?

Me   No. Not until you mentioned it.

Jim   (making fun of me to get the message across) I'm going to start waving at you to see if I can get you to pay some attention to me. You can wave back. . . . I didn't feel like you were attending to me.

Me   It's hard for me to attend to you and answer your question at the same time.

Jim   Why?

Me   I have difficulty thinking and responding at the same time. You surprise me. On the one hand I enjoy it every time you do it and on the other hand it's unsettling for me and I . . . sort of an approach-avoidance kind of . . . (I see Jim frowning at me) no text book stuff.

Jim   Oh, please. No textbook stuff.

Me   I feel OK until you ask me to do something and then I start thinking about how to do it.

Jim   So any time that I make a request, you then have to formulate some response. You feel you can't just be here.

Me   Exactly.

Jim   (Taking me off guard again–while poking fun) OK, no more requests. That wasn't a request. That's a statement. (Jim had the tenacity of a bulldog in pursuing his objective of not letting me become so preoccupied with myself that I excluded him and others).

Me   (not liking his poking fun at me and not taking me seriously) I was thinking the issue is of major concern to me.

Jim   That issue being?

Me   Wow . . . when you make a request I trip out, or try to find the answer that will sort of give you what you want to hear as opposed . . . not fully give you what you want . . .

Jim   Right, yeah.

Me   You're noticing the delight I had when I said that.

Jim   You bet.

Me   It's going to be a short week. (Meaning what I was saying but at that time wishing the hell the session was over).

Jim   That's what I thought. You said you hadn't decided on whether you'd stay at the motel, or stay here at the house. You keep one foot out there and one foot here. It's difficult for you to be with both feet here.

Me   The feeling I have is wanting to have all the possibilities covered and what I do is cover them sparsely.

Jim   You look like a first base coach. (Jim gets up and stretches one leg in one direction and one leg in the other so he will be able to identify how I experience that stance in the world.) (inaudible material) I feel stretched and pulled and, ah, hurting, as I try to stay in two places at one time.

Me   My body often feels beat up–almost like when I get through a day I'm ready to zonk out.

Jim   That's what happens to me when I don't get any nourishment. When I'm working with somebody that gives nothing back I feel drained at the end of the day. If they give something back, if there's a give and take, I feel good at the end of the day. Good tired, rather than good zonked out.

Me   I don't feel tired from my therapy hours. I feel tired from my other hours.

Jim   What are those?

Me	I write a lot and I don't get as much nourishment as I need in my personal relationships. I have been getting more in the last year than ever before, but I find it hard to ask people for nourishment.
Jim	(Comes scooting over to me and lies his back up against me so I am in a position to hold him) What's going on?
Me	(Caressing his head in a very gentle way) Well, I was noticing your head and I was wondering what you were thinking?
Jim	(Sort of joltingly) Oh!
Me	You're not shy. You know, for all those ladies that want to run their fingers through your hair, they better hurry.
Jim	Which ladies?
Me	(I was stunned again. My wit usually gets me out of discomforting situations when I get too close). Oh, I was making a joke.
Jim	Oh, why?
Me	I felt discomfort with you there.
Jim	And you weren't going to say you felt discomfort?
Me	Right.
Jim	That's too bad. I know what that's like to make a joke instead of saying what you feel (very emphatically).
Me	Yes. You look like you know.

Jim	Instead of making jokes, talk to the other guy. I was leaning on you. You were running your finger through my bushy eyebrows and I got startled when you said something about ladies. You got me off balance.
Me	Now that my discomfort is out in the open I still don't think I would feel anymore comfortable about being close to you if you were to lean on me again.
Jim	Are you saying that you have no way of expressing your discomfort and getting unstuck that you know about?
Me	I have one. My wife. The reason I married her was because . . . .
Jim	Look at her and say that.
Me	(Pretending my wife was in empty chair) The reason I married you is because you're very soft and very nurturing and you seem to know how to give me what I need, even when I don't ask you for it.
Jim	She's not very helpful.
Me	(Stunned. His comment helped me to create a much fresher relationship after the workshop.) I never thought about it that way.
Jim	She's teaching you to not ask for what you want.
Me	At the same time it feels good.
Jim	Sure. It's a helluva way to go through life. Getting very stuck with one person.

Me   When I let myself feel what goes on I feel an underlying sadness and I hear my voice quiver some and I feel my mouth drooping.

Jim   What I hear is that your voice is relatively high pitched and has a quality of, not quite . . . but just on the edge of complaining and whining.

Me   That's an improvement.

Jim   How?

Me   From complaining and whining. It's only the past year that change has taken place.

Jim   And as you're able to acknowledge what you're feeling, sadness, and other things–

Me   I get on the verge of feeling things, some sadness, some of this, some of that, then I go into my head.

Jim   Is that what you're doing?

Me   Yes. Fast enough to stop me from making any changes in a big sort of way. I feel challenging toward you. There is a part of me that wants to challenge you, but it doesn't serve my own purposes.

Jim   What are your purposes?

Me   To get unstuck.

Jim   I'm fascinated with your avoidance techniques.

Me   I'm fascinated and startled with how fast you picked up on them.

Jim	I look for something out here that interests me and I'm very interested in where you go, you're looking away, and I'm interested in your voice.
Me	I'm glad you're interested in me. You have a very warm, accepting look about you when you say that and those are things about me that I readily accept.
Jim	Right.
Me	So you surprised me. I would have set up an agenda of change for myself, and then sabotaged it. That's why I'm so tired.
Jim	WELL, I HAVE A HOPE FOR YOU. MY HOPE IS THAT THIS WEEK YOU DO SOMETHING ABOUT BEING MORE SIMPLE. MY GUESS IS THAT YOU ARE SIMPLE AND YOU TRY TO BE QUICK. THEN YOU FEEL LIKE YOU'RE OUTCLASSED.
Me	I'M AFRAID BEING SIMPLE WILL SLOW ME DOWN.
Jim	YOU'LL WORK EVEN FASTER. AND IT IS SO MUCH EASIER TO BE SIMPLE. AT LEAST THAT IS MY EXPERIENCE.
Me	It's a new thought for me.
Jim	Before you compute that, do something simple. Anything.
Me	You still surprise me (simple).
Jim	I like the way you look right now. You turned pink and you're beginning to look alive, and I like that.

Me   I can feel a flush.

Jim   So, see what you can do about being simple without
                      planning it too much.

Me   Thank you.

While I had been developing the tender side of me in working with Erv, I got to working on developing the solid side of me the following day with Jim. I was experimenting with requesting, demanding and manipulating. *Jim said he was surprised that he was willing to give me what I asked for when I was demanding.* I felt that I was harsh when I was demanding. He experienced me as solid, that is, when I came straight out and said "I want- - -." He dismissed my wants when I manipulated or requested. Jim thought I had an ideal story how my voice should sound which distracted me from paying attention to how people reacted to me–and that I was *getting stuck with my own preoccupation.* As the session went on, Jim commented that I was taking and not giving back. There were quite a few interchanges where I contacted him. There were also quite a few interchanges while we were not working in group, but in the house, where I could tell I rubbed him the wrong way. It was difficult for an only child to learn how to live in a family in a week. For a few days I began to feel a dread while driving from my motel, about a 30 minute drive, to Jim's house. One night I was feeling a tremendous heaviness in the room and had been feeling a headache for about two hours, when Jim complained about his eyes burning and his head hurting. All of a sudden he turned to me and said, "Len, I don't like you. I think you suck." He was referring to my only taking and not giving to him.

I got the full impact of how I affected someone when I wasn't talking directly to them. It was a remark engraved in indelible ink, and which I thought of often. The pattern I had to change was to talk directly to people instead of talking to myself in front of them, thinking I was giving to them while I was draining both their energy and my own. Strangely enough I was relieved after Jim said what he said. It was as if the heavy mist cleared right out of the room. My headache went away. His headache went away and his eyes stopped burning. He had said what I feared he would say, and I had both learned from his impact and survived what he said.

When the group was coming to an end I felt free and made a great deal of contact. Jim looked very surprised at the difference. I was not surprised because I had often experienced myself using full power without being fearful. However, I found it much easier to do so when I was the therapist in my office, than when I was the patient in Jim's training group. With someone as powerful as Jim, who tended to work from the same judging of absolute authenticity that I did, I triggered my own fears and became frozen.

At the very end of the week's experience, Jim's last comments to me were that something didn't make sense between us, in referring to the contradiction between my potency and my fear. Then he smiled and said, "So you want to fill my shoes." I looked him straight in the eye. He knew I was serious. When I was leaving he said, "Do it man, do it." With all his toughness he certainly commanded my full respect, especially with his last comment. He was encouraging me to be his equal, even though there was a strong part of both of us that enjoyed the guru spot at the top while at the same time struggling to relate both with humility and equally. The last thing I said to Jim in the group was that some day I hoped I would like him as much as I appreciated and respected him. He thought for a moment, and said, "That would be rare." I felt a sadness when he said that. I was very thankful there was a Jim who could train us therapists to get that straight with ourselves–who could rattle our cages at the primal level. Yet, I knew all too well what he meant when he said that would be rare. It is difficult for people to approach such paradoxical love–that is love that doesn't feel too good when it's happening–with appreciation and a return of love. When therapists take patients on in their primal stuck spots, therapists can expect all the hell patients can give them. It was that feeling that made me interested in learning how to reach people with honey while I could still be a tough guy when I had to.

When I look at the differences in style between Erv and Jim I see Erv demonstrating so flowing and unfolding of experience that he could work with most anyone. Erv's work unfolds into a cathartic high for the patient. Jim's work also unfolds into high and accentuated experiences; however, his toughness and crispness with game-playing may leave the other person with an empty, awful feeling that lets one know the full price of their facade. Both Jim and Erv do many of the same things that Miriam and Erv did with the difficult patient whose work moved the entire group unexpectedly. We have seen different types of existential moments take place–one is the unfolding that comes with the absorption at the end of Erv's work and the flush I felt at the end of my first piece of work with Jim when he suggested I move in the direction of simplicity. Another existential moment was when Jim said to me, "I don't like you Len, I think you suck." This is the interpersonal, "I-Thou" encounter.

Of course, the reader must realize that when Jim hits as hard as he does, he is working with a psychologically sophisticated group of therapists who are so fast at picking up on what others are doing that they can con themselves at the same rate of speed. The effect Jim's response had on me was that I now am concerned about whether I am giving or taking, and whenever there is any doubt, I hear his words go through my head, "I don't like you Len, I think you suck." It is like a magic message to keep my relationships progressing in a positive direction.

Both Erv's work and Jim's first piece of work had a lasting impact on me. "Absorption" and "simple" keep coming back to me. Existential moments are valuable because they become imbedded and can be used repeatedly to help people change their behavior. Therapeutic judgment will flow naturally from the well-seasoned therapist. The choice of honey or salt will be a spontaneous one. Existential moments will be aroused from either of the two. However, the less mature therapist needs to be more cautious to know when judgments are his or her own projections. It is important to be able to say what flows and what will impact others, but it is also important to be able to own what you, the therapist, are doing during that process. In this way existential moments are more likely to happen from a general arousal.

IMPACT: THE KEY TO RESPONSIBLE ACTION WITH COUPLES, WITH DR. WALTER KEMPLER, M.D.

Walt Kempler is perhaps one of the most unheralded therapeutic geniuses of marital and family therapy that the profession of psychotherapy has yet to experience. He currently spends most of the year in Holland, where he trains psychotherapists from many European and Scandinavian countries, and therefore is not in the mainstream of American therapists' conversations these days. However, his wisdom reaches depths of authenticity that are indeed rare. He consistently gets "the job" accomplished at the most primal levels. I strongly urge that therapists become familiar with his book, *Principles of Gestalt Family Therapy* (see References).

For the month or two that Walt returns to California each year, I continue to enjoy and profit greatly from whatever training experiences he offers. In addition, I enjoy his banjo playing very much!

Therapists need to say and do things with enough power to set the wheels of marital interaction into responsible motion. This was Dr. Walter Kempler's major contribution to my thinking in terms of helping couples to reach existential moments. I had always felt that marital therapy was something I loved doing. My particular style lent itself to this kind of work. My quickness on process helped me to rapidly pick up the intricacies of what each partner was doing. When I stood behind one or the other of the couples and spoke what came from my guts, I knew I made an impact because I could sense and clarify what people were implicitly communicating to each other. However, there was still something missing and I wasn't quite sure what it was. So I decided to go to a three-day workshop given by Dr. Kempler. From my brief experiences with him, what I had read of his writings, and a tape recording in which he was speaking–one word kept coming to mind– DYNAMITE! That is how Walt would describe his focus on potency and impact.

DYNAMITE–POTENCY–IMPACT: It is the therapist's responsibility to deliver the message in a way so that patients *will feel the therapist's power* (with *teeth*) thereby helping them implement changes needed in their lives.

No mistake about it. That was Dr. Kempler, and it became quite apparent what was missing in my work. Walt knew how to implant the dynamite into the relationship that would help people get through the impasse. Each time he worked there was a sense of movement. It was not only the kind of movement that happens when one does good therapy, but it was the kind of movement that left patients feeling they had a way to live their lives more effectively, and they had a clear direction of exactly what they needed to do to get the ball rolling. He was active and engaging throughout the work, and delivered his messages with conviction and accuracy. While this in principle appears quite contrary to people finding their own path in life, Kempler's forceful reactions point to natural paths that patients might neither have found nor taken if left to his own devices initially. Further, his reactions force patients to find their reactions. He has reached a level of authenticity within himself, in addition to a very fine-tuned conscious experiential flow, an extraordinary ability to pay attention to details, and a wisdom that comes from years of experience. He hits at the precise points where people are stuck, and with such involvement and potency that people feel enough of their own power and hopefulness to do the things which were preventing them from living happy and healthy lives. There is a pragmatic quality to Dr. Kempler's work. He spoke of feelings–anger, depression, anxiety, and other emotions with which people use to keep themselves crippled through self-defeating behavior. He felt that therapists by and large waste their time working through these feelings with patients, and that patients need to be able to live more effectively–*regardless of those feelings*. It is in this context that Dr. Kempler used an authoritarian approach delivered in a direct manner both elegant and eloquent in style. Within a one- to three-hour session he could effect a firm resolution that resulted in major breakthroughs in a couple's lives.

Once, working with a mother and a couple of family members he asked the mother why her husband and other family members were not there. She said that they did not want to come and that her husband was working and basically felt it was a waste of time. Walt told the woman to call her husband and tell him to get the rest of the children and bring them to the session. This was a demonstration before about forty professional therapists. The woman said it would take about forty-five minutes for him to get there if she could reach him. The looks in the room suggested that there was no way Walt could get her to bring the husband and the family in that day. He just as quickly responded by saying that he could wait forty-five minutes and that he would go to the telephone with her while she made the call. Everyone, including the woman, was stunned. His *tenacity* was remarkable. When they came back the woman reported that she couldn't reach her husband. At that time Walt either said or implied there was nothing more to be done with her alone, and that he wanted her to bring her husband

and all her children to a session on the following day at 4:30 p.m. She said that she could not get them to come. He said that it was her job to get them to come. It was her responsibility to herself, her husband and her family. He pointed out how their absence was having negative consequences for the boy that came with her and again said that it was her job to get them there. He told her it was about time she used her power in a constructive way. Walt told her to either come with the entire family, or not to come at all. That was the dynamite needed to get her to move. If she did so, the entire balance of power in the family would be shifted–and so would the possibility for change. That was the existential moment of impact.

Quite a few people felt that Walt was too tough on this woman. All sorts of questions came in the discussion period, after she had left. What would happen to her? Would she come back? What if she didn't? Would Walt be responsible if any harm came to her as a result of his tough treatment? I was fascinated at his instantaneous capacity to do the unexpected–such as waiting forty-five minutes, telling her to leave that session and not to come back unless she brought her husband and the entire family.

There was much talk in the group as to whether she would come back that Sunday. Sure enough, at about 4:20 p.m. she appeared with her husband and about six or seven children. The group was spellbound. I felt my entire body charged with emotion when I realized that he had accomplished most of the therapy with the woman before the session ever started on that Sunday.

He had picked up on the woman's power and had found a way to structure the situation so she could use power to move the entire family. She had it in her all along. But it was Walt's genius that had helped her turn her power loose for constructive purposes. Walt's work with the wife continued until the husband stopped feeling hopeless about her, and impact he might make in the family. Walt showed him how to get back into the family, and showed the woman how to use her power in a direct way instead of passively complaining to be powerless. He felt their new way of interacting would help them provide more effective parenting although he didn't necessarily work on this in front of the children. I sensed that he felt if the power lines between mom and dad were working in an active and engaged way, that they would do their parenting job in a way that was both helpful and hopeful. Walt did work on the children's communication with the mother, because they had also given up.

Walt felt that therapy must be relevant to be potent. There is no way to play at therapy, as demonstrated by Walt's jumping right into people's immediate problems. In this way, people could quickly come to grips with their existential crisis–and can get on with their lives. When Walt practiced his therapy, I was aware of an anxiety that moved from slight to great when I was in his presence. Yet, there was a feeling that no matter how the therapy came out, all parties concerned would be in a truer place, with themselves, with their partner and/or other family members. There was a session between a couple in which the truth that evolved was painful for both parties. Although both partners were reluctant to openly confront the truth, the session proceeded as follows.

The couple was not married, but had been living together for some time. The woman seemed to hang on to her boyfriend, and he showed an unwillingness to further the relationship. He had a desire to move on to what he anxiously felt might be greener pastures.

Walt worked with the couple and the couple's therapist in this session. He stated things so directly and clearly that the couple was forced to acknowledge the truth of their situation.

Walt   (To the therapist after talking a bit with the couple). She doesn't know that liking someone is not enough for a long-term commitment. She wants to know why he doesn't have those intentions. I like my car, but I'm not commited to it (existential moment).

Walt did not try to make things better between the couple. He picked up that the man did not show enough interest to stay, and in no way disaffirmed his position. On this basis the session proceeded. Initially, he commented that the man did not appear to be inspired by her. She didn't touch his life in a way that left him feeling that he could not live without her. While talking to the other therapist, he said she didn't turn him on, and saw sound commitment in a relationship as a consequence of irresistible desire, something beyond.

Walt   (To the woman) You are passionless when you talk to him. (Turning to the man) And you put up with it. That's not love. (To her) The person he's going to choose isn't going to put up with that.

(Walt tries to arouse her from her passive position. Then, continuing to the woman) It gets a little cold outside sometimes, so he likes to come in out of the rain. In his friendly way he's telling you, "I haven't got it for you, baby doll." (To the other therapist) Sometimes things need to be said in a hard way.

Man   (Sighs)

Walt   (To woman) What's missing for me is your reaction to his confirming sigh. I am afraid you are going to be calloused and bitter. It's better to go to the pain instead of your apparent and seemingly easy acceptance. I'm more interested in your pain than in your eagerness to learn things from me. I want to hear the pain, however you want to tell it to me.

Woman   It's painful not being needed. Knowing that I am not the number one person. (She stopped–almost after she began)

Walt   I don't think you have reached the end of your pain.

Woman   I don't want to be unsettled.

Walt   I'd like you to say goodbye to him, however you would like to say it. Being brave doesn't count. (She looks away from the man) You're looking the wrong way (While nodding toward the man).

Here is the dynamite again. Walt captured the essence of the couple's relationship with each other, and pushed for them to let go of a relationship that had died. He later commented that if there was *any hope* that the relationship could revive, it would come in part out of experiencing what was–in this case, for her, knowledge of the grief over the separation and a realization that he cared for her less than she hoped.

The man looked like he was going to start to cry.

Woman   If I said goodbye what kind of feelings would you have?

Walt   (Interrupting) That's not important. You do what you have to do.

A long period of time goes by.

Woman   Goodbye (Very weak).

Walt   You're not able to say it. Are you?

Woman   (Very weak) Yes.

Walt   It appears as though you are doing it for me.

Woman   I'm doing it for me and what kind of life I could have. (More feeling in her words).

Walt   You look like there is something you need from me to make it final.

Woman   It's final. It's been on the verge for quite awhile.

Walt   (To woman) I would feel it was more finished if I saw your grief. What's missing is there is no release in your words.

Woman   The crying has already been.

Walt   I think there is more. I don't see relief in your face.

Woman   But I feel it.

Walt   (To man) You know her better than I do. Do you feel she means it?

Man   Yes, but it doesn't have a bearing on my truth.

Walt   I'm sure you'll have more reacting in the next ten days. Your grief is blocked. If you get to the real crying of it, then you'll be better able to let him go. Otherwise you will have bitterness, cold anger. You're losing somebody who has been precious to you for a long time. (Turning toward the man) Do you want to say anything to her?

Man   Not now.

Walt   You have more to say. If you don't want to do it here, maybe we can get you a room.

Man   (To her–crying) It's really not your fault or mine. The truth I know is something we have to deal with. It's not going to go away. I was trying to avoid it to not go through the pain. I want to apologize, but there is nothing to apologize for.

Walt   I wonder if you wish that she could have captured you?

Man   It never occurred to me.

Walt   SOMEWHERE IN EVERY MAN THERE IS THE DESIRE THAT SOME GOOD WOMAN WILL COME UP AND CAPTURE HIM SO HE WILL HAVE SOMEONE ELSE TO LIVE FOR BESIDES HIMSELF. IF YOU MEET THE WOMAN AND IT HAPPENS TO YOU, YOU ARE GRATEFUL FOR THAT.

Other Therapist (To man) Is there anything left?

Man   Only sadness.

Walt   I think you are both entitled to that sadness. I'm
                       glad you have the sadness without taking it on as a
                       guilt. You are both losing somebody good.

End of session.

In the aftermath one of the workshop participants posed the question, would they have been able to work through their problems so they could have had a satisfying relationship? Walt responded by saying that it was a real separation issue for the two of them, and the issue should not be confronted. Hope can only come out of truth–not the therapist's reasons. Walt went on to comment that joining and separating both involved grieving.

Walt, My wife at the time, and Me

My wife and I were having some difficulties so we went to a three-day weekend workshop for couples given by Walt. The way in which we accommodated each other was responsible for a lack of freshness between us. My wife at the time was bitching about my flicking a cigar butt in the sink without cleaning it. I said that her request sounded reasonable. Walt asked if that is what I really wanted to do at that time–clean the cigar butt. I said no, that frankly it was the last thing on my mind. He told me to tell that to My wife at the time. We had used so many methods to come to agreements with each other that we were having one hell of a time sharing our differences in a lively and engaged way. Rather than My wife at the time developing herself, she would turn it back on me by blaming me. And I would try and do better? I would accommodate. My wife at the time was also quite insecure and kept her wants unknown to both herself and me. The result was a relationship in which at times I would feel tortured just walking into the room. My wife at the time had a sugar-sweet way of responding, and I felt tortured when she wasn't getting her needs met. I was too narcissistic to stop to try and figure out what her needs were, and she took no great pains to tell me. She always had a feeling that I shortchanged her–that she didn't get enough from me, while I always felt guilty–that I always owed more to someone who was depending on me.

An interesting exchange took place between myself and a woman at the workshop. She said that knowing the things I did, she wouldn't want to be married to me. I was trying hard to figure out what she meant in the way only a true obsessive can do. Suddenly I burst out, "I don't want to be married to you anyway." Walt laughed and said, "Now isn't that easier?" I never forgot that exchange because of its simplicity and the freshness I felt when I said it. My wife at the time got the message too. We began to talk to each other more simply. I want. I don't want. I want you to do this for me. We were beginning to feel each other as separate people. Things were getting better, but not great. I still had the feeling of being tortured. I still had the feeling that a large vacuum cleaner was sucking at my guts. I could actually feel My wife at the time doing it when she was in the kitchen below my study. I felt as if I were going to be sucked right through the floor. Some nights, without a word being said, I would feel as if little darts were being shot into my head. Sometimes I would really get angry and one of us would sleep downstairs. Neither one of us knew what to do about the impasse. We decided to see Walt for a private session.

We had a two and one-half hour session and were able to break our deadlocks so I never again was in doubt regarding my commitment to our marriage. It was the first time I ever felt that clear. When I felt the sucking feeling, Walt asked My wife at the time what she felt. She said that she felt insecure. However, her insecurities weren't coming from what I was doing with her. They were coming from the catastrophic fantasies she gave to herself. Len was going to leave. It wasn't going to work out. Things weren't going well at school. She would feel so insecure and tortured that even her presence would torture me.

Walt suggested I tell My wife at the time that I understood that she needed reassurance at that time. I hesitated, saying that I couldn't see any reason why I should reinforce her inability to deal with existential anxiety. Walt said that he understood my sensitivity to that issue and that if I did so it would not help My wife at the time grow. He said, however, that I did not have to do anything beyond telling her that, I *understood her need for reassurance.* This was alright with me because it took the feeling of obligation or demand off me (an existential moment for me).

After an hour and fifteen minutes we took a ten-minute break. Walt asked us if there was anything else we wanted. I said there was.

I still felt as if we couldn't break clean. We couldn't separate. I felt that My wife at the time was still hanging on which made me want to run away from her. Walt asked My wife at the time what she was feeling. She complained that I wasn't giving her enough, and felt deprived in both specific and non-specific ways. So did I. It seemed all she would do was nag at me. Walt suggested to My wife at the time that *all we both wanted was love and affection, and that we both felt deprived. He then told her she could say to me, "I've got an extra hug. Would you like one?"* (Another existential moment for me.) In that way she would be offering me something, and I wouldn't feel any need to respond to a demand, or perform. And I had a free choice to accept or reject her offer of a hug. Without telling me directly, I also got the message. To this day neither one of us has rejected that extra hug, and both of us continue to enrich each other's life. That's a hell of a lot for a little over one weekend's work! He made it possible for the generosity in both of us to appear.

Another issue I brought up with Walt was anger. I told him I was a bit disappointed that he had mellowed, because I wasn't sure if he could still help me with anger. He asked me what the problem was. I said that when I had been in different group situations, people would occasionally say they felt I was sitting on a lot of anger. However, that I thought I had been irritated, not angry. Walt said that he knew me well enough to trust my judgment on the matter, and the real problem was that I was making myself a patsy. He said I was appropriately fearful of those who were saying this to me because they had the anger and I was defenseless. I said I needed to challenge them on the matter, rather than just accept what people said about me as being the truth about me (existential moment). He said that I might want to begin experimenting so I could include strong anger responses into my repertoire, but that I might just prefer to stop making myself a patsy and not worry about it. Since that time I have challenged people much more when I feel others are projecting on me.

My Work With a Couple

I was seeing a man for individual psychotherapy and hypnosis. He was eating too much, drinking too much booze, and not exercising enough. As he had had seven years of analysis before coming to me, I sensed that he wasn't the type who was going to take control of his life. I thought of Walt and the idea that it was partly the partner's responsibility to stop someone from self-destructive behavior. I demanded he bring his wife into therapy.

During the session I told her that Jimmy was incapable of stopping himself from abusing himself mentally, physically, and sexually by overeating and drinking and that it was her job to stop him and to wake him up. She was angry. She said that he was a grown man, and that he was responsible for himself. I said that he obviously couldn't do it himself. I told her that it was her job to stop him. Maybe she felt it wasn't worth it, and there wasn't enough in it for her to take on such a big job. But if she wanted a relationship with him, that was her job. She moaned and bitched, complaining that he was an adult and that she feared such conflict. She also said that everytime he went near the refrigerator she told him to stop eating. I remembered what Walt had said in a similar situation, so I told her, "All you do is make him feel bad. You don't have to say anything to him. Just take the food and smash it all over his clothes. Or take the booze and pour it down the sink!" She looked shocked and even more fearful of such conflict. She said he probably wouldn't come home from work, that he would go drinking before he came home. I told her to meet him at the office or whatever she needed to do to get the job done. This was Walt's concept of responsible action, what one partner needed to do to help the other who was stuck due to their own passivity. I also told her that it was her job and responsibility for his erection; and that it was obvious that he was fearful and that he couldn't get it up. I told her to go after him, even if he said he didn't want sex, and even if he rejected her. I sensed that it was more a matter of fear on his part than not wanting sex.

The woman felt so threatened by the responsibility that she didn't come to the next session. I asked the man where she was and he said in an apologetic way, "She didn't feel like coming." In an aroused and almost screaming voice I said, "I don't give a shit if she feels like coming or not. Your life depends on her being here and it's your job to get her here. Don't come without her next week, even if you have to carry her over your shoulder."

Knowing that she had to come the next week, I expected that her anxiety would keep building. I had a hunch from her later report that she would rather take responsible action with her husband than face me if she hadn't. In any case, when she came in she said,

> I grabbed his bottle of wine and threw it down the
> sink. He got so mad he took his dinner and smashed
> it all over the floor. However, to my surprise his anger
> vanished quickly and he was quite pleased that he hadn't
> overeaten and he wasn't bombed out from drinking. On
> top of that our conversation was so stimulating that
> neither of us used the excuse that we were too tired to
> avoid sex.

The above example illustrates how partners can take responsible action. That is the *job of a partner.* Otherwise, *why would a person need a relationship*–that is, if that person could do everything by him or herself? And there is a job that each partner resists doing. That is a good deal of what marital couples therapy is about, as I have yet to meet a completely whole person. Of course, the responsibility becomes greater with obsessives who are insensitive to their partners' needs and with those who are stuck more into passive, dependent symbiotic roles. This is where "dynamite" becomes crucial. In the area of sex, I have found that sometimes assigning the responsibility for the man's erection to the woman, in any way she sees fit, has worked out very well in getting the couple sexually involved. Once the man doesn't feel threatened, and is assured that his woman will get him aroused, even when he has done his best to tire himself out by his obsessive behavior, he can begin to enjoy sex again. I tell women to go after their man even when he says no, that he really wants you to go after him, even when he rejects you. The kinds of dynamite I have described have helped couples move toward resolution in much quicker periods of time.

One woman described her reaction to the assignment of taking responsibility for her husband's erection in detail. My instructions were to go after him even if he tried to avoid her, not to take any of his rebuffs personally, and not to expect any cooperation on his part. When you go after somebody in an area in which he needs to be stopped, all you can expect is flack coming back at you. That's part of the job. She reported,

> For the first time I felt it was all right to be sexually
> assertive. What I want is all right. I had a sense of humor
> about it and didn't take any of his avoidances personally.
> I felt like going for it and had fun going through all the

resistance. One time I chased him all over the house, and finally chased him right onto the toilet seat, and we made it there. Ever since I found out it was all right to go for it, I didn't feel the same pressure about having to have sex. I didn't have any tension and I wasn't feeling sorry for myself. I used to get wrapped up in my own feelings instead of paying attention to my husband's reaction (narcissistic involvement with self as opposed to having sex with partner in an involved way). I now feel freer to feel my own sexuality. I opened the gate and said I can be what I want to be. There is something nice about being responsible for my husband's reaction, but in general it took the pressure off because I don't want to fail (it reversed the pressure point in sex. It's usually on the male). I feel a lot freer and we are both enjoying sex more without pressure.

(Perhaps the pressure technique I suggested helped the woman empathize with her husband's pressure on himself.)

I had found that telling people what they ought to do to live more effectively, when indeed I did not know what they ought to do at either conscious or unconscious levels, or in specific behavioral terms (behavioral prescriptions) was not an abuse of power on my part but a presentation of a hope founded in the reality between patients and therapists, and that it indeed gave patients the opportunity to resolve major issues in their lives that had been preventing them from living as fully as they might. These moments of impact are existential moments.

CREATIVE EXPRESSION AND SENSORY PERCEPTION, WITH BOB MARTIN, D.S.W.

I have always viewed one of the goals of gestalt therapy as coming as fully alive in the moment as one dare. In this context I had the good fortune to experience Dr. Bob Martin, in a weekend marathon. It is my hope that this section will provide the reader with some feel for the sense of creative expression, vitality, joy, and sensitivity I experienced in working with Bob.

He is able to respond to his highly developed sensitivity in a split second while almost simultaneously helping the client respond, too. He provides the opportunity for clients to experience joy much of the time, by facilitating creative expression. He encourages people to act in ways that their self-images would never permit–until they once again experience the joy of living.

I had worked with Bob years before, but personality differences had caused a strained relationship, although I had always respected him as a mentor. How we came to work together after seven years was strange in itself. I was part of an ongoing training program in gestalt therapy and the group elected to have a weekend marathon with Bob. I did not vote. Part of me was stubborn while the other part was secretly glad that I was going to have the opportunity to work with him again.

The marathon was at a motel suite in LaJolla. I drove to the wrong motel at first and was one-half hour late. How's that for resistance! When I walked in there was a tension in the group. They knew of the bad blood between Bob and me. Bob began by asking people what they wanted for themselves and I was seated in a way where I was out of his view after having come in quietly. When his attention came around to me, we stared at each other. There was a look of hatred, fear, and wariness in his eyes that left me feeling he could have killed me at that moment. Later Bob verified my assessment. I thought, "It's going to be a long weekend!" However, in the very next moment Bob was able to transform himself and I knew that he knew I was in a much different place with myself than seven years before. I also knew that he had changed, seeing him switch from hate to warmth. We had both been on the path to become more compassionate people.

He asked me what I wanted. I told him I wanted to see how he worked with creative process and how he integrated that into gestalt therapy. Then he stunned me for the second time. It was as if he were inside my head, because he started to turn away but came back and said, "And is there anything else you want to say to me?" in a way that he knew there was. I replied that I also wondered how we were going to get along this time. A woman in the group asked me if I had a bad experience with Bob in the past. Although it was bad at the conscious level, at the unconscious level I felt it was a good experience, so I said, "No, it wasn't bad, but let's just say it was very provocative." She said, "Oh, you mean you provoked Bob the way you provoke us." The entire group laughed. At that moment everyone knew the rest of the weekend would go well. But no one knew how well!

There was another time that first evening that Bob looked at me and said, "You want to ask me some things in the group and you want to ask me something in private." I was shocked; there was indeed a very personal issue that I was thinking about asking him privately.

He would say and do things like that throughout the weekend. It was eerie in a way. I began to feel I couldn't keep a secret from him even if I wanted to, but that level of communication and understanding felt so clear that I found my risk-taking level and willingness increasing rapidly. He had developed his sensitivities to an extraordinary level. The other phenomenon was that the group continued to increase to higher and higher levels of vitality. There were times when I felt so much vitality that I could jump right out of my skin. Bob's sense of aliveness was catching.

Bob was working with one fellow who was deadening and took great unconscious pride in hanging therapists out to dry. Bob gave it his best shot and wasn't getting anywhere with the fellow. He turned it around beautifully. He got up and began to dance around the man in a circle singing, "I dunno what to do with you. I dunno what to do with you. Oh, I just dunno what to do with you." The entire group was laughing. Even the patient himself was laughing–knowing that he had met his match, and that his match had actually gotten to him with playful joy. Bob made a difficult situation look very easy because he, for the entire weekend, gave himself permission to do the absurd, the foolish, the unheard of. I was admiring of his creative play. While working with me he began to sing something about my having the disease of seriosity. Yet, how could I maintain the disease with Bob dancing, singing and playfully spoofing me when I was unconsciously attempting to make myself joyless? He encouraged me to sing in a high-pitched voice while I was dancing. My eyes became much brighter, the ground looked much closer and I lost my fear of falling. I have had more fun in all of my sessions and my life since that weekend. I find myself singing, dancing around, willing to risk making an ass of myself. Patients love it. I love it too. Thank you, Bob!

Bob not only had a sense of aliveness in himself that was beautiful to experience, but he helped all of us provide it for each other. In many ways each of the group members had particular idiosyncracies that we preferred to avoid displaying in public. Bob helped to set a situation in motion that let each member of the group break through the stultifying death of living up to their self-images. At the end of this group experience, I felt the freest I had ever felt in my life and the freest I have ever felt with a group of people. The situation began to unfold between Bob and another psychologist who was a trainee in the group.

Bob	I'll bet you're really weird. (Of course, this comment must be taken in the context with which Bob said it. The group had been together for some time, and we were not threatened by such a comment.)
Psychologist	(Pausing, making his eyebrows come together in a frown for about thirty seconds before answering) I am really weird.
Bob	I'll bet you have the weirdest stuff in you I could ever imagine.
Psychologist	(Another long pause with eyebrows frowning) You're right. I do have the weirdest stuff in me you could ever imagine. But I would never show those parts of me to anyone.
Bob	I'll bet you could become the director for the maddest play this group will have ever imagined or experienced by casting each of the group members.
Psychologist	(An even longer pause, then jumps to his feet with a twisted face and shriek that made Boris Karloff seem tame)

Half hunched and crouched, in a weird voice he began to approach people in the group, giving them instructions on the roles they were to play. This psychologist had a brilliant and creative unconscious, but often depressed himself by avoiding going with his unconscious. It was obvious that he feared his own weirdness and was making his life joyless by doing so. That is, it was obvious after Bob picked it out of thin air.

The psychologist was really getting into it. Of course, the things he asked people to do were acted out symbolically, and not actually done in reality.

The psychologist ran up to a woman who had beat around the bush about her sexual desires in the group. He told her he wanted her to be a nymphomanic. She was to fuck men, women, tree stumps, anything and everybody she could find.

He went over to a psychiatrist and told him he wanted him to lie down in the middle of the floor and masturbate. What an eye the psychologist had! For when the psychiatrist was stuck in his communications, they did have a masturbatory quality.

He went over to the first lady's boyfriend and asked him to be the most beautiful woman in the group, using a pink scarf to seduce men and women. The man was given an opportunity to symbolically act out his bisexual fantasies publicly. Perhaps this is an issue that most people never get the chance to deal with, yet, I have seen very few patients whose sexual makeup was either all male or all female. However, they must be all one or the other to fit into society's mold–thereby hampering their creative expression.

The psychologist asked Bob to continue to roll around the floor as if he were a ball. My hunch about Bob is that he is so sensitive and alive that stability becomes a problem for him.

He asked another woman to pretend she didn't see anything. To just sit there and be catatonic while all this sinful, evil, weird and immoral behavior was going on. This was similar to the passive behavior in which she engaged, the rage she denied.

He told a physician in the group that he wanted him to be god and to take care of all his people. This was precisely the issue this internist was struggling with in his daily existence, being severely overweight from taking care of all but himself.

He asked another woman to be a tiger and crawl around the floor leaping on people while she was using all her power.

He asked another woman to be a little mouse, who near the end of the play could turn into anything she wanted to, even a beautiful woman. At the end of the three-year program she did indeed turn into a beautiful woman.

Another woman was asked to be a madonna-whore, who while she acted lustfully kept the expression of a madonna on her face.

A man who had paranoid tendencies and nearly always was more interested in looking good than in expressing himself was told that while everyone else in the group was engaging in this sinful and weird behavior, he was to be the only sane one. At the end of the mad play, this fellow was the only one who didn't have a good time and didn't enjoy his role, but that was therapeutic, for he could see where his lack of self-expression left him in life.

Another fellow, who had so much oppression and poison in his system, despite his good intentions, was asked to go around behind people when they were acting out their madness, stab them in the heart, and kill them. This was tantamount to what he had been doing on a psychic level.

The psychologist then approached me and told me to stand up, and while all these people were engaging in this sinful, crazy, weird and evil behavior, that I must become their minister, and preach to them and convert them (a familiar but embarrassing request).

Well, everyone began acting out their roles. But while I was preaching to the psychiatrist who was in the middle of the floor pretending to masturbate, the woman who was requested to be a nymphomaniac came up from behind me and started rubbing her breasts and her crotch into my backside while her boyfriend came up from the front and began twirling his pink scarf around my head. I must admit I was rapidly losing enthusiasm for the preaching. Especially when a man came up from behind and stabbed me in the heart.

As you can see, there was some unexpressed part of our characters that was keeping us joyless, and Bob set up a situation in which the other psychologist could tap into his extensive unconscious potential and help get to that strain in each of us.

The result: High vitality and joy!

Thank you again, Dr. Bob Martin.

Although they have differences in style, we have seen five extremely well-balanced therapists, with a wide variance in responsiveness, make an impact on me and others in both similar and different ways. Miriam, Erv, Jim, Walt and Bob are all stylistic therapists. Each has great range in reaching the extremes of human emotional development. Each has the capacity to work from an "I" or "Thou" frame of reference, and to flow with whichever is appropriate at the moment. Most important, each leans toward ways that are congruent with their own personal nature. This is vital to remember when developing a personal and effective style of working. What is presented in this chapter and throughout the book are ways of learning about different methods experimenting with them until the right style of working becomes second nature. In this way, each therapist will find his or her personal style and way of making the greatest impact possible to help patients change their lives at the more primal levels of human existence. And it is in this way that therapists can best help patients experience existential moments that become imbedded in patients' minds and can be used over and over again to help patients change their behavior.

Walter Kempler, M.D.
Original Gestalt–Experiential Family Therapist

My major professor at University of Southern California (USC), Dr. Bill Ofman, said, "Hey, you ought to look up Walter Kempler. I think he would like you." Around 1977 I was building a private practice and I called him. We met. He said "If you ever want to see me again you will have to pay me." I thought I had written him off permanently after that but something tugged at me and I went to a family therapy workshop he gave in Phoenix in 1977. After seeing him work I understood why he said what he said. He thought I did not give him enough credit for the experience and differences between us at our respective stages of career development. So began a nine-year training experience in gestalt–experiential family therapy as well as a friendship in which he accompanied my mandolin on his tenor banjo.

Walt gave me a picture of himself taken in front of my home where he was holding up a rose and smelling it. He was a "natural" and no matter what kind of therapy I do or did his spirit is always with me—he was a creative genius going outside the box and never giving in to the projected hopelessness of patients or for that matter letting them give into it.

Walt would not see individual patients. In the Phoenix workshop he persuaded the wife to

get the whole family mobilized, which included her husband, their children, and their grandchildren—nine people in all. He was excellent at utilizing the naturalness of children as a healing resource from which the family could build and heal itself. His book *Principles of Gestalt Family Therapy: A Gestalt–Experiential Handbook* (1973) is magnificent.

As I matured in my work I developed the ability in some cases to evoke "an existential shift" in family members in one to three sessions. Prior to my knowing that I had any ability for this kind of work, Kempler was always chastising me for not curing patients in one session. Before I knew that shifts in family dynamics could happen that quickly, I thought he was just giving me a crazy idea as one-upmanship. He was serious!

He thought of family therapy as the therapist's therapeutic use of self, "warts and all, as giving patients something to rub up against, and *that* authenticity then had a healing effect on the family by showing them that they each and every one could be themselves and have something of value to contribute to the family as a whole." So it wasn't so much his technique that affected me for the rest of my life, it was his "naturalness" in his attitude toward and use of himself in the work, and in the way we hung out together.

However, in terms of technique, he did work smoothly like a Rolls Royce engine. He did not see each family on a regular basis. He charged a healthy fee at the time, $300 an hour, to provide a one-of-a-kind service. He would work for two to six straight hours until he gave the family something to work with that was considered to be a resolution to the problem. That way, the family might never have to come back again, or if they did it was rarely before six months, as they had a lot to work with.

Walt believed that family members—the not being able to live with them and the not being able to live without them, and the unbearable pain all that causes—was the only true motivation for therapeutic change, and he did not want to waste his time doing anything else but family therapy. I was fortunate to have known him and to have been trained by him.

LEN BERGANTINO, a Clinical Psychologist licensed in California, Arizona, and Hawaii, and Diplomate in Family Psychology, American Board of Professional Psychology, is currently working with families in their homes or telephonically 310/207-939".

ENDNOTES

1   Erving Polster, "Stolen by Gypsies," in Twelve Therapists, ed. Arthur Burton. (San Francisco: Jossey-Bass Publishers, 1972), p. 155.

2   Ibid.

3   Erving Polster and Miriam Polster, "Therapy without Resistance: Gestalt Therapy," in What Makes Behavior Change Possible? ed. Arthur Burton (New York: Brunner/Mazel, 1976), p. 263.

4   Ibid., p. 273.

5   Miriam Polster, conversation with author, 1978.

REFERENCES

Kempler, Walter. *Principles of Gestalt Family Therapy* (published by the author, 1973). For each copy, send $10 to The Kempler Institute, P.O. Box 1692, Costa Mesa, CA 92626.

***I WILL PAY FOR THE TELEPHONE CALL. YOU PAY FOR THE SPEAKERPHONE WITH THREE GENERATIONAL FAMILY THERAPY. GRANDPARENTS CAN BE PLAYED IN FROM STATES OTHER THAN CA, AZ, HI!!!

Polster, Erving, "Stolen by Gypsies." In *Twelve Therapists*. Edited by Arthur Burton. San Francisco: Jossey-Bass Publishers, 1972.

Polster, Erving, and Polster, Miriam. "Therapy without Resistance: Gestalt Therapy." In *What Makes Behavior Change Possible?* Edited by Arthur Burton. New York: Brunner/Mazel, 1976.

Polster, Erving, and Polster, Miriam. *Gestalt Therapy Integrated.* New York: Brunner/Mazel, 1973.

Simkin, James S. *Gestalt Therapy Mini-Lectures.* Millbrae, Calif.: Celestial Arts, 1974.

PsychDirectory   About Us | Basic Listing | Sponsored Listings | Contact Us   » Submit New Listing

» Psych User Login

Mental Health > Psychology > Psychologist in West Los Angeles

Home Page   Psychology Psychiatry Psychoanalysis Psychotherapy

Directory Index | Mental Health Professionals | Psychology | Psychologists

Mental Health Professionals

Education and Training

***I WILL PAY FOR THE TELEPHONE CALL. YOU PAY FOR THE SPEAKERPHONE AND THE TWO OR THREE GENERATIONAL FAMILY THERAPY. GRANDPARENTS CAN BE PLAYED IN FROM STATES OTHER THAN CA, AZ, HI!

Directory Search

[ ] find

Find a Psychologist
Advanced Search

Psychological Testing/Evaluation

Psychology Psychiatry Psychoanalysis Psychotherapy

Directory Index > Mental Health Professionals > Psychology > Psychologists

Mental Health & Social Services

Organizations Centers & Institutes

Mental Health & Psychology News

»» Job Search Mental Health Jobs

THREE GENERATIONAL INTERSTATE TELEPHONIC FAMILY THERAPY / TRAINING / SUPERVISION-DR. LEN BERGANTINO

Name/Company: THREE GENERATIONAL INTERSTATE TELEPHONIC FAMILY THERAPY / TRAINING / SUPERVISION-DR. LEN BERGANTINO premium updated

Description: DR. BERGANTINO – A LICENSED PSYCHOLOGIST IN CA, AZ & HI
DIPLOMATE IN FAMILY PSYCHOLOGY – AMERICAN BOARD OF PROFESSIONAL PSYCHOLOGY
THREE GENERATIONAL INTERSTATE TELEPHONIC FAMILY THERAPY WAS TAUGHT TO ME BY WORLD RENOWN PIONEER CARL WHITAKER, M.D.
IDENTIFIED PATIENT MUST RESIDE IN CA, AZ OR HI, BUT OTHER COLLATERAL FAMILY MEMBERS CAN BE IN ANY STATE OF THE FIFTY
THIS KIND OF FAMILY THERAPY HAS A CHANCE TO:
1. Create a shift so that what does not work in a family now works (sometimes in 3 sessions)
2. Evoke a psychosexual heat among the married couple in the nuclear family
3. Teach each family member what his/her value is to the family as a whole-as in gestalt family therapy the whole is greater than the sum of its parts
4. Give grandparents a way to contribute to the family's well-being without being a burden and to die with a clean slate between them and their children
5. Utilize the spontaneity of the grandchildren to bring value to the entire family
CALL AT 310-207-9397

Country: United States

State: California

City: West Los Angeles, CA

ZIP / Postal Code: 90025

Phone: 310-207-9397

Contact Person: Dr. Len Bergantino

Map / route: View map / route

E-Mail Address: Send message

URL / Website: http://s1.webstarts.com/lenbergantino/

Classification(s):

- Mental Health Professionals | Psychology / Psychologists
- Mental Health Professionals | Psychotherapy / Psychotherapists
- Mental Health Professionals | Psychotherapy / Other

What the Reviewers Say:
Psychotherapy, Insight and Style
The Existential Moment
by Len Bergantino, Ed. D., ABPP

_The book sells for $26.95 / Send check to _1215 Brockton Ave. #104, Los Angeles, C_ 90025_
Interested? Contact Dr.Bergantino / (310) 207-8818

Dr. Carl A. Whitaker, M.D. Professor of Psychiatry / School of Medicine, University of Wisconsin

"The plethora of how-to books is increasing. Barbara Betz stated that the dynamics of psychotherapy is in the person of the therapist. Abraham Maslow stated the the peak experience lasts two weeks. Winicott insisted that if you haven't been hated by your psychotherapist you have been cheated. Ehrenwald has stated that psychotherapy is the effort to evolve an existential shift.

Len Bergantino is trying to expand this operational territory by stretching the psychotherapeutic geology He succeeds. Describing the therapist as a person of liberated wisdom, he dares to the chaos and anxiety of not knowing; he opens a gate to see and make the impact of psychotherapy more clearly. His description of beingness as a process is reminiscent of Paul Tillich. His grasp of responsible involvement with the patient as a discipline of self shows his own search for creative options. He makes no pretense of camouflaging the psychotherapist as a wounded healer. Furthermore, Len makes crucial the pattern of the therapist's search for his own healing and successfully validates the authentic trickery of the psychotherapist as a liberated spirit. The approach to his own craziness, the freedom from the culture bind, and the discipline of self each emerged as obtainable goals of that professional parent we call the psychotherapist.

Further evidence of his own search is illustrated by his impersonalized impressionistic response to the other searchers he uses as models. Simply reading his book leaves me feeling it would be meaningful to join in his search for his beingness. Though he would be enjoying himself and enjoying me as a patient, he would not be doing things to keep from being himself and thus I could be more fully myself."

Dr. Donald Rinsley, M.D., F. R.S.H. Fellow, American College of Psychoanalysts in his

review of Dr. Bergantino's book published in Bulletin of the Menninger Clinic, Vol. 47, No. 5, September, 1983 wrote:

"The book reflects the personal odyssey of a trained, disciplined yet openminded professional psychologist who has drunk at the wells of an number of acknowledged healer-therapists whose work he has carefully studied and evaluated, among them, Viktor Frankl, Wilfred Bion, the Gouldings, Frederick Perls, Milton Erickson and Carl Whitaker. A unique feature of Dr. Bergantino's presentation is his detailed accounts of these therapists' hour-to-hour work, drawn from his own personal experience and from verbatim descriptions provided by their students and analysands, offering fascinating and instructive insights into the therapeutic labors of admittedly gifted treaters."

Dr. Martin Grotjahn, M.D., Training andSupervising Analyst Emeritus, Southern California

Psychoanalytic Institute, in a pre-publication review wrote:

"Dr. Bergantino is obviously a gifted therapist ...Most cases as reported in the literature describe the patient's associations and productions while the therapist remains hidden in the mystery of darkness unrevealed. Dr. B is an exception: the great advantage of his work is the openess and frankness with which the author reveals his experiences when treating patients or when accepting himself as a patient of another therapist.

Dr. Walter Kempler, M.D. The Kempler Institute - Costa Mesa, CA

"Len's writing is intelligent and lucid...engrossing......
I think his book is valuable...an interesting and propelling work...His ideas ride the crest of current thought in the field, provides clean reviews of popular modes, formulates in the popular jargon of the day using traditional interpretions and terminology. His personal touch is enchancing."

Dr. James S. Simkin, Ph.D. American Board of Examiners in Professional Psychology - Big Sur, CA

"Professionals could benefit directly from this book in that Bergantino describes how it is possible to integrate a variety of psychotherapeutic approaches."

Dr. Ernest Lawrence Rossi, Ph.D. Diplomate in Clinical Psychology - Los Angeles, CA

"A deeply moving flood of insights and approaches to becoming oneself as a psychotherapist....It is a highly readable record of (Bergantino's) development as a therapist via his personal contacts and training with a variety of current-day psychotherapists...a new understanding of what it means to be a creative therapist continually living in the present's potential for change and transformation...
....focuses on the precise and often provocative and shocking techniques that are useful in helping patients break out of their learned limitations to realize their potentials for creative change."

*This book is being republished by Jason Aronson Publishers Inc. as part of The Master Classic Series under a new title, Moments of Impact in Psychotherapy: How The Masters Interrege

LEN BERGANTINO Ed. D., ABPP
In-Depth Family Therapy • Ericksonian Hypnosis
American Board of Professional Psychology • Diplomate in Family Psychology

Foreword
Making an Impact in Therapy:
How Master Clinicians Intervene

Len Bergantino, Ed.D., Ph.D.

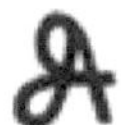

JASON ARONSON INC.
Northvale, New Jersey
London

The plethora of how-to books is increasing. This is not one of those. Barbara Betz stated that the dynamics of psychotherapy is in the person of the therapist. Abraham Maslow stated that the peak experience lasts two weeks. Winicott insisted that if you haven't been hated by your psychotherapist you have been cheated. Erenwald has stated that psychotherapy is the effort to evolve an existential shift.

Len Bergantino is trying to expand this operational territory by stretching the psychotherapeutic geology. He succeeds. Describing the therapist as a person of liberated wisdom, he dares to the chaos and anxiety of not knowing; he opens a gate to see and make the impact of psychotherapy more clearly. His description of beingness as a process is reminiscent of Paul Tillich. His grasp of responsible involvement with the patient as a discipline of self shows his own search for creative options. He makes no pretense of camouflaging the psychotherapist as a wounded healer. Furthermore, Len makes crucial the pattern of the therapist's search for his own healing and successfully validates the authentic trickery of the psychotherapist as a liberated spirit. The approach to his own craziness, the freedom from the culture bind, and the discipline of self each emerged as obtainable goals of that professional parent we call the psychotherapist.

Further evidence of his own search is illustrated by his impersonalized impressionistic response to the other searchers he uses as models.

Simply reading his book leaves me feeling it would be meaningful to join in his search for his beingness. Though he would be enjoying himself and enjoying me as a patient, he would not be doing things to keep from being himself and thus I could be more fully myself.

Carl A. Whitaker, M.D.
Professor of Psychiatry
School of Medicine
University of Wisconsin

7

The Somatic Therapy of Stanley Keleman

S TANLEY KELEMAN IS a therapist and author residing in Berkeley, California, and is associate editor of *The Journal of Biological Experience*. His concern is with body process as the basis for how individuals form themselves and their worlds. Using a combination of physical and psychological approaches, his focus is on the language of biological process, the differing states of excitement and feeling, and the way these find expression in image and action. He has published five books: *Your Body Speaks Its Mind, The Human Ground/Sexuality/Self and Survival, Living Your Dying, Todtmoos,* and *Somatic Reality.* He is director of The Center for Energetic Studies in Berkeley, California.

Body therapy focus is on increased experiencing. Body therapy certainly falls within the realm of existential therapy and philosophy by adding its existential moments in a therapy that can help people to reclaim themselves and to unify themselves. Body therapy is a way people can learn to reduce the three kinds of lies–lying for oneself, lying for others, and lying in the world (described by Keen earlier in the book). Although I had done much to reduce these lies in myself at an intellectual level, which is useful in more talk-oriented therapies, I had not been able to do so physically. The body therapy process got me started in a more physically honest direction, and is truly existential in its goals of pursuing unity within people, unity of *head* with *body*, and of body with *heart*.

From an existential point of view we will have an opportunity to observe Stanley staying with me one step at a time, while he was responding and being with me, having had the courage to be with himself physically at very deep levels. We will see him respond in a confrontive way when he refuses to work with Clara, and how that refusal had a variety of therapeutic consequences for her. Stanley's concern was on being all that he could with her, and there was a trust that she would do what she needed to do for herself. This trust in her unconscious processes is congruent with existential and other therapies that help people take responsibility for their own lives.

As my exposure to body therapy has been brief, this chapter has only been written so that those practicing body therapy may profit from existential philosophy and what existential moment may offer them; and so that those existentialists who are having difficulty reducing the physical tightenings of the body that have been a result of the dehumanization process since birth may reunite their bodies with their heads and hearts, and by so doing become truly existential. This physical unity will also make for truer levels of responding. The ideas and experiences which I write about are taken from two one-day workshops with Stanley Keleman.

Through Stanley I was able to grasp how to shift my focus of attention out of my head and into my body, a major breakthrough. Also, I was able to learn to behave in ways that would actually reduce the tension in my right shoulder, stress that I had lived with for several years. Although the process of body therapy was new to me, the step-by-step process was similar enough to gestalt therapy to integrate it into my style. The difference between the gestalt focus on one step at a time in following the patient's process, and Stanley's following one step at a time, is that Stanley's focus was primarily on what people were doing and how they were doing it with their bodies. The focus on body process was keener than I had ever seen before, and can give people a new kind of awareness. If people know exactly what steps to follow in their thinking and body movements in order to change destructive patterns, they certainly are in a much better place to begin to experience more.

The end result of Stanley's work with me was a feeling of pleasant relief that was an existential moment. Gestalt therapists might refer to it as closure, the difference being that the closure was an actual relief of bodily pressure. The tension was actually gone in my right shoulder and I had learned how to keep the shoulder loose both in bodily function and thought process. This same process might also happen in gestalt therapy, but it would be more by chance than by design.

As I am writing a book about existential therapy, and existential moments, one might ask how I see body therapy fitting into this framework. First, Stanley made it clear that for him to work with people they must talk about things in the context of their lives. So there was a focus on how people constructed their existence. Second, Stanley could touch people in a way that was comprised of existential moments–person-to-person–direct communication. Third, the focus on increased physical awareness is necessary if people are to give meaning to their existence that is rooted in their experience.

Let us take a look at that work itself and you will begin to see how the process unfolds and how the principles I describe appear in the work. Throughout the work Stanley's thrust was toward helping us become familiar with our somatic reality; to grasp the experience of how our bodies function.

Stanley gave the group a clear picture of what he wanted from the people with whom he was working. One woman, Clara, said she wanted to work but just waited. It looked like she wanted Stanley to work without her taking responsibility for herself. Stanley told her he didn't think she was ready to work and he wanted to go on to someone else. Their subsequent interaction created an existential moment between them.

Clara   I really resent what you just did. I'm unclear about what it is you want.

Stanley   I said that the only way I knew how to work that made sense to me was for people to put whatever they wanted to work on in the context of their lives. Are people dealing with their situation in life? When a person says they want to enter the process of working individually and are not prepared to do that, I take it as a sign that the person is not ready. It's been an extraordinary indicator to me about where therapy goes and where the therapeutic situation goes, as well as the relationships between people. I notice whether people really have something going on in their lives that's scaring the hell out of them, and if they want to get down to business. When this does not take place I would prefer not to deal with the situation. I don't see that you are prepared except in the most, "Well, I would like to work at it," and I don't feel that attitude is sufficient. You may resent me. There's nothing I can do about that.

Clara

I still feel confused.

Stanley

(Giving her another chance to stop playing at being confused) I said that I would be happy to work with people individually; however, in order to put the work situation in a context which I can handle I need to know where you stand in relationship to your life. That's what it means to work physically. You can't just say here I am. I have a pain in my back. What does it mean?

Clara

And I thought I said to you, do you want me to tell you what's happening with me right now in my life? And you said bullshit!

Stanley

I still feel my judgment is right. (Stan responded very quickly from his intuition, but he was right in the fact that the woman was more interested in proving he was wrong than in beginning to tell him about her situation.)

Clara	I feel like I don't belong. (She gets up and leaves the group room.)

To this point we have seen Stanley deal existentially with Clara. He did not let himself get bear-trapped into working with someone who wasn't going to do anything for herself as a result of her confusion game. Following these interchanges I worked with Stanley for about a half hour and another woman had been working about twenty minutes when Clara came barging back into the room and screamed at Stanley at the top of her lungs.

Clara	Stanley, I want you to know I think you are an arrogant, pompous, inconsiderate ass. And for you to–
Stanley	Thank you.
Clara	Call whatever it is you do therapeutic, it's crazy.
Stanley	Thank you.

Although Stanley was interrupted by the woman he thanked her for her genuine communications. The extreme reaction surprised me, but she was behind her words for the first time. Now for a look at the process that was so helpful to me.

Me	My dilemma is that I am so driven by my work that I don't pay attention to my body. About once every couple of months I just collapse. I get sick. Then as soon as I feel better, I'm back at it feeling as if I need to make up for lost time. I wonder if I'm going to give myself a heart attack and I'm scared about that.
Stanley	About the collapsing or the disconnection?
Me	Both. I feel a lack of richness in my life when I don't feel me. I know it intellectually, but that doesn't seem to help me know it experientially. I

feel a lack of substance. A lack of solidity about myself. I feel that the way I go about things in life is impoverished, and yet I have a way to trick myself so that I don't feel the body pain until I collapse. If I can't feel my body motivating me to do otherwise, I feel stuck. My head and my images rule me.

Stanley   How do you feel that you are impoverished?

Me   When you said that there was just a little sensation in my gut, but not much. Not much feeling.

Stanley   How do you think you do it to yourself?

Me   I think all my focus of attention is in my head.

Stanley   How does it get there?

Me   I think about everything. I'm blank. Nothing's coming.

Stanley   What is the image of thinking that you have?

Me   If I think about things hard enough, all the answers will come.

Stanley   But how is that? What is the acting process that you are in?

Me   I just heard what you said and now I'm sitting with it and I'm thinking, well, if I spin around what Stanley says long enough, something's going to come up for me that's important.

Stanley   What's spinning around?

About this point in the work you can begin to see how Stanley stays with me step-by-step in dogged pursuit of my bodily process.

Me	I put the information in my head and try to make something of what you said in terms of . . .
Stanley	How do you try to make something?
Me	I try to fit something that is meaningful from my frame of existence.
Stanley	How do you do that?
Me	I don't know. I don't know. I'm blanking.
Stanley	You have a process in which you think that if you agitate one set of emotions with another set of emotions, that if you pair them, you will undergo a process of deduction that will let you come up with certain answers. That's what you mean by working hard. Now I want to know how do you get your head to function?
Me	I concentrate.
Stanley	What is it that you have to do to yourself to commit that activity?
Me	I have to put total concentration–all my energy . . .
Stanley	No, concentration is a physical activity. How do you do it?
Me	I tighten my shoulders.
Stanley	Thank you.
Me	I tighten my neck.
Stanley	Thank you.

Me   And I strain.

Stanley   It sounds like you're taking a shit. (Laughter) Sorry, I just couldn't resist that part. OK, let's back up now. Tighten your shoulders.

Me   Yes, I am tightening them.

Stanley   You tighten your neck. And you strain.

Me   And I strain (while straining).

Stanley   This is the attitude of thinking. The action you make. Let's start again. Len is going to think. Right? Tighten your shoulders. What does that do for you?

Me   I'm attending to the pain in the shoulders and I just . . .

Stanley   Wait a minute. There's no pain there.

Me   I'm tightening pretty tight.

Stanley   You don't have to hurt yourself. Just tighten. Let me know what it does for you.

Me   It makes me feel alert. Ready to . . .

Stanley   What part of you feels alert?

Me   Right from my toes, up, like I could spring.

Stanley   OK. Next step. You're tightening your throat. And the back of your neck. Now let's see what that does for you.

Me   I'm feeling very weary.

Stanley	What does that do for you?
Me	Not much.
Stanley	All right. Tighten your neck. I understand the arms and shoulders, now, but I haven't understood the neck part. Don't think about it, do it.
Me	When I produce that kind of tension, it makes me at least believe that I'm more alert. (I'm doing it)
Stanley	Now what does that give you?
Me	Pain. Pain in my shoulder and my neck.
Stanley	What else? What's the end product of what it gives you?
Me	A sense of feeling safe. I can move in any direction quickly.
Stanley	Only your shoulders. What does that do for you inside? What does that do to your excitement? Your feeling?
Me	All my concentration is on the shoulders.
Stanley	What does that mean?
Me	There's no concentration anywhere else.
Stanley	Thank you. Now tightening up. What does that do for you inside?
Me	Even less concentration from the shoulders down. All the concentration is on my discomfort.
Stanley	Strain. Now what?

Me

I feel like it's going to be a long day. (Group laughs)

Stanley

There are a couple of things that are going on. Everything that you've done has isolated the head from the body in a series of degrees with escalating intensity. Concentration, preparation, isolate the head from the body. OK. (He pauses to make sure I have integrated what he said.) Statement number two is that the first statement of readiness is what you call alertness. Getting ready. Now how do you take that state of readiness for alertness and transfer in that way? That is, divorce it from body feeling and keep it in the brain?

Me

By the tightening.

Stanley

The tightening is the attitude of alertness. Now you're ready. You now have an alert pattern. A readiness to attack. To deal with something. Right? But you're not going to do this physically. You're going to do it mentally. Right? How do you do it?

Me

OK, I figure you're not going to do anything physically, so all I need to do is figure you out.

Stanley

We're talking about figuring the problem out.

Me

But I make you my problem.

Stanley

I'm not going to do anything to you. Now what?

Me

I was keeping the tension, but your reassurance makes me feel I don't need it anymore.

Stanley

But then you won't be able to think.

Me

It feels that way. I mean when I just let go, I fogged out again.

Stanley   Maybe you're not a thinker. (Group laughter)

Me   Well, I can think when my body is tight.

Stanley   I understand that. You're ready to fight.

Me   Yeah, and as soon as I let go I had no answer for what you said.

Stanley   You'll never make it up in the world without a dream, right?

Me   Right. I have to be at constant attention all the time. I loosened up and I just fogged out. Boy, that's frustrating.

Stanley   But now wait a second. You think that creation is the result of good thinking and figuring things out. That's not the way I see things. I feel that stipulation comes in, it goes through a process of digestion and assimilation, and then one has something, you and your life. OK. You keep things in a closed circuit auditorium. We're talking about being now impoverished. We are looking at the mechanism of impoverishment somatically (in terms of the body). One of the things that comes up along the way is are you in fact a thinker or do you see the brain as the problem-solver, the question/answerer, and everything else that has been dismissed? Or are you a thinker, a feeler, a senser, or a dreamer, or an imaginer, or a pleasure-seeker? Or are you turning yourself into another cog in the mind term machine? You may be a thinker. I don't know that you're not. I'm simply asking the question. Are you?

Me   It doesn't feel natural. It feels like hard work for me.

Stanley Well, thinking is hard work. But there's all kinds of thinking. And I think that you are restrained by a particular model of thinking.

In the last few paragraphs Stanley is educating me about some childlike misconceptions of thinking and childlike behavioral habits that are limiting. Stanley views educating, as well as working on process as being a valuable part of therapy. He feels that one without the other makes an artificial split that diminishes peoples' humanity.

Me (Referring to Stanley's statement about my particular model of thinking) Which is?

Stanley Digging things out, sorting them through different categories, recording them–not giving information enough chance to become rooted in your experience. Letting the information grow and letting it present you with more internal information that you could then recategorize. This is just one other model you may want to consider.

Me I feel scared, right in the pit of my stomach.

Stanley You may not make your mark in life if you pursue this.

Me Yeah. That's where I'm ambivalent about changing. I feel like I'm sitting on a dime right now.

Stanley I don't blame you for that. I'm just trying to have you see the stakes in the game.

Me You know, it feels to me as if I have to do what I am doing to make it, and yet, up here I also know that what I am doing is getting in my way.

Stanley Ideally, you would like to make it and not hurt yourself.

Me	Right.

Stanley	What do you want to make? Be famous, making money, or just simply be successful and live. Making money? Being known?

Me	How about all of the above?

Stanley	It depends upon which one, though. Your order is to be famous. Make money. And not get hurt. An *alternative order* is to *enjoy living, be successful*, and *maybe make money*, and *maybe be known.*

I thought the way Stanley put this was brilliant. He was meeting me where I was. He wasn't saying I had to give up anything. He was just giving me a new hierarchy with which to pursue my objectives. I did not feel threatened and was able to use this structure to change my pace of living. This was one of the keys that helped unlock and free me.

Stanley	Ready? Get ready. Tighten your shoulder, your neck and strain. Welcome to your life. (Long pause) Are you willing to pursue your goals with respect to establishing another kind of order?

Me	Yes.

Stanley	Then I've just given you the beginning of the tools. It's no more complicated than the three stages of the process that I've just given you. You've got a start. Recognizing the three stages and beginning to deprogram yourself when you think, when you lecture, and when you're with people. And then we'll see what comes out of that. Then we can go to the next step. Thank you.

Me	(Appreciatively) Thank you.

Three months later I spent another day with Stanley in which I again had the privilege of working with him in a large group setting. His topic was the connection between the head and the body. In the three months that went by I no longer had tension in my right shoulder and my body was much looser. Stanley asked me to strip down to my shorts, common practice in body therapy. He asked me to turn one way, then another, and then another. He got a good look at me from four different sides and then went to work. He asked me to lie down on my back, to raise my knees and to begin moving them, first one and then the other, almost the way a person would walk. However, he told me to focus on my inner bodily pace while doing this. His suggestion was very difficult for me to follow, because initially I could barely recognize an inner pace. However, as I continued doing this for fifteen to twenty minutes, my inner pace became clearer and clearer. The pace felt like a metronome that was ticking at about one-third the speed at which I usually moved. I never forgot that experience or that pace, which was a second major step in helping me (the first being the work with my right shoulder). Toward the end of the work other group members were asked to stand over me and look at my face. All of them were saying that I looked ten years younger. This was an existential moment.

REFERENCES

Keleman, Stanley. *Somatic Reality*. Berkeley: Center Press, 2045 Francisco Street, Berkeley, CA 94709, 1979.

Keleman, Stanley. *Your Body Speaks Its Mind*. New York: Simon and Schuster, 1975.

Keleman, Stanley. *Living Your Dying*. New York: A Random House Bookworks Book, 1974.

Keleman, Stanley. *Sexuality, Self & Survival*. San Francisco: Lodestar Press, P.O. Box 31003, San Francisco, CA 94131, 1971.

8

Behavior Modification: Cognitive-Emotive Therapy

THE REINFORCEMENT OF EXISTENTIAL MOMENTS, WITH GEORGE BACH, PH.D.

GEORGE BACH, PH.D., is an author and clinical psychologist. He is a fellow of the American Psychological Association. He lives and practices in West Hollywood, California, and is the author of one of the basic texts in group psychotherapy; *Intensive Group Psychotherapy.* Among his many books is *Creative Aggression,* which he co-authored with Dr. Herb Goldberg.

While existential moments certainly provide the impact necessary for change to occur, behavior modification can supply the continuity and reinforcement that make such change probable. People engage in self-destructive behavior patterns which are not easy to change. While patients may very well have excellent experiences during the therapy session, there is no guarantee that they will know how to follow up on their therapy experience, or that they will do so even if they know how. Behavior modification can be quite useful in manipulating the environment so that patients will have opportunities to experience personal growth and behavior change.

Changing old feelings and behavior patterns requires constant repetition. For example, in gestalt therapy the patient achieves a closure. In clinical hypnosis the patient may experience a feeling from the unconscious mind, or a relaxed sensation through visual imagery. With behavior modification patients are asked to remember the particular feeling, sensation, closure, etc., and use the memory of that positive existential moment to help them change. For example, patients may be asked to practice and remember a relaxing scene by a fireplace with logs burning and flames creating a warm feeling throughout the patient's body. A gestalt patient having difficulty saying no may be asked to remember the surge of power and energy that went through his or her body when screaming, "No, I won't!" to other members of the group.

Another type of reinforcement is homework assignments. For example, when I wanted to work more on developing my capacity to feel my emotions, Dr. George Bach suggested that I write down a historical development of what made me have difficulty experiencing feelings. When I brought this homework into the group the following week and read it aloud, I was quite touched and so were the group members. George suggested that I read what I had written aloud each day, and that reinforcement would be one way to help me to continue to experience my feelings at deeper levels. I was able to profit from the existential moments in the group over and over again.

Reinforcement is also used with obese patients. They may say to themselves, twenty seconds each hour, "For my body, overeating is a poison." "I need my body to live." "I owe my body this respect and protection."[1] It is the reinforcement of the suggestion as well as the reinforcement of the satisfying relaxation that helps obese patients to experience enough rewards to help them over the hurdles of the great deprivation in losing weight. The existential moments that obese patients learn to provide for themselves may be all they have to push them forward each day.

Positive and negative reinforcement is also important when doing marital and couples' therapy. Many couples come in engaging in very punitive and self-destructive behavior. Oftentimes, they are so vicious with each other that therapists can tell that one more scar may be the one that causes a permanent separation. Therapists cut off such behavior between couples and begin to give them positive options to practice. They can deal with negative behavior by using the empty chair in a gestalt framework either when the partner is not present, or once the partner has understood that the anger is a working-through of a projection. This is not to say that aggressive behavior shouldn't be expressed between couples, but only that behavior that would possibly cause a permanent severing of the relationship at the beginning stages of marital therapy should be cut off–with the provision of positive options. Such suggestion can come by paying attention to what both partners are doing with each other and then making an intuitive suggestion that is acceptable to them. For example, if spouses are blaming and criticizing each other, the focus may be shifted by having them compliment each other. If they revert back, the therapist can cut in to refocus the dialogue in a positive direction.

While attending a marathon of another behavior modifier, I noticed that her responses were pretty straightforward instances of positive and negative reinforcement. She would reinforce authentic behavior–existential moments–positively, and negatively stroke the patient's self-defeating behavior. She could gauge precisely how much to stroke and how much to hit while she was working.

Behavior modification also provides an excellent opportunity for continuity. Patients often go from one session to the next without any sense of continuity about their objectives. Transactional analysis is probably less guilty of this error than other therapies I discuss in this book because patients traditionally have long-term therapy contracts. Psychoanalysis also provides reinforcement through continuity by the very fact that the patient meets with the psychoanalyst four or five times per week.

It may be suggested to patients that they keep a diary and record each day how they have worked on the particular behavior they wish to change, as well as other significant events in their lives. Patients can refer to this record when they need to confirm they are both beautiful and changeable.

Therapists may suggest that patients consider certain themes during the course of therapy. When therapists provide a bit of structuring, patients may find it easier to get to the heart of their problem. For example, while working on the development of my creativity, I dealt with the theme of being a reactor as opposed to an actor. The therapist suggested I come in the following week with something I wanted to do for or with the group.

One of my male patients was complaining about his daughters' behavior. He said they never cleaned their dishes from the table after the meal despite the fact he asked them to do so each evening. I suggested he tell them that if they did not do it that evening, they would not be able to dine with the family the following evening. While this can be seen as straight behavior modification, it helped the man deal with the issue of setting limits, which helped him to provide good, firm contact with his children.

Another patient was a writer. He wanted to be able to finish a screenplay, but was in the midst of a writer's block. It was going to cost him dearly in terms of professional opportunity if he did not meet the deadline. I asked him how much money he had in the bank. He said he had five thousand dollars. I told him to make me a cashier's check that I could donate to his favorite charity if he did not complete the screenplay within two weeks (a realistic period of time in which he could complete the assignment). Needless to say, his finished piece of work was excellent. He experienced an existential moment when he completed the work. His sabotaging behavior was stopped, and he experienced both joy and success. So behavior modification is also important in modifying the environment of patients, so they will be able to experience existential moments that help them create permanent changes in their lives.

I remember hearing a story about Dr. Milton H. Erickson. He was treating two adults who wet the bed every night. His recommended treatment was to have them kneel over the bed and urinate before going to sleep each night. He was using the double-bind technique of instructing them to do what they were already doing. This suggestion cut right through their rebellious behavior and helped them provide a different kind of environment which led to the cessation of the bedwetting within two weeks. This was an uncommon suggestion for sure, yet still within the range of behavior modification technique and resulting in the experience of accomplishment of the objective for the patients.

In group therapy Dr. George Bach suggested each of the patients write down what they were thinking privately to themselves about other members of the group, and make a commitment to share these feelings and thoughts with those group members the following week. This commitment encouraged both a caring attitude and genuine communication regarding things that people might ordinarily find hard to say to each other. Such caring and commitment built into the group structure can help to create existential moments between the group members. Dr. Bach referred to this as the "Telling people to their face what I usually say behind their backs" part of the group.

When manipulating the environment of patients, it is important to shift their focus a bit. For example, the issue should not be whether they will try a new behavior, but would they rather try it now or later, this week or next week. In this way people are presented a choice, but the only real choice is to live happier, freer, and healthier lives. *The real art of behavior modification, especially in relationship to existential philosophy, is to make behavioral prescriptions that will help patients deal with and move beyond the existential crisis in their lives.* People are stuck. Choice is difficult because of internal conflict. Knowing how to manipulate the environment so people will be able to choose beyond that impasse is part of the art of behavior modification, and is a tie into existentialism and the creation of existential moments because the behavioral prescription often captures the essence of patients' lives and all that they are grappling with. The therapist's aid in helping patients move beyond their deadlock opens up the path for free choice in the future.

I remember hearing about a psychologist who was particularly good with adolescent patients who were on heavy drugs and for all practical purposes had dropped out of society. He told their parents he wanted an advance of so much money–usually as large a fee as they could possibly afford, usually in the thousands. He then told the parents that he wanted complete control of the situation and full possession of everything that was valuable to the adolescent. He would take possession of their television sets, allowances, etc. When he controlled all the contingencies, sooner or later the adolescents were able to see that their rebellious behavior was not working out as it had in the past, and that they were losing more than they were gaining. I remember hearing that he chained one adolescent who went back on drugs to his piano overnight. He had some extreme methods, but was very successful in helping adolescents who were felt to be hopeless cases turn their lives around into well-adjusted human beings. This therapist's methods surely produced existential moments for those adolescents, because they had great impact in helping these patients learn to take charge of their lives by changing self-destructive habits–even though they had to be forced to change them.

Structuring Situations to Create Movement

Often patients feel hopelessly stuck and are not able to change. Awareness alone does not seem to help. It is with such patients, in his group therapy marathons, that George Bach resembles a maestro conducting a symphony. The following describes both the personal style of Dr. Bach as well as the way he structures situations to create movement in patients.

Much of what I am going to describe took place at a marathon therapy experience that lasted from 9 a.m. Saturday morning to 1 a.m. Sunday morning, and resumed at 7:30 a.m. Sunday morning, until 5:30 p.m. that evening.

The marathon took place at Dr. Bach's home in the Hollywood Hills. He is not only a charismatic, but a dramatic figure as well. He is about five feet, eight inches tall, wore brown pants with unusual zipper patch pockets and a blue western style shirt that had the same sizzle as his personality. He brought his flare for acting and drama into the therapeutic situation, and while therapy was occurring I could not help but be interested, fascinated, and entertained at the same time. These personal qualities of Dr. Bach were particularly important to me since my mind had a tendency to wander. George felt that he was good for me while I made the transition, but that I should not come to depend upon his charismatic personality for my own growth.

When the marathon began George came in with a pair of dark sun glasses. With his German accent I could not help but think of him as a field marshall. Only instead of being a field marshall to create war, George was a human engineer who could create situations whereby people would have major breakthroughs in their lives–even if George wasn't physically present while it was happening.

My wife, and I both attended this marathon. It was her first interactive therapeutic experience, that is, her first experience where she would be dealing with herself, me, and other people, in a therapeutic environment.

While I had had a great deal of individual and group therapy, I had always given my wife mixed messages about pursuing personal growth. Part of me wanted her to change. The other part feared her changing, primarily because I had been stuck in certain areas throughout my life. At this point, though, I was feeling both strong enough and frustrated enough to give my wife a straight message about coming to the marathon.

In the group session prior to the marathon, George mentioned that he heard through the grapevine, that my wife was scared. I told George that I was bringing her to the marathon because our relationship had problems. We were not experiencing each other either as interesting to talk to or to make love with. George said, no wonder she is scared about coming, and he gently reproached me not to push her.

When she came in, George immediately, in his charming and roguish manner, went up to her, hugged her and kissed her in an outgoing and affectionate way, telling her that he heard she was a little afraid. But he did it in a way that put her at ease and made her feel that she was immediately among friends in a safe environment. It was that quality of reaching out and demonstrating all the charm he had on first sight that I wished to emulate.

I can remember one of my first group sessions with him. He quickly zeroed in on my ambitions, abilities and frustrations.

GEORGE   (TO ME) HOW DOES IT FEEL TO BE AMONG THE NINETY-NINE PERCENT OF THE MASSES? (HE PAUSED AND LAUGHED AT ME, IN A WAY WHERE I COULD TELL HE WAS REALLY ENJOYING HIMSELF). WOULDN'T YOU LIKE TO STICK YOUR HEAD ABOVE THE CROWD–JUST A LITTLE BIT?! WOULDN'T YOU LIKE TO BE AMONG THAT ONE PERCENT?! (EACH SENTENCE WAS EMPHATIC.) OF COURSE, IF YOU STICK YOUR HEAD ABOVE THE CROWD A LITTLE BIT, YOU MIGHT GET YOUR HEAD CHOPPED OFF! (HITTING RIGHT ON MY

FEAR OF IMMEDIATE SELF-EXPRESSION IN SOCIAL SITUATIONS). OF COURSE, (BEGINNING TO PAT HIS HAND ON HIS NECK) YOU COULD ALWAYS MAKE YOUR NECK A LITTLE TOUGHER! (THEN HE LAUGHED UPROARIOUSLY, TELLING ME THAT ONE OF HIS GREATEST ASSETS WAS HIS WILLINGNESS TO MAKE A FOOL OF HIMSELF.)

While part of me didn't like what he was saying, I couldn't help but find myself enchanted by the way he said it. In any case, his message was loud and clear!

Back to the marathon. George's instructions were to have a working lunch. Six of us gathered together at one table. The objective was for each of us to convince the other five that we should be *it*. To be *it* we had to convince each of the other members at the table that our problem was the most important. This was the first structured experience that had great impact for me. Each of us, including my wife stated our problems, but one fellow monopolized the floor. I found myself becoming more and more frustrated, and thought to myself, this son of a bitch doesn't care if anyone else gets any time. He isn't being fair. Then I felt anger. Finally I blurted out, why the hell don't you shut up and give someone else a chance?! He said, "Look, the name of the game is to be *it*. That's what I'm doing. If you want to be *it*, then you had better be able to take the floor from me." I experienced this insight as a shocking existential moment because I never saw my passivity. He backed off to give me the opportunity to be *it*. I felt a great difficulty in mobilizing all that was within me and saying it in an articulate way. Now things were becoming clear regarding my difficulty in becoming one with my own charisma. Although I never thought of myself as passive, I was clearly faced with my reacting instead of taking positive action on my own behalf. Out of six of us at the table, my aggression level was about third; my wife's unwillingness to be aggressive left her sixth, as she did little more than express her needs. I was beginning to feel both responsible for and resentful towards her. It was also becoming clear why we did not have a great deal of interesting conversation between us. I used half my aggression, and copped out on the other half. She used less than me.

So when I was stuck, things would become deadly boring between us. My wife and I both realized this, and that weekend we began to change life-long behavior patterns.

She said she was passive because she was afraid of my anger. She referred to a time when I got angry and stormed out of the room, swearing at her. Dr. Bach's co-leader suggested that when I was angry I just tell her *I'm very angry about her doing that particular behavior.* His suggesting that I stay with my feeling of anger and relate it to a particular behavior gave me a specific way to reach a resolution with her about our problems. I began to see that the behavior modifier's emphasis on specific behavior was very valuable, especially with couples. Otherwise, things could easily become too vague, as couples might very well express their feelings clearly to each other without knowing exactly what to do to change the undesirable state of affairs. I experienced a feeling of freedom that was an existential moment when there was a focus on specific behavior.

She and I both made strides from that time onward. She volunteered to host the dinner party and she was very assertive and caring, while becoming the primary person in the work of another woman in the group. She was showing me sides of her personality I had never seen before. I, too, was making much more aggressive and interesting contact with people by bringing up my inner feelings and expressing myself to people. I was reaching out much more instead of waiting to be approached. The good feelings I got from reaching out were existential moments.

A second impactful situation came about as a result of the structured nudity experience. There were about eighteen people at the marathon. George suggested that we break into three groups of six for the nude body imagery work. The first group was called the "eager beavers." The second group was the "reluctant but conflicted." The third group were the "unwilling." She and I were in the third group.

While I had been to a nude marathon in 1970 as part of my doctoral training and had been to a marathon that had nudity as a part of it in 1972, there were other issues that were far more prevalent to me—although they happened to center around the nudity. I had that really stuck feeling, as if I consciously knew I should do something other than what I was doing, but I either couldn't or wouldn't budge. Yet, intellectually I had positioned myself in a marathon where nudity would provoke those emotionally stuck feelings and where I would have the opportunity to perhaps break through the stubborn, childlike feelings. Here's how it went as I began talking to Dr. Bach's co-leader. Everyone was undressed except my ex-wife and me.

Me   I've been to a couple of nude marathons. Nudity isn't the primary issue. I'm comfortable with all my clothes on. The sauna bath is outside. It's cold outside. I feel sleepy, like I don't want to bother with the whole damn thing. Also, I don't want her taking her clothes off in front of anyone else.

Therapist   (To her) How do you feel about what Len is saying or telling you not to do?

My wife at the time   Well, I'm making my decision independent of him. He is the only person I have ever taken my clothes off in front of.

Therapist   (To me, offering options of taking all my clothes off; going in my shorts; having her go in bra and panties.)

Me   Didn't you hear me! I don't want to do it. And neither is she! (While I knew what I was doing intellectually, I was being a stubborn childish mule. I stuck with every bit of stubbornness because that is where I was stuck both with the relationship and with myself.)

There is another important aspect to all this. This is exactly how I feel some nights when we don't have sex. I get sleepy. I nod out. I don't do anything. She often gets stuck in the same place.

At this point I guess it was too much for her to bear. She took a stand (her taking a stand was an existential moment of relief for me and our relationship), telling the therapist to get a towel. She went to the sauna in bra and panties with the towel but I did not know exactly what she was going to do at this time. My feelings at the adult level were those of relief. At the child level I was angry, jealous and mistrustful.

Me   Well, if she is going I will go so I can keep an eye on her (I stayed with the feelings all the way).

Therapist   That's not a valid reason to go.

Me   It is for me.

The therapist was missing the issue at this point. The issue was that movement had taken place. She had taken a stand, something she had been unwilling to do in our relationship. Her unwillingness to take a stand was partly why I had lost some interest in her. Well, I was now interested, along with a lot of other emotions! I moved. Although I did not move independently, which was the therapist's complaint, I did move in response to her and this was a step. About this time George walked in telling us that we were running behind schedule and to hurry up into the sauna. The other therapist complained about my motives and George told him that I could either stay or go, but that the group must go now. In the sauna, which was pitch black, I talked of my feelings and that I saw the need to take independent action. I told them that if I had trouble taking action when she didn't take a stand. *I could imagine or fantasize that she did take a stand and then take action based on that fantasy or image.* In either case I was setting myself up to be an actor instead of a reactor, which was my "growth edge" with beginning the group. I felt very good about this major breakthrough for me and for her. The group said that I looked far more alive and colorful after returning from the sauna. She felt very good about herself sexually as each of us stood before a mirror and talked about our three physical "uglies" and ended with our three physical "beauties." Each of us received a group hug at the end of the nude body work and the intimacy between her and me rapidly returned.

The third major growth experience for me at the marathon came from George's initial instructions. He said that people would often let themselves get distracted due to the length of the marathon. And when they became distracted, they would become uninvolved. He said that if we let this happen we would probably be very bitter and frustrated about the marathon.

After supper that evening I was feeling groggy and distracted, and had to force myself to pay attention for another six hours. It felt incredibly burdensome and almost painful to stop myself from nodding off. Since that time, however, I have had more vigor. I was able to push through a bad habit and force myself back into the land of the living.

George referred to this as "a slough of despond" which every group sooner or later must confront–a feeling of being stuck or going backward, a time of no real revolt. He did not take the group off the hook, as he felt group therapists should let the group experience the SLOUGH OF DESPOND with all its LOW ENERGY, DEFENSIVENESS, AND SLEEPINESS. The slough of despond is what teaches people to revolt back into life! It helps people to learn to avoid sitting on their aggression–and making themselves sleepy. The slough of despond is mismanagement of aggression.

More specifically, George made recommendations to the group on the following day. *He said we should look for something we can't do that is a strength in other people, and let ourselves become fascinated with them.*

Before the marathon came to a close there were two final structured situations. The marathon was defined as a transition between the way we were and the way we were going to be. The therapists suggested that the fullness of the marathon would be most realized after it ended, and that each of us were to select a growth buddy with whom we would keep in contact for two months, and who would help us take specific steps from the marathon to the outside world. We would keep in touch with our growth buddy once a week to make sure we were fulfilling our contract.

While I felt I had the general knowledge of how My wife at the time and I were going to make ourselves interesting to each other, both verbally and physically, my growth buddy and I began to work out the specifics in contract form. He had the things to work on with his wife. Our contract read as follows:

1. Goal: To revitalize my marital sex life.
2. What will I do to bring about that change?
    a. Tell my wife what I want sexually in very specific terms.

b. Be specific even when feelings of embarrassment attempt to block my doing so.
c. Let my wife know when I feel turned on.
d. To have a sexier relationship all the time rather than just during love- making.

About this time George's co-therapist came by and began to get even more specific. He asked questions such as:

1. When are you going to do it?
2. How often? How often are you going to ask her for sex?
3. What happens when she gets sleepy?
4. What happens when she says no?

He made a variety of suggestions that included seducing our wives, deciding not to be tired, avoiding any alcoholic beverages before bed, avoiding wine at dinner until the new habit patterns were well entrenched. He checked things out in a way that would enable us to deal with any initial rejections that might occur, so we would be successful. Being specific writes success into the contract and will help to insure that patients get what they need for themselves–especially between marital partners. The positioning of people in situations where they are forced to deal with their passivity, and to break through into healthy aggressive behavior also provides the opportunity for existential moments to occur.

The final situation involved feedback from two group members of our choice. They were requested to give us homework assignments which we could not refuse to do. One woman suggested that I keep my body more active, possibly through dance.

I felt as if my partner and I had gotten much more than we came for, in attending the marathon. When we got home that evening there was a committed, intimate, interested feeling between us that pervaded both our conversation and our sexual activities.

Post-Marathon Experience

Prior to the marathon, Margie, a woman in the weekly group session of which I was a member, talked of her desire to leave her husband. She was fooling herself into thinking she had done all she could do to make her marriage work. The group was quite frustrated with her and chose to let it drop. At this point I came on very tough and told her that she was fooling herself. I told her that it was her job to get her husband to the marathon, and that she had the power to do it if she really wanted to do it. This was amidst several protestations that he was an uncooperative husband and that she knew that he would not come. I insisted that she was doing little more than complaining, seeking to rationalize a decision she had already made without really giving herself, her marriage, or her husband a fair chance. She agreed to apply pressure to bring Sammy to the marathon.

Sure enough, Sammy appeared at the marathon. He looked like a man who belonged in the early 1950's and was out of his time zone. He wore brown pants with white socks and wore his hair very short and slicked back. Nevertheless, Sammy had more courage than anyone thought he would have from Margie's description of him. He stayed right in there and dealt with his feelings about himself and Margie. He had a remarkable sincerity and willingness to change because he realized that with or without his wife, he was leading a stultifying life. He ended by crying, hugging people, getting closer to reality.

While all this was happening, I still sensed that Margie's decision was already made. So I confronted her. I told her that I thought the real issue was that she was ripe for an affair, and that she already had her mind made up about leaving Sammy. Several members of the group felt I took a harsh potshot at her. However, she looked at me, and told me that what I said was true. So she and her husband had the opportunity to deal with their sex lives out front. When the marathon ended Margie looked surprised about how much her husband had changed at the marathon, in terms of becoming a responsive and aggressive man. He was beginning to make himself interesting. Yet she remained quite decisive and still leaned toward divorce.

Two Group Sessions after the Marathon

Margie was looking rather spent. Dr. Bach asked her what was the matter. She said she just got back from a vacation in Hawaii with her husband that was like a honeymoon. She felt sexually exhausted from having sex as often as she did, but was quite pleased with both herself and her husband.

She said that the first day after the marathon she realized she liked her husband but was still planning to leave. On the second day, she was on the way to the store when he grabbed her hand. One thing led to another. She never made it to the store, but instead wound up in the bedroom! The group was delighted with her success story.

She gave me a very heartfelt and warm thank you for being tough with her in two respects: pushing her to bring her husband to the marathon, and confronting her about wanting to leave. She said that I had made it clear to her that she wasn't giving it a fair shot, and that she was very happy that she did.

Thus, in addition to my own experience, my way of thinking about marital relationships was also validated by Margie and Sammy, who each gave themselves and their partner their best effort to make the relationship successful. If couples have that level of *responsible commitment*, and can see past their own feelings of hopelessness, in many cases they can work things out.

So, in terms of reinforcement of existential moments, continuity of therapeutic experience, manipulation of the patient's environment, and positive and negative reinforcement of authentic moments, behavior modification can provide a useful adjunct to all of the therapies I discuss in this book. It can help patients make permanent changes in their lives. Without repetition of experience, permanent change from self-defeating behavior becomes much more difficult. While the impact of powerful existential moments is likely to stick with patients, and remembering of these moments if likely to facilitate change, a contractual reinforcement scheduled with the particular therapist-patient contract increases the likelihood that patients will achieve more permanent results. This also makes existential philosophy a hopeful philosophy.

When I was a graduate student, I studied the polarized differences of behavior modification and existential philosophy. I do not think they need to be in opposition. People can freely choose their existence, and if a behavior modification technique helps them to be able to choose freely–all the more power to them. It is important to experience the ongoing process of life. Nowhere do I hear behavior modifiers deny this importance. Yet, existentialists often claim that behavior modifiers want to help people "fix it." They claim behavior modifiers are repair men and women who really are unwilling to grapple with the meaning of life and the nature and predicament of the human condition. While these philosophical perspectives may be true at times, I suspect they are true less often than philosophers would like to believe. It seems to me that the support of the repair man, if the behavior modifier be referred to as such, can be quite important in helping the existentially oriented patient create an existence that is both meaningful and hopeful. In this way behavior modification can help existentialism develop itself beyond the depression and despair with which it is often identified. Behavior modification can help existentialism become a philosophy that is positive in nature–and that people can utilize in living better lives. Otherwise, existential philosophy may often be considered so vague that it has little practical value for people in day-to-day living. Philosophically, while the existentialists feel that existence precedes essence, the techniques of behavior modification can help make choosing a positive experience, as opposed to choosing responses that are stuck in old script behavior.

Dr. Milton H. Erickson told a story about a patient who had very little control over her bladder. He suggested that she go to the bathroom, and urinate, but while she was doing so, to imagine a strange man broke into the bathroom. He then asked what she experienced. She said she froze immediately, and the urine stopped. He then suggested that she knew how to do it. She was very pleased. Dr. Erickson then discussed with the group the common claim of symptom substitution, for which behavior modifiers are often attacked. He said that the patient indeed was suffering from symptom substitution. She was now coming to him because she couldn't make up her mind about what she should pursue as a major field of study in college!

I remember visiting a state hospital that was treating retarded children. Here again, I was convinced that behavior modification was the most helpful and most expedient way to help these children to learn the principles of self-care and self-grooming. I am sure that such learning added meaning to their lives.

However, as the key word in psychotherapeutic treatment may very well be balance, I can also see where the behavior modifier may stretch his or her boundaries by studying, experiencing, and profiting from existential philosophy, existentially-oriented psychotherapies, and some of the experiential psychotherapies I describe in this book. The augmentation of ongoing experience is quite important. Sometimes behavior modifiers put an over-emphasis upon the use of suggestion, and upon specific behaviors, and not enough emphasis upon experiencing life. Gestalt therapy and some body therapies are particularly good counterbalances since they take the patient step-by-step in the here and now and gradually lead that patient to a working-through of experience so the patient will be able to experience richer and more amplified contact with self and others. This is different in quality than just positive or negative reinforcement. Yet, when reinforcement can be added to that type of experience, the result is dynamite!

Therapists must be open to stretching their boundaries, to use all of themselves and their knowledge to help patients. The existentialist who neglects behavior modification, and the behavior modifier who neglects other experiential modalities, are both guilty of bad faith. I am referring to therapists choosing to stop their own personal growth and therapeutic knowledge because they have been trained in a particular modality, or because they have found a style that is comfortable. The real issue is one of balance. Balance of the therapist's personality, balance in terms of having options available to help patients that range from the experiential to the cognitive. And balance in philosophy and perspective about life. It is with this view of therapy, reality, and the human condition that I see existentialism and behavior modification providing each other with something of value!

RATIONAL-EMOTIVE THERAPY WITH ALBERT ELLIS, PH.D.

> People are disturbed not by things, but by the views
> which they take of them.–Epictetus, first century A.D.

Albert Ellis, Ph.D. is a clinical psychologist who created rational-emotive therapy and has written extensively for both professionals and the lay public. Among his books are *How to Live With and Without Anger,* and *A New Guide to Rational Living.*

He is director of the Institute for Rational Living in New York City and is a fellow of the American Psychological Association.

I have placed rational-emotive therapy in the chapter on behavior therapy, because in my view, it is a cognitive approach to the restructuring of emotions and behavior. This is also my view of behavior therapy.

What I have attempted to capture in this chapter is both the rational-emotive approach to therapy and the way it can be potent in helping people change, and when combined with a unique personal style such as Ellis manifests, can be a lot of fun for patients. And if patients can get better while they are enjoying themselves, I am all for it. While I feel that I have captured some of Ellis' personality, it would be nearly impossible to capture the full essence of the permission he gives himself to be *outrageous in attacking irrational belief systems and helping people change their basic philosophy of life.* In terms of the themes of this book–the existential moment, potency, and personal style in doing therapy, Ellis and RET are an interesting and, in my opinion, mandatory inclusion into therapeutic repertoire. I say mandatory because unless therapists are able to get to patients' irrational beliefs and philosophy of life, those patients aren't likely to free themselves from their self-torture or for the self-expression sought by those interested in therapy for personal growth.

I first saw Albert Ellis do a demonstration of rational-emotive therapy in 1968 when I was in my first year of graduate school. I remember buying his books, *A Guide to Rational Living,* and *Sex Without Guilt.* Speaking of resistance, I left the second in the trunk of my car for a couple of years. About the first time I saw Dr. Ellis I was studying the different modes of therapy. My professor dismissed rational-emotive therapy and Ellis by saying all he did was point out the idiocy of peoples' ways. When I saw him work it *appeared* he was only pointing out the idiocy of peoples' ways, and this oneupmanship quality plus my naivete permitted me to dismiss Dr. Ellis for several years.

Melvin Powers, a fascinating man who is president of the Wilshire Book Company, called to tell me that he liked my style of writing. He invited me to visit with him. When I arrived he took out two books: *A New Guide to Rational Living* by Albert Ellis, and *Psychocybernetics* by Dr. Maxwell Maltz. He told me that both of these books have sold over one hundred thousand copies a year for over ten years. He suggested that I read them and go to the introductory meeting of EST, then call him back to chat again. He felt such experiences would help me as a writer. Melvin Powers wasn't the sort of fellow one would take lightly.

For example, when I walked in, he was playing his guitar and played a beautiful tune around the Italian version of my name, Leonardo Bergantino. By the time he finished the song, anything he said was deeply imbedded in my mind.

Also, a woman who was a client along with me in George Bach's group told me she thought I worked like Albert Ellis. So I thought it was probably time to stop being so stubborn about the idiocy of my ways and check out what Dr. Ellis had to offer first-hand. I took a one-week workshop in rational emotive therapy, and had two hours of personal therapy with Dr. Ellis.

In 1968 I listened to Albert Ellis and felt enraged at some of the things he said and did. In 1979 I was fascinated. He had a brilliant mind. He would have made a great lawyer if he had not chosen to make his contribution to the field of psychotherapy. He had a way of barking out the most outrageous things in a New York accent, with an emphasis on the words which he particularly wants to impress upon peoples' minds. He is the kind of speaker I could listen to all day long and still continue to learn from while enjoying myself. An example of something he said was, "Transmigration od Souls! Bullshit! If it's not in the New York Times, it doesn't exist!" However, with statements such as this one, any supporters of this belief would immediately begin to argue with Dr. Ellis, and after they lost the argument, would probably contend that he was an opinionated asshole who just happened to be bright enough to defeat most anyone at any particular argument he chose, no matter on which side of the fence he happened to be. But Dr. Ellis does a lot more than meets the eye with his personally provocative style. He wakes people up and forces the passivity, the anger, the depression, the anxiety, to the surface very quickly. He challenges peoples' irrational beliefs in ways that help people think more clearly. He then teaches them to dispute their own irrational beliefs in ways that produce nearly instant relief, in ten to twenty minutes. It's no small wonder that he sells 100,000 copies of *A New Guide to Rational Living* each year. Ellis made a major contribution by giving psychotherapists permission to argue with their patients. That is, to argue more powerfully against the patient's craziness, or irrational beliefs, than the crazy part of the patient is arguing for them. Only Ellis is more powerful because he shows patients that they have lived their lives based on a particular irrational belief that has no foundation, and that has caused them much suffering. After people see there is no evidence for their belief, he teaches them a more rational belief that has a freeing emotional consequence. Depression, anxiety, anger, are relieved quite readily. So while in 1968 I naively mistook Ellis for pulling a oneupmanship trip and showing people the idiocy of their ways, I now see that he has created a very hopeful and effective method of therapy that helps people feel better quickly. Furthermore, it should probably be the first method considered for patients who are severely disturbed, because it teaches them how to challenge the self-torturing part very quickly.

Another flaring argument Ellis got into was when he barked out at a woman that most transvestites are very seriously disturbed, while she was trying to argue a more humanistic, non-judgmental viewpoint. However, she was very angry and I had a sense that she was against Ellis's provocative statements due to many of her own problems that she would just as soon leave unchallenged. She practiced the kind of humanistic therapy that would probably leave people feeling good without changing. Thus, I believe Ellis' brand of therapy, although it may sometimes appear quite rough, is very humanistic in that it helps people to change themselves and get relief quickly.

I remember the first group supervision session where another trainee was doing therapy with me. Ellis began to yell out, "And you think that you *should*, and you *must*, and you *should*, and you *must*, etc." I was shocked. I was engaging in far more self-torture than I had realized. Every other sentence that came out of my mouth had an implied *should* or *must* behind it.

I did not find the other trainees at the workshop particularly artistic or creative therapists. I emphasize this point because I was particularly impressed with the training. It helped average members of the helping profession to do very effective work in a one-week workshop. Here is the method.

Rational-emotive therapy is as simple as *ABCDE*. *A* is the *activating event*. For example, a patient told me that she was going to give a speech to a group. RET then quickly goes for her *C (consequence)*. That is, what is her emotional problem–anxiety, depression, anger, self-pity, feelings of worthlessness? The speed at which it goes for the *C*, and teaches people to think about how they create their own disturbed emotions (problem) cuts out much of the irrelevant drivel that often occurs in therapy. She said the problem was anxiety. Once we have an *A* and a *C*, an activating event and an emotional problem, the therapist can ask for the *B*. *B* is her irrational belief. What is she telling herself that makes her feel anxious? The dialogue may go as follows:

Patient

If I am not interesting, or I forget what I was going to say, people will think I am a jerk.

Therapist

Why *must* people think well of you?

Patient

People must think well of me because if they don't I will feel bad.

Therapist

What *evidence* do you have to support the *belief* that people *must* think well of you in order for you to *accept yourself*?

Patient

Because if people don't think well of me I may never get another speaking engagement; it may affect my livelihood, it may affect my style of life, etc.

Therapist

Yes, but even if it does, why *must* other people think well of you as a condition for you to accept yourself and for you to try to be as happy as you can be? What *evidence* do you have to *support* the *belief* that you can *only* accept yourself and value your existence by getting *others* to approve of you? (Ellis would unleash his sing-song style of challenging by emphasizing the italicized words.)

Patient

(Sooner or later the patient usually realizes): I have no evidence to support the belief that people must think well of me for me to accept myself. (This may come after tracking down a step at a time each of the moves patients make on their irrational journey, but the key words are *must, accept yourself,* and *evidence.* Therapists will find the job easier if they quickly look for the *must* in people's beliefs, and then get to what *evidence* they have to support the belief that they *must* do so and so or else they are totally unacceptable *to themselves*.)

At this point Ellis would probably explain the *elegant solution*–that the issue of self-esteem is a moot point because people are neither worthwhile nor worthless based on their action, and that people merit self-acceptance on the basis of being members of the human race. This is Ellis's way of teaching people unconditional positive regard so they can use it to enjoy themselves rather than thinking they have to *prove* themselves and so that they *rarely upset themselves when faced with undesirable conditions.*

D stands for *disputing.* And *disputing* had better be vigorous because the irrational beliefs are easily invented and sustained over the course of a lifetime. For example, "What *evidence* do you have to support the belief that people must think well of you or you are a shit?" is a vigorous dispute, and the RET therapist unrelentlessly pursues it until the patient comes up with a more rational belief that will help him/her live a healthier life.

E stands for the *new rational belief.* "It would be desirable if people liked me and thought well of my public speaking. It might have desirable results I would enjoy. But I'm not worthless if I don't do well. People don't *have to* like me and *I am still acceptable because I am a member of the human race.*"

Once people have integrated the new rational belief the pressure is off. They feel freer and have relief from symptoms of anxiety, depression, or anger, and they are then able to engage in behaviors that help them expand themselves instead of crippling themselves. For example, once she removed her anxiety, my patient felt much better about giving a speech, because her entire worth as a human being didn't depend upon the outcome. The particular section of work I described took twelve minutes. Another patient had one year of therapy with a more non-directive therapist and claimed she was turned off with therapy because she didn't accomplish anything during this year. Her *A* (activating experience) was that her boyfriend would leave her alone for a period of time. Her *C* (emotional consequence) was that she felt so *depressed* that she didn't even want to get out of bed when he wasn't there. She felt her life wasn't worth living without him. I asked, "Why *must* he be with you all the time for you to feel worthwhile!?" Her bottom line after about five interchanges was that she learned it from her parents. I questioned their authority as psychological experts, and further noted that she was complaining of feeling absolutely miserable about her life, and that this would probably continue unless she were willing to take the action needed to both dispute the irrational belief and substitute a rational belief based on the elegant solution which would permit her to live a happier life. I taught her how to do it herself, the ABCDE RET Method, and she left with a feeling of relief that she could begin to take control over her life. And so we see that existential moments occurred with the freedom that accompanied the loss of irrational belief of time. In addition, both patients were provided with tools they could use to make their life healthier and happier.

RET is particularly effective with obsessive-compulsive patients who are used to having a multitude of problems by which they overwhelm themselves and other people thereby keeping themselves feeling hopeless. However, with the degree of potency the therapist uses in *disputing*, and especially by single-mindedly disputing one disturbed emotional consequence (c) at a time, this type of overly toilet-trained patient can be stopped from self-destructive behavior and given a new lease on life. This is not to say that RET only works with this kind of patient, but it is to say that it is one of the few approaches that reaches this difficult population when the disputing is done powerfully.

I had a two-hour private therapy session with Dr. Ellis toward the end of the workshop. He asked me why I wanted to see him and I told him that I thought his experience and ability in the field could help me both therapeutically and with my writing skills. I got a lot more than I bargained for out of this two-hour session because in addition to what I asked for I also became freer in a way that left me, as a patient, able to experience more, and as a therapist, able to experiment more creatively. The problems which Dr. Ellis uncovered included those I tended to project onto my patients and thereby interfered with my acting more adult-like and less critical of them. RET can be as valuable to the personal growth therapist as it is to the therapist who works with more severely disturbed patients.

The session began with Dr. Ellis going to the couch and lying down while removing his glasses. I was in a chair sitting up straight taking notes. One of Dr. Ellis's assistants knocked on the door to see what time he would be finished so they could plan dinner. She looked at us and shook her head saying, "I don't believe this." Then it hit me. It appeared as if I were his analyst. The session had that kind of twist to it from beginning to end. Al began by asking me about my training. I said I had trained in existential therapy, gestalt therapy, clinical hypnosis, transactional analysis, and bioenergetic therapy. I mentioned that I had first-rate trainers. Then he went about getting my attention. He was bellowing out,

> No wonder you are having trouble. Gestaltists rarely have a rational thought among the entire lot of them. Clinical hypnotists often tell people that if they dig up what they have in the hidden recesses of their unconscious minds, that will automatically give them what they need to live happy and healthy lives. Bullshit! This kind of hypnotic therapy does nothing to challenge people's irrational beliefs; and if their unconscious beliefs are crazy, they will be just as crazy after hypnosis as they were before. Transactional analysis includes antiscientific reification–that your parent, your adult, your child nonsense–instead of much more clearly and accurately defining peoples' childish ideas. Bioenergetic therapy is an offshoot of Reich, who was overtly psychotic much of his life and who carried his psychosis into orgone therapy.

Taken out of context one could interpret what Al said as a putdown of all other therapies except his own. However, at a deeper level he knew that I had a lot of experience and that he needed to catch my attention. He certainly did that.

When he began working with me he picked up that "I must succeed" on the top end of things, and that "It is too hard to do the work required to succeed," on the other end. These two simultaneous beliefs caused me to be much less effective in every aspect of my life, including my writing. I left the session with more rational beliefs. It would be nice if I succeeded in publishing a book, but if I didn't I would still be an acceptable person. And it may be hard to write that kind of book and do some of the other things I was setting out to do, but in fact *it is not too hard*. It was critically important to challenge the irrational belief that it was too hard because that is how the person with *low frustration tolerance* keeps him or herself from turning away from the tragic corner in his or her life. Al used the example of the overweight patients who keep telling themselves that it is too hard to lose the weight when in fact it would be much easier than the suffering they bring on themselves by continuing their current eating habits. Obesity can affect sexual attractiveness, physical stamina, physical health, work performance, etc. Changing patients' perspectives so they see that it is not too hard to uproot their self-defeating behavior patterns has been very important to many people.

A third impasse was my "problem about the problem." I engaged in the *process of "self-downing."* For example, at first I might be depressed about not having a contract to publish a book, but then I might be depressed about being depressed. I would tell myself that a fellow with all the therapy I had should have his act together so he didn't feel depressed. Ellis then challenged, asking me what evidence I had to support the belief that I must not feel depressed, or else I was unacceptable as a person.

Simple RET formulas that I have made up for myself are to check for pressure at the top (e.g., "I must succeed"), and at the bottom ("it's too hard"), along with any tendencies toward self-downing. Hit 'em high and hit 'em low, and any other place that works. This kind of pursuit makes it difficult for patients to escape into their defensive "freedom."

"Shame attacking exercises" are another way Ellis reaches people who have boxed themselves in through the self-critical part of the mind and the irrational belief system. He told a story about a woman patient who agreed, as a self-freeing shame-attacking exercise, to "to walk a banana on a long red leash in New York City." He reported that as she and her husband strolled along the streets with the banana on a leash some 200 people looked the other way because they were embarrassed to look at this "crazy" woman. Finally, one child pointed at the woman and said, "Hey, look mommy! That woman is walking a banana!" Another such exercise was to have a person walk into a market or a bank, point his arm at the clock on the wall, and yell out at the top of his lungs the time–e.g., "It's 10:22." Then, when everyone turns around to look, just walk out. A third shame-attacking exercise Ellis mentioned was to enter an elevator, face the back of the elevator with a crowd of people on it, and say, "Would someone please push the 7 floor. I can't see the buttons." Such a homework approach has unlimited possibilities. And Ellis is a firm believer in homework.

Shortly after Ellis talked about shame attacking exercises he presented another interesting way to spoof irrational belief systems. He began to sing, in one of the most awful voices I have ever heard, to the tune of the Yale Whiffenpoof Song, one of his rational humorous songs:

WHINE, WHINE, WHINE!
I cannot have all of my wishes filled–
Whine, whine, whine!
I cannot have every frustration stilled–
Whine, whine, whine!
Life really owes me the things that I miss,
Fate has to grant me eternal bliss!
And if I must settle for less than this–
Whine, whine, whine![2]

Al had the entire group of therapists sing the second chorus with him before whipping out a tape of him singing other songs on a cassette with a harpsichord background. It sounded so funny and gave people the feeling they too, could be foolish, have fun, and enjoy life. A second rational humorous song Ellis composed was sung to the tune of "After the Ball."

MAYBE I'LL MOVE MY ASS
After you make things easy,
And you provide the gas,
After you squeeze and please me,
Maybe I'll move my ass!
Just make things soft and breezy,
Fill life with sassafras!
And possibly, if things are easy,
I'll move my ass![3]

Al and Joanna–Working with Guilt

Joanna would feel guilty over what to me appeared to be the most inconsequential things. For example, she was feeling guilty about taking two days off so we could have a long weekend and visit out of state.

Joanna	My guilt makes me feel rotten.
Ellis	Any rotten person would have to be rotten to the core, wouldn't she?
Joanna	And do everything wrong.
Ellis	So therefore she would have to do everything rotten. Well, is that likely?
Joanna	No.

Ellis set Joanna up for the course of the work in his first comment. If she accepted his premise that to be a rotten person she would have to do everything in a rotten way, she was taking an indefensible position. Ellis would prove this over and over to her in a hundred different ways. Joanna, in retrospect, felt that Ellis was so humorous in the way he went about doing therapy that it was like working with Woody Allen. Also, as soon as Ellis asked a question he answered it, and Joanna was left in a position where she could only agree. For example, he said, "So therefore she would have to do everything rotten. Well, is that likely?" Joanna agreed, "No." From here Ellis sets Joanna up by comparing her to two people who would most be thought of as rotten, and even goes about proving that they were not totally rotten. I could not help but laugh when Joanna, who was playing hooky from two days of school, was being compared to Hitler and Nathan Leopold, a murderer of a teenage boy who killed for thrill.

Ellis	Even Hitler didn't do everything rotten, did he?
Joanna	Well, I guess he was a pretty good housepainter.
Ellis	And he did some other things. Actually his intentions were honorable. He wasn't really trying to do that

badly, even though his deeds were heinous. He was vile to Gypsies and Jews because he wrongly believed that he was thereby helping the human race. So he wasn't rotten to the core. And you don't have to *only* do and *always* do rotten acts. Well, is there really any such person as someone who exclusively does bad acts and who could thereby be called totally rotten?

Joanna   No.

Ellis   But let's assume for the sake of discussion that *you or Hitler only* and *always* did rotten acts. That would be very phenomenal! You'd be the only one in history! Such a person, to be legitimately labeled as a *bad person* would have to have another trait, and that would be *damnability*.

Ellis then went on to prove that it was impossible for a human to be damnable, before returning to another example attacking Joanna's rotten person belief.

Ellis   And we also have the famous case of Nathan Leopold. In one sense he was really worse than Hitler. He killed for thrill. He killed an innocent thirteen-year old boy. He was convicted for his crime but his famous lawyer, Clarence Darrow, saved him from the electric chair. If he had been rotten to the core, as you are saying you are, he couldn't have done what he later did. He stayed in jail for about thirty-five years, read books, permitted medical experiments to be performed on him, and when he was pardoned, moved to Puerto Rico. He married, became a social worker, helped many people, was a fine father, and died very loved and respected. If he were totally rotten, how could he have done those things?

Joanna   He couldn't.

Ellis   And he murdered a boy for a thrill. That was about the worst crime of the twentieth century. And even he wasn't a rotten person. He was a person who acted rottenly in those respects. Now in your case, you can't even prove that your acts are that bad, and you certainly can't prove that you are wrong, rotten or a damnable person. But when you feel guilty, that is what you are saying: (1) My acts are reprehensible, and (2) I am a no-good. *Prove it.*

Joanna   I can't.

Ellis   When you really feel guilty, self-downing, lousy as a human, that's what you are really saying. You had better give up those beliefs and change them to: Maybe my acts were bad, but even if they were, I am never a louse, and never a nogoodnick.

Ellis was asking Joanna to prove that she was rotten because she couldn't live up to her idealized image. Her inability to defend this position throughout the interview left her with the feeling that her belief must have been mistaken. The result was that she has been able to become a good deal more assertive without feeling guilty.

Later on in the interview Joanna presented a tricky problem.

Joanna   I feel more silly than guilty.

Ellis   Your primary symptom is guilt. At "A," the activating event, you are doing something you consider wrong. At "B" you're telling yourself, "I *should* be a fucking angel!" and at "C" you're feeling guilty. But then you take the guilt, and you make it into a new "A." You then say to yourself, "I see that I feel guilty." Then at "C" you feel silly about your guilt. You are putting yourself down for feeling guilty, so you feel guilty about your guilt. Because at "B" you are saying "I *shouldn't* feel guilty!" Why *shouldn't* you? You *should* feel guilty. Do you know *why* you should?

Joanna

No.

Ellis

Because you *do*. Whatever you feel you feel. It's a mistake for you to have yourself guilty or self-downing instead of merely sorry about your guilt. But if you are mistaken that's the way you are mistaken! So you'd better *accept yourself with your guilt*. Tell yourself, "I am acting stupidly for feeling guilty, but it's only a stupid *act*. I am not a shit, though my *act* is shitty!" Then, when you do that, you become unashamed of your guilt and are finally able to work on ridding yourself of it. But while you are putting yourself down for feeling guilty, you really won't work much on eliminating it. You have two symptoms for the price of one! So first accept yourself with your guilt, and then go back to work on eliminating the guilt. You can do this by telling yourself: "The act of staying away from school is wrong and I'll eventually find a better solution to this problem. But in the meantime I'll live with wrongness. I won't be an archangel."

Joanna came out of the session with a feeling that she was entitled to make some human errors and began to consistently give herself greater permission to do what she wanted to do. I was stunned quite a bit with her "No," but at worst I was angry for a few moments and then forgot about it. It was difficult for her to forget Ellis' message because he thoroughly dealt with a few basic themes until Joanna arrived at and stuck to more rational modes of dealing with her problem and unconditionally accepting herself. While the marital work Joanna and I did prior to working with Ellis helped Joanna get started in the right direction toward becoming more assertive and saying no, Ellis gave her backup philosophic reinforcement that she could use effectively.

Summary

Albert Ellis has made a major contribution to the field of psychotherapy. Rational-emotive therapy helps people change their basic philosophy of life. It teaches patients to think clearly and gives them the knowledge whereby they can take control of their conscious and rational faculties, and reduce the number of occasions where they fall victim to their own irrational thinking. In addition to therapeutic interventions giving people faith in their ability to change, RET educates them by showing them precisely how to effect these changes. It can help people experience relief in a short period of time because its therapeutic potency is notably increased through the vigorous, disputing, argumentative style of which Ellis is one of the pioneers. It is such potency that leads to the creation of existential moments that help people take charge of their lives.

DIRECT DECISION THERAPY AND THE REBELLIOUS PATIENT, WITH HAROLD GREENWALD, PH.D.

Dr. Greenwald is a clinical psychologist in private practice and also Distinguished Professor of Clinical Psychology at United States International University and chairman of the university's program in Humanistic Psychology. Dr. Greenwald has authored many books and articles. Among his books are *The Call Girl* and *Direct Decision Therapy*.

I learned some very important things about doing psychotherapy as a result of being present while Dr. Greenwald did a demonstration with a twenty-six-year old female patient before a large group at the Direct Decision Institute Associates workshop in San Diego.

First, I learned to look for the decision behind the decision. For example, while it appeared that this patient made a decision to rebel against everything her mother suggested she do, Dr. Greenwald was able to pinpoint that the real decision was to cooperate and comply with her mother by avoiding connecting with her father, and other men, particularly Jewish men, in her life.

Second, I learned how Dr. Greenwald became the kind of person that the patient had trouble with in her life, and in a sense smoked her out by acting like that person. In this case, he acted as he thought the girl's mother might act, whom the girl mistakenly felt she was rebelling against. While transactional analysis deals with the issues of the rebellious and compliant Child ego states, Dr. Greenwald's psychodynamic way of combining learning theory with a here-and-now brand of existentialism similar to Albert Ellis's RET, takes you right into the patient's life.

Third, I learned that while Dr. Greenwald speaks of helping a person have the free choice to make a decision, he lays things out in a rational way when it is obvious that a continuation of the patient's present behavior would be foolhardy and crazy. Thus, the only real choice he leaves the patient is rational living.

Fourth, I learned how Dr. Greenwald continually used his psychoanalytic training to keep tabs on the evidence the patient gave him, and how he used such evidence as a way to confront the patient so the movement would be in the direction of rational living.

Fifth, I learned a *basic truth that runs through rebellious patients, that they must ask themselves whether they are free to choose what Mom or Dad wants them to do, even if the patient wants to do it.* This awareness has proved to be liberating in many patients since my attendance at the workshop.

Sixth, I learned how to experientially help a patient correct the damaged situation by rewiring the parental connection. For example, this patient was requested to really pay attention to her Dad while ignoring the opportunity to rebel against her Mom.

Seventh, I learned the unique ways that Dr. Greenwald views payoffs behind the past decisions that are destructively being lived out in the present tense. For example, the payoff for withdrawal is to avoid anxiety and to express hostility.

Eighth, I was interested in Dr. Greenwald's view that therapists get themselves in trouble when they demand that people live up to their potential, that they self-actualize. Dr. Greenwald emphasized that people need not live up to their potential unless they want to. There is a paradoxical twist to accepting what a patient is doing. I feel this even pertains to what a patient does on a moment-to-moment basis. For it is when a therapist has a difficult time accepting a patient's behavior on a here-and-now basis that therapists sometimes get feelings that they don't want to work with that patient or even that they don't like that patient. But if therapists put their own demands aside in those situations, more is likely to happen, therapists are likely to feel better about the patient, and in turn the patient may feel better about him or herself. Such acceptance is critical in the treatment of narcissistic and passive-aggressive personality problems.

Dr. Greenwald feels that when therapists tell people to do what they are already doing, many people can choose *not* to do it. Conversely, he feels they cannot make the choice not to do it as long as therapists tell them to do what they are not doing. Therapists who keep these principles in mind are much less likely to impose their own judgmental standards on patients. This is Dr. Greenwald's way of paradoxically accepting what the patient is doing.

The steps of Direct Decision Therapy are highlighted in the following case. The steps are:

1. Ask the patient about the patient's goal
2. Find out what the problem is that prevents the patient from reaching the goal
3. Examine the past decisions which helped to create the problem
4. Examine the payoffs for the decisions that are behind the current problem
5. Explore new options that are not based on old and no longer functional decisions that are responsible for the problem
6. Help the patient make a new decision, realizing that the patient will not be perfect in carrying out the new decision and that the decision will have to be repeated over and over to be effective.

G (Dr. Greenwald) If you were coming to see me now, what would be your problem? (This is the first step of direct decision therapy–'DDT'–asking the patient to state the problem. He was also subtly disarming by saying, "if you were coming, etc." when she was there in front of him.)

M (Marianne) To not rely so much on outside acceptance; especially in terms of my family. And to feel good enough about myself that I don't need to satisfy my parent's expectations.

G   What prevents you from doing that? (Second step of DDT is to ask the patient what gets in the way of her accomplishing her goal.)

At this point Dr. Greenwald begins to ask Marianne for specific examples and the dialogue reveals that Marianne was raised in New York from a Jewish background. She feels a basic conflict in values in that she views her parents as materialistic and success-oriented. She said they disapproved of her husband, who was a Southern Baptist farm boy who went into the Navy to fly planes.

G   You obviously needed your parents approval very badly. (Humor is used to confront the incongruity and rebelliousness of her behavior. HE RECOMMENDS HUMOR BE USED TO CONFRONT ONLY WHEN THE THERAPIST LIKES THE PATIENT, OTHERWISE IT LEAVES A BAD TASTE. He then pushes for step three of DDT–understanding the past decision that is at the root of the problem.) And they couldn't understand your choice? How about you? Could you understand your choice?

Marianne saw her problem in terms of striving for *differentness*, but Dr. Greenwald brought it back to the family dynamic. Marianne felt defensive, saying she loved both parents.

G   . . . mother, father, you didn't have to choose when you were young, growing up. (Telling her that she didn't have to choose was a sophisticated way to bypass the obvious resistance and Marianne's need to be fair and be seen as loving of her parents.)

Marianne described a difficult time with her mother when she was growing up. She said she was very close to her father and jealous of her mother, but that now she was close to her mother and her father was off the pedestal.

G   What does your father do?

M   He's a Jewish jeweler.

G   How come you didn't marry a Jewish jeweler? (A stunning type of question coming from a strong intuition.)

G   (Later on in the dialogue) Suppose you find somebody that's interesting and then you find out they are Jewish? What happens to your feeling?

Marianne reported that she is not sexually attracted to a man who is Jewish. Dr. Greenwald then begins to indirectly focus on how this past decision gets in the way of the patient reaching her goal when he says,

G   It's a good thing, too.

M   Why?

G   Because your mother would kill you. (He humorously hits right at the primal fear.)

M   You've got me cold.

G   From now on you can do the rest yourself (affirms her power which is important for the rebellious person to whom power is an issue. As Napoleon said, "Power is never ridiculous.") It's a decision.

However, Marianne is not ready to accept the interpretation, and after clearly stating it, denies it, but Dr. Greenwald is quick on his comeback.

M   What you are trying to tell me is that I am not attracted to Jewish men because my mother would kill me for being sexually attracted to my father, no.

G   Would she have liked it? (A beautiful question to challenge the denial.)

In the following interchanges Dr. Greenwald used the evidence as she continues with her denial by telling him the interpretation doesn't fit.

G   No, of course not. But you were very close to your father and you didn't get along with your mother.

M   When I was younger, yes. (The evidence leads to a *yes* response, which is an important step in working with rebellious patients.)

G   OK.

M   Why does it have to be sexual?

G   (Again, very sharp in remembering the evidence.) Who said?

M   You.

G   No, I didn't say that. You brought that in. I was trying to find out how come when it was so important for your family and when you love your parents so much, how is it if it was so important to them that you marry somebody that's Jewish, that you haven't found yourself attracted to a Jewish man. You said, I don't find them sexually attractive. After explaining that you were very close to your father and hated your mother. Now you don't have to put this together if you don't want to. It's alright with me. (After presenting the evidence he gives her permission not to put it together, or to continue doing what she is doing, which leads through the passive block to movement. It is the use of paradoxical acceptance of what she is doing.)

M　　The reason that I didn't and I'm not attracted to Jewish men generally is because of my dislike for my mother when I was growing up. It is out of my disrespect for her. I don't respect my mother's values because I don't respect my mother. And those values are real important to her–that he is Jewish, he's a doctor, and he's rich. (She makes a switch here. As the sexual interpretation was too threatening, and as she was *given permission not to put that together*, she now talks of values which would broach her problem in a more delicate way. It is easier for her to accept herself as a moral person concerned about values rather than as a daughter lusting after her father.)

G　　So there's a negative identification with your mother. (Fourth step in DDT is exploration of the payoff. In this case there is a reverse payoff in that negative identification gets mother's covert approval.)

M　　Yes.

G　　And you'd figure out what your mother wanted and you would do the opposite.

M　　Right.

G　　And yet with all that you expect her to like this? You came up saying the real problem is you don't feel accepted by your parents. And now you are claiming that you make it a point to do the opposite of what your mother wants. (The contradiction of the evidence she has presented about a past decision that dominates her life in the here and now.)

M　　I guess so, yes. (Reluctant acknowledgement)

G   And that you were going to have completely different values, so that actually in your bid for independence of your mother you have become completely dominated by her. (He slyly hit her with this interpretation while beginning to talk about the issue of values. This sneaky, fast way of moving from a non-threatening situation to the dynamite was tantamount to shock therapy. Further, it both paradoxically used her rebelliousness to point out that by Marianne's own past decision, she has been defeated by her mother, and it demonstrated the absolute craziness and absurdity of continuing to act upon her past decision. From this point on Marianne's only real choice is rational living.)

M   (A begrudging acknowledgement) I guess so, because even three thousand miles away, she comes into play in my indecisions. (This was an unconscious slip–she meant to say decisions.)

G   So you are still deciding on the basis of the negative–that you are not going to do anything she wants you to do. You know what the terrible thing is, you were fooled.

M   (Very sad voice) Explain that to me.

G   You've done everything she has wanted you to do. (What a shock for someone who thinks she is rebellious! Again, he points to the craziness so blatantly that her only choice is to decide to be rational.)

M   How?

G   Your mother saw you as a very formidable competitor. Not necessarily sexually. Your father was very interested and very close to you. She was cold and disapproving. This is the way you have described it, right?

M   Yes.

G   Now, she, like many people–I'm guessing, it's a pure guess, therefore, to make you into a bad person would be very much in her favor. (Dr. Greenwald's comment points to a universal truth of the rebellious person really winding up being the patsy as a result of letting themselves be fooled, both in the original decision, and over and over.)

M   If I was a bad person, then justifiably I couldn't be close with her.

G   With your father, too. You are now much closer to your mother than you are your father, you said. So she was worked very well. She wasn't consciously doing this to be scheming or anything like that, but the amazing thing is, that you thought you were reacting against her in your decision to be very different from your mother, but you are really playing out a scenario that she unconsciously had in mind for you. (Dr. Greenwald was careful to say the mother had no conscious awareness of this so Marianne would not cling to the victim position that would be filled with vengeful hatred toward her mother.)

At this point Marianne showed a great deal of sadness. Dr. Greenwald was empathic and caring, but also tried to capitalize on her pain as a motivation for change.

G   How do you feel about having devoted your life under an illusion?

M   The reality of it isn't integrated in me. I'm not feeling anything. (Two basic problems that her denial bring her: a lack of integration with reality and a sense of being cut off from her genuine feelings apart from rebellion and anger.)

Dr. Greenwald retraces his steps, telling her that she made a conscious decision to do the exact opposite of what her mother wanted her to be, and that by doing that she was very much in charge of Marianne and her life was still dominated by her mother, whether it be positive or negative.

Marianne acknowledged feeling trapped. It is here that Dr. Greenwald begins the exploration for a new decision and new options (fifth step of DDT) by asking her how she is going to get out of it. His comments continually were in the directions of decision and action after she acknowledged the trap and the desire to change.

G   *Even if she wanted you to do it, would you be able to do it?* (This is the key–the way out of the trap for the patient suffering from the rebellious illusion. The patient must finally decide to begin paying attention to what she thinks and feels and to what she wants to do.)

G   Now, to be really free, wouldn't it also be important for you to be able to choose what you want to do whether they want it or not? (This comment struck both a rational and an emotive chord because it appealed to the rational mind while freeing the emotions from the trap. And while it looked like Dr. Greenwald had given Marianne a choice he did not. When things have been so rationally clarified, how could she choose the decision not to choose what she wants? Perhaps it is such work on the part of Dr. Greenwald that has been responsible for him being compared to Dr. Ellis and his brand of rational-emotive therapy. For Dr. Ellis, too, while presenting the illusion of choice to the patient, makes it perfectly clear by attacking the irrational beliefs in so many ways that the patient is almost forced to make a rational change or say, I am going to choose to be crazy in the face of overwhelming evidence.

Dr. Greenwald began to lay out the steps for Marianne's new decision: first, to be free to do what she wants whether they want it or not; second, to check her own motivation occasionally when she says, "Oh, no, I couldn't do that," to see if her decision is really hers or if it is an automatic reaction not to do anything her parents want her to do.

G   (Referring to earlier part of their dialogue) And when I asked you even a simple thing like "Repeat out loud," you wouldn't do it. And it's OK, but what I'm indicating to you is, that you were able in this situation to decide to do what you wanted to do despite all my power, my prestige, my position. You still challenged me to do what you wanted to do. (A rebellious situation is turned around into a victory for her, and thereby a victory for him–stroking the resistance.)

Dr. Greenwald then admitted to trying to deliberately push her around, and that she did demonstrate the capacity to choose what she wanted. (This is the way he used himself in the role of the feared object–Mom.) When Marianne acknowledged feeling her power in the face of Dr. Greenwald pushing her around, he, almost in the voice of a warm, gently nudging Jewish mother said, "Now, when are you going to start changing?" Marianne felt supported with this comment.

Then Marianne made a decision that she was going to go back to her sister's wedding in New York, not because her parents wanted her to go, but because she was curious and did love her sister. It took some work on Dr. Greenwald's part to help her to this realization, but she did begin putting her decision into action immediately by focusing on what she really wanted to do. In the process of helping her recognize her true wants a humorous confrontation took place.

M   I know you are fishing for why I want to go.

G   No, no. I'm not fishing for anything. I'm not your mother. (Group laughs, but this was a point of therapist denial because, as I indicated earlier, he did begin responding like a Jewish mother. However, he was very quick to own this behavior in the very next statement, which is all that is required of a therapist when a mistake is made.) The resemblance may be striking. (Group cracked up with laughter, acknowledging they, too, thought he was responding like a Jewish mother at this point in the work.)

G   You can enjoy the trip even if your parents want you to go.

M   God, I can't believe how much there is of an adolescent rebel in me. I don't know . . . .

G   OK. This is something you will have to work on for awhile. (The sixth step of DDT is to reinforce the idea that this is an area that is going to take a lot of practice, and that she shouldn't have either magical expectations or disproportionate disappointments as a result of her desire to be perfect at the task and a low frustration tolerance.)

Then Dr. Greenwald ended the session with a stroke of genius by helping the patient rewire her family connections, which also had implications for a sexual rewiring.

G   When you go home, you want to have some fun?

M   Yes.

G   Whenever your father and mother are around pay great attention to your father. Be sweet and kind to your father and pay no attention to your mother. (Group laughter) How does that feel?

M   I think my father would get upset.

G   That's his problem. How would you like doing that? (Dr. Greenwald intimates that Dad fell down on the job in not stroking Marianne's womanhood as she was growing up.)

M   I'd like to see what would happen.

Marianne agreed to try it. She later gave him a post-session report that she had enjoyed the wedding and that she met two attractive Jewish men.

After this workshop I did therapy with a surgeon who lived in a mansion, had an extremely lucrative practice, and had all that money could buy. While there were certainly some other problems in his life, the realization that he wasn't free to choose to enjoy what he had because they were his mother's values left him sabotaging himself to the point he wanted to either give up his fortune or unconsciously set himself up to lose it. When he realized that he could choose to want what he had, and enjoy it, even if his mother wanted it for him, it was certainly an existential moment that put his life in an entirely different and freer perspective. He had the freedom to decide!

ENDNOTES

1 Herbert Spiegel and David Spiegel, Trance and Treatment: Uses of Hypnosis. New York: Basic Books, 1978, p. 223-224.

2 These two songs and several others are written on a one-page paper that Dr. Ellis gave to the group. Copyright 1977 by The Institute for Rational Living, Inc. Those interested may write to The Institute for Rational Living, Inc., 45 East 65th St., New York, N.Y. 10021. A cassette and songbook are also available.

REFERENCES

Bach, George, and Goldberg, Herb. *Creative Aggression*. New York: Doubleday & Co., 1974.

Bach, George. *Intensive Group Psychotherapy*. New York: The Ronald Press, 1954.

Ellis, Albert, and Harper, Robert. *A New Guide to Rational Living*. 1978, Wilshire Book Company, 12015 Sherman Road, North Hollywood, Calif. 91605

Ellis, Albert. *How to Live With and Without Anger*. New York: Reader's Digest Press, distributed by Thomas Y. Crowell, 1977.

Ellis, Albert. *Sex Without Guilt*. 1969, Wilshire Book Company, 12015 Sherman Road, North Hollywood, Calif. 91605

Greenwald, Harold. *Direct Decision Therapy*. San Diego: Edits, Publisher, 1973.

Greenwald, Harold. *The Call Girl*. San Diego: Decision Books, 1978.

Maltz, Maxwell. *Psycho-Cybernetics*. 1978, Wilshire Book Company, 12015 Sherman Road, North Hollywood, Calif. 91605

Spiegel, Herbert, and Spiegel, David. *Trance and Treatment: Uses of Hypnosis*. New York: Basic Books, Inc., 1978.

9

Clinical Hypnosis

Into each life some confusion should come . . . also some enlightenment.–Milton H. Eri9ckson, M.D.

AN EXPERIENCE OF THE HYPNOTHERAPY OF MILTON H. ERICKSON, M.D.

DR. MILTON HYLAND Erickson, known for his innovative approaches to psychotherapy and hypnosis is considered the father of medical hypnosis. Dr. Erickson published extensively in addition to several books being written about his work. Among them are *Uncommon Therapy: The Psychiatric Techniques of Milton H. Erickson, M.D.*, written by Jay Haley, and *Hypnotherapy* written by Dr. Erickson and Dr. Ernest Rossi, Ph.D. Dr. Erickson was born December 5, 1901, at Aurum, Nevada, and died March 25, 1980, in Phoenix, Arizona.

Dr. Erickson was a pioneer in both behavior modification and clinical hypnosis. Among psychotherapists, Dr. Erickson was known for his unusual approaches to both psychotherapy and clinical hypnosis. His unique synthesis is called *hypnotherapy*. While a great deal has been written about Dr. Erickson, his work has not been approached from an existential viewpoint. Yet, it was Dr. Erickson's uncommon methods of clinical hypnosis and behavior modification that helped this existentialist to experience life, in a much fuller way than I had previously known. To say the very least, Dr. Erickson provided one experience after the other that most of the time pleasantly surprised me, sometimes unpleasantly surprised me, yet always made an impact on me. He provided a series of accentuated, peak existential moments that became imbedded in my unconscious mind and helped to stir up much of me that lay dormant. Once again enlivened, I found my unconscious to be a trustworthy and creative companion.

Dr. Erickson was primarily concerned with the uniqueness of each individual. It is from his *astute perceptions*, on *many levels*, of the *uniqueness of the individual*, that Dr. Erickson found ways of *entering the world of the individual* and *setting it in motion with the laws of nature*. He had said that his enemies often called him a manipulator, but he felt that manipulating the individual *helps that person* to take new action *(in either direction)*, to further new actions that may eventually lead to more satisfying living. He felt such manipulation is one of the basics of doing effective hypnotherapy.

While every human being has limitations, Dr. Erickson presupposed a view of consciousness that has unlimited possibilities and did his best to provide the kind of open-ended environment so his patients could expand their possibilities. He did this by helping to create experiences in which patients were able to let go of conscious control and begin to trust in their unconscious processes and their inner wisdom.

Although this chapter runs the risk of oversimplifying the creative genius of Dr. Erickson, I want to emphasize the simplicity that was at the heart of his creative genius. By practicing the principles mentioned in this chapter I have been able to develop my style of doing hypnotherapy.

I am writing my particular view of how Dr. Erickson influenced me and there is not a great deal of attention given to how Dr. Erickson may have perceived situations that I describe. Nor is there a great deal of attention given to the accuracy or inaccuracy of exact words used by

Dr. Erickson. My basic concern is with the general impact his unique hypnotherapy had upon me and on others with whom I have seen him work. It is this impact that resulted in existential moments. As the years went by, I added attention to direct words in my creation of "REVERSE ANALYSIS."

I will attempt to give the reader a personal flavor of Dr. Erickson–and the extent to which this personal flavor was creatively and dynamically injected into his work. His techniques supplemented his person, but it was his person that initially presented an awesome sense of presence. By presence, I refer to therapists' ability to respond immediately as a result of an implicit trust in their own unconscious minds and what will flow from them. Thus, manifesting presence is an active process. It is not mere words.

Distracting the Conscious Mind

PART OF DR. ERICKSON'S CREATIVE GENIUS WAS HIS AMAZING CLINICAL ACCURACY, SPEED, PERCEPTION, AND HIS DOING THE UNEXPECTED. The therapist's basic task is to evaluate the patient as quickly as possible, and then, through whatever common or uncommon means that flowed through the therapist's unconscious mind, to distract the patient's conscious mind so the therapist can work with the unconscious mind and have the patient's cooperation.

By distracting the patient's unconscious mind, I am referring to the therapist's ability to *surprise* the patient–to get the patient off balance–to have the patient willing to listen to the therapist in a way that will permit that therapist to bypass much or all of the patient's conscious defense mechanisms. When the therapist is able to do this, the patient will regress to a childlike state in which that patient is then open to the authority of a new parent–the therapist–who may then be able to facilitate a curative experience. I include here my initial experience with Dr. Erickson to illustrate how he surprised me. Then I shall give a few other examples.

I telephoned Dr. Erickson. He asked me when I wanted to come to Phoenix to work with him. I said the first weekend he could see me alone. He quickly blurted out that people were coming the next two weekends but that I should come next weekend because I would get what I wanted. I was stunned! I didn't want to share my time with anyone, yet, I was intrigued by his assurance that I would get what I wanted. Who knows what he knew? I said I could come. He hung up. I was frustrated at a twenty-second telephone call in which I wound up going somewhere without knowing what time I had to be there or the address of my destination. I called back. He said, "Eleven a.m. and call Mrs. Erickson from the airport. She will give you directions and tell you what motel is nearest." Click. I was frustrated again. I called back a day later to ask about his health. I didn't want to go to Phoenix if he wasn't well enough to work with me–a mistake a colleague made a couple of months after I had gone. (Dr. Erickson's voice sounded very feeble on the telephone. I did not know it at the time, but his lips were partially paralyzed). In another ten second call he said, "Call me the day before." Click. I had all the information I needed but was still frustrated. In retrospect I believe this process had a great deal to do with the outcome of the session. Let's just say I was ready to change by the time I arrived.

My wife, drove me to Dr. Erickson's house and said she would come in to find out what time to pick me up. She had never been in therapy and never expressed any desire to do so. Mrs. Erickson answered the door and told us to go around to the side of the house, where the office was located. It was a strange looking office, about one hundred square feet and most humble in its appearance. I couldn't quite put my finger on why it affected me as being strange.

Mrs. Erickson wheeled Dr. Erickson into the office. In addition to my wife and me, three other people were present. Dr. Erickson handed each of us a piece of paper and told us to write our names, age, occupation, educational background and marital status. He peered intently at us while we did so. There was no escaping from his eyes. I felt like I was in grammar school again. The other thing I noticed was that my wife wasn't leaving the office and that she did fill out the paper. I was beginning to think I was in the twilight zone.

Dr. Erickson began to talk to me. "So you have come all the way from California and you are avoiding the hot seat." He paused for a while. I could have told him I didn't know which seat was the hot seat because they all looked the same to me, but I had a thought that he would think I was just dodging the issue. I felt frozen. His next response, "Now that I have mentioned it I see that you are still avoiding the hot seat." I told him I was ambivalent about taking it. I then moved into the chair next to his desk. His third statement, "So you're a clinical psychologist. I'll bet you don't even know why I am wearing purple!" I thought to myself, he has picked up on my lack of environmental awareness already. It hit me in a flash. His office was unusual because it had so damn much purple in it. He had a purple telephone. A purple cloth hanging from the wall. Two of his published books had purple covers and all his clothes including his socks were purple. He was an awesome sight. I said, "You are wearing purple because that is just part of Dr. Erickson's style." Although this was also a correct answer in retrospect, at the time he said, "I am wearing purple because I am color blind! It's the only color I can see!" However, he said it in a way that left me feeling extremely foolish. He had established his point, that he was the teacher and I was the student.

Although Dr. Erickson did not limit himself to any particular method to put patients off balance and catch their unconscious mind's attention, he chose to use an authoritarian attitude with me. Also, I never heard him use the words "hot seat" with anyone else. He was tapping into my prior gestalt training and speaking to me in my own language. This is an extremely important point in Dr. Erickson's success in communicating with a wide variety of patients, and certain patients in particular that would have been diagnosed as untreatable by many therapists.

He was quickly able to communicate with patients in their own language, their own way of viewing the world, and once he did this he then interjected the surprise elements to take patients off balance so they would regress and through their unconscious, highlight the particular feelings, thoughts and actions that would help patients creatively break through the impasse in their lives.

He took a woman off balance to get her attention when he asked her if she would tell him all the possible ways she could physically move from his office to his waiting room. She said, "I can walk, I can crawl, I can slide on my stomach, or I can ask other people in the room to carry me." Dr. Erickson said, "I asked you to tell me all the possible ways you could physically move from my office into my waiting room." The woman, playing hotshot, was taken aback. She thought she had done what he requested, and his repeating the question indicated that she did not. She repeated her thoughts on the matter and then Dr. Erickson said something that alluded to people's limitations. He looked at her and said, "You couldn't even think of walking into the room backwards!" She was left with the impression of her limitations and he now had provided an environment that got the focus of her attention. He intimidated her by being a trickster, doing so with an authoritarian attitude.

Also of interest was that after Dr. Erickson had used an authoritarian approach to get my attention, he induced hypnosis by a very passive and simple method. The emphasis was not on the technique, but on the fact that he had my conscious attention diverted by demonstrating, in an intimidating way, that *I was limited,"* and *"I could learn new ways."*

Changing Belief Systems

With Dr. Erickson's therapy, once patients were put off balance, and had regressed to a childlike state, they could seek some resolution to their discomfort and confusion. At this point patients were in a position to search for a new resolution, as opposed to defending themselves against new input.

However, Dr. Erickson didn't always make changing their belief systems easy for them. They were often left to search for the new resolutions to their problems. After all, Dr. Erickson said he is just an old man who tells stories. However, it is through the use of this indirect suggestion via stories, anecdotes, and metaphors that patients are given the opportunity to search for new answers. These answers do come. Dr. Erickson would sit there, telling one story after another for three or four hours. Every now and then, the punchline slips right through the unguarded conscious mind into the unconscious mind and frees that unconscious mind to utilize this new stimulus to continue to build on its own talents to enhance creative and happy living. The message the patient's unconscious mind needs to experience bypasses the conscious defenses because there is no way to foretell what the message will be, and the patient's confused, off-balance, childlike state makes it a strain to come up with the relevant message from the story. In most therapies, therapeutic progress is delayed because patients are in full control of their conscious faculties, and are not taken off balance; they would dismiss the same suggestion they had searched for in one of Dr. Erickson's stories if it were told to them directly.

The following is an example of such a story, as I remember it, which I am sure leaves out many of the details that Dr. Erickson included, but nevertheless is still quite forceful and gives a feeling for his style:

(The story is told at a very slow, monotonous pace. The phrases that stuck in my unconsciousness and that were responsible for my changing are in italics. They hit me at a symbolic level like red neon signs flashing across my mind.) I remember a patient named Pete. Pete was an *ex-convict*. He had lived *most of his life in jail*. But he has been *out of jail for the last seven months*. He was living with a girl, had a job as a bartender, and was *drunk every night* for the last seven months (just about the time he would say *drunk* Dr. Erickson might turn toward someone in the group, or around at several members in the group, and look at them in a very intimidating way). His girlfriend got sick and tired of him. She threw him out. He walked eighteen miles in the *blazing hot desert sun* of Phoenix to get to my office. When he got to my office he asked me for my help and I gave it to him. He became angry, got up, slammed the door (long pause after each comma), and walked another eighteen miles back to town in the *scorching sun* of Phoenix, Arizona. He talked his girlfriend into taking him back. He resumed his job as a bartender. And he was *drunk* every night for another two weeks. His girlfriend got *sick and tired* of him again and *threw him out* (long pause while Dr. Erickson would turn his head about looking at people in a very intimidating way). Pete, feeling *more desperate* than he had the first time, walked *another eighteen miles* in the *blazing hot desert sun* of Phoenix, Arizona. He got to my office and asked me for my help. I told him, Pete, you asked me for my help and I gave it to you. You told me to shove it so I shoved it. (A good time for a few intimidating looks.) And if *you want my help "NOW"* (as he stretched the word out in a droning fashion) you're going to have to *beg me to take your boots*. That is the convict's *code of honor* that he really *means business*. Well, Pete, understanding the full nature of the request, became angrier than he was the first time. He got up, slammed the door, and walked *another* eighteen miles in the *blazing hot desert sun of Phoenix, Arizona*. He got back to town, talked his girlfriend into taking him back, resumed his job as a bartender, and was drunk every night for another week and a half. His girlfriend got fed up with him. She said it was for the last time. She threw him out. Pete, feeling the *most desperate* he had felt yet, walked another eighteen miles in the blazing hot sun of Phoenix, Arizona. He got to my door, knocked on the door, *took off his boots* and begged me to take his boots. I said, Pete, come on in. *All I want you to do* is go out into my back yard, you can stay as long as you need, there's an old mattress out there you can sleep on, if you get cold at night you can ask Mrs. Erickson for a blanket, but I don't think you will because it's summertime. If you get hungry you can tell Mrs. Erickson and she will give you pork and beans, and *think about what you want to do with your whole life*. (This is how Dr. Erickson might slip in suggestions amidst the monotonous details of his story.) Pete had been there awhile. It was my birthday and my daughter and granddaughter came to visit on a Sunday afternoon. They asked if they could go out and talk with Pete. I agreed. Everyone had a most enjoyable afternoon. At the end of the day Pete told me that he never knew that women and girls like that really existed. A short time after that Pete asked for his boots back. I heard from him a year later. He had a job that was enjoyable. He was involved in a relationship that was meaningful, and he was dry.

Through the use of indirect suggestion via stories, patients were able to take in suggestions that might otherwise take years to incorporate, if ever.

He was a master in using *double binds:* a method in which the therapist will set up the situation in a way so that the patient will use their resisting behavior to promote their cure. Dr. Jerry Tepperman, a clinical psychologist in the Los Angeles area, provided me with an interesting example of a double bind he uses with chronic pain patients who are involved in litigation. They have so many secondary reinforcers, such as their lawsuit being contingent on maintaining the pain, that such a group is most difficult to reach. Dr. Tepperman tells them, "The average patient in your condition that comes to see me doesn't have any success with hypnosis. It would take an extraordinary patient to have any success at all. But I'm willing to give you twelve weeks of my time. If you were to make any subjective progress I would be the most surprised."

The object of the double bind in the above example is to give the patient a setup to reinforce the symptom, so the patient will either rebel against the therapist and rid him or herself of the pain, or follow the therapist's suggestion, thereby removing the masochistic secondary gains that accompany the patient's sabotage in trying to help themselves. Either way there is a change.

Dr. Erickson relied heavily upon the power of expectancy to help people change their belief systems. He acted with a supreme sense of self-confidence, implying that it would be foolish for patients to even imagine they could not use all of their unconscious potential to bring about the changes they want to effect in their lives.

Occasionally he would demonstrate this power of expectancy through the use of hypnosis and trance ratification. Although he departed from using traditional hypnosis in later years in favor of an anecdotal approach (except for the fact he had everyone's undivided attention and in that sense we were in trance), Dr. Erickson did give one demonstration where I was able to see many of the techniques demonstrated. He challenged a woman about whether she was in hypnotic trance. He asked her when she first stopped hearing the traffic noises, then chuckled at her, giving the impression it would be ridiculous for her to even imagine she were not in trance. Then he asked her if she could move her arms. She said no. He asked her if she thought she could stand up. She said no. Each time he looked at her as though it would have been ridiculous for her to even attempt it. Finally it appeared to the woman and the group that he had brought her out of trance. Then he asked her if she thought she was now awake. She said yes, and he reached over very quickly, giving her arm a quick flip at which point it stayed in a raised position.

The same power of expectancy demonstrated by Dr. Erickson's words and actions were also demonstrated in his attitude. He had a powerful expectancy that people have all they need within their unconscious minds to lead happy and healthy lives. He viewed his task as helping them tap into their unconscious roots and creativity. However, his power of expectant belief in the unconscious provided a belief for me in my unconscious mind that did not exist before. It also provided the same belief in the trustworthiness of the unconscious minds of others. It is this belief that first helped me to believe in myself and change my own self-destructive belief systems in a relatively short period of time (one eight-hour weekend with Dr. Erickson) and helped me to instill those same beliefs in my patients; to trust their unconscious minds and even use the same behavior that was previously considered self-destructive to their advantage. For example, an obsessive compulsive patient who exemplifies self-destructive behavior that might lead to a heart attack eventually, could instead use that same obsessive behavior to take good care of his health.

Once patients' belief systems have been altered in a way that leaves them open to new experience, they become open to the creative genius of their unconscious minds. They realize they have the capacity to change their lives around. The remainder of the therapeutic work after this point is to carry out new behavior which they now believe in. In most patients this will not be too difficult a task. And in the highly rebellious patient, Dr. Erickson used the double bind technique. For example, a patient went to work with Dr. Erickson. His wife became jealous and she too telephoned. She said that although she was not a training therapist she would also like to see Dr. Erickson if her husband was going to see him. She was interested in working on weight loss, but told Dr. Erickson that she did not think he could hypnotize her. He told her that was not a valid reason to try to hypnotize her. However, quickly picking up on her competitive spirit with her husband, the following day he told her husband that he was going to hypnotize him and proceeded to do so. Well, not wanting to be outdone, she followed the same directives that were given to the husband and became hypnotized. When her husband had awakened he was surprised to find his wife in trance, and Dr. Erickson made fun of her a bit by telling her that he had indeed hypnotized her. At this point she was a believer, and one of the stories Dr. Erickson told stuck in her mind. He told a story about a girl who was trying to lose weight. He said that he told the girl to get a bottle of cod liver oil, to put it in the refrigerator, and if she wanted to eat between meals, that was perfectly all right, as long as she swallowed two teaspoonfuls of cod liver oil first. The moral of the story is that our doubting and resistive patient has come back to California, put a bottle of cod liver oil in the refrigerator, and lost six pounds in the first week. The bottle of cod liver oil is still unopened!

I spoke to Dr. Erickson about people changing self-destructive behavior. He said that although people might change certain ways of responding, they would revert right back to the ways in which they were behaving if put back in their original environments. If he were back on the farm where he grew up, he said he would easily remember and use the behaviors that became part of him at that time.

Dr. Erickson had an optimistic view of people. People could take charge of their lives either by utilizing old behavior patterns in new ways, learning new behavior patterns, or by drawing on parts of unconscious learning not previously highlighted. However, Dr. Erickson also had a deterministic viewpoint–that the past is the past, and those learnings for better or worse are forever a part of our existence.

Getting to the Heart of the Matter

While he had your attention, Dr. Erickson would continue to tell story after story. He described his work in the context of telling stories about his family, which could not but help stimulate unconscious fantasies about patients' families, or told stories about his work, which stimulated unconscious fantasies about patients' own careers. It might have been my own unconscious way of working, or perhaps Dr. Erickson's intention–I am not sure which; however, I experienced themes that traveled throughout life and death–and dealt fully and comprehensively with the nature of the human predicament.

For example, Dr. Erickson told a variety of stories about the different jobs he had held. There was an intimation that he accepted each job with the idea that it was a good opportunity and that it might very well be a lifelong career. In each instance some unforeseen event happened and Dr. Erickson was forced to move on. Some of these situations were very painful. He told the stories from his unconscious mind, but also from his heart and his experience of those people in the room. The theme that kept going throughout the stories was the theme of the unexpected, and that Dr. Erickson throughout his life had to continually come to grips with learning how to "let go." The theme of letting go flashed like a neon sign before my unconscious mind, letting me know that I couldn't experience much of life's surprises if I did not become more willing to let go. His stories focused on the universal insecurity feelings of all people.

Series of his stories sometimes centered around one or several themes. However, they went deep–right to the core or center or people and how they choose to exist or be in the world. They confronted people with their existential predicament in the world, and gave them the opportunity to consider the possibility of choosing an existence that has greater meaning. In addition to the stories, as a behavioral task to capture the essence of their existence one couple at the weekend session was asked to climb to the top of Squaw's Peak, and to arise at 4:30 in the morning to do so. The man had been forced to make many adjustments in his life. His wife had formerly been a bored housewife who had become a lawyer. She became interested in power and money, the same two interests of the man. Their existence was now structured around their competition for power and money. The man said his wife had the problem. Dr. Erickson accepted the man's statement and began working with the wife. However, his stories traveled to all corners of the room. The suggestion to climb to the top of Squaw's Peak gave them the opportunity to climb to the top together, if that was what they were set on doing. However, they came back before noon and said they had driven around for hours and not been able to find the entrance to start climbing Squaw's Peak. This had many implications regarding the peak they were trying to climb in their personal lives. The man reported to me that he had been depressed for three weeks after his visit to Dr. Erickson regarding his climb toward money and power, and that he and his wife were planning on setting out on a new path–a path that had compassion and heart–a path that left them both enjoying each other and much richer in their capacity to love others.

Touching Their Souls

Dr. Erickson, besides talking from his unconscious, had the ability to talk from his heart in a way that made deep contact with a person. During the training session one of Dr. Erickson's patients needed to see him and had a session in front of the training group. She had asthma and complained of not being able to sleep. She went into trance during which time he gave her suggestions about peace, restfulness and sleep. When she came out of trance it was apparent that she still wasn't quite satisfied. Dr. Erickson said to her in a spry, bubbly way through half-paralyzed lips, "Take it from a seventy-five year old authoritarian fellow like myself that you have very kissable lips and think about that when you go to sleep tonight." Well, you should have seen this woman beaming. You could tell that no one had ever told her anything like that in her entire life. She came alive. She looked delightful. The change in her appearance was amazing because upon arrival she looked lifeless, drained of energy and exhausted.

Dr. Erickson had captured the moment and created a moment between them that was to be cherished, an existential moment. He had reached in and touched her soul. However, she had been hungry for so long that she still felt unsatisfied. After she enjoyed what he had said to her for a few minutes, and as she was getting ready to walk out, she said, "But how will that help me sleep and stop coughing tonight?" Dr. Erickson, in another fully human moment, began to sing, something like "the lip bone is connected to the cheek bone, the cheek bone is connected to the neck bone, the neck bone is connected to the chest bone," etc. While she was still listening and walking out he told the rest of the group that he knew she would sleep very, very well that night. Thereby, he used all his power to set up an expectation for positive health behavior. It was quite touching to see such an awesome figure as Dr. Erickson turn into an adorable little old man singing the kind of song that couldn't help touch his patient's heart as well as her chest.

Therapy Is Just a Part of Life

Most therapists maintain a certain sanctity about the non-interruption of the therapeutic hour. This was not true of Dr. Erickson. Throughout the day I watched Dr. Erickson answer telephone calls and carry on business when his wife came in with messages. There was no special reverence given to the therapy session as something that should be separate from everyday life. During these times he would occasionally tell indirect stories or make comments about the *value of interrupted learning*. I moved into a new office shortly after returning home from Phoenix. The dentist next door played his stereo very loud. I felt incensed, and told him so; he nodded his head in acquiescence but I knew he wouldn't do a damn thing about it. Then I remembered the value of interrupted learning and changed a lifelong pattern about disturbing myself with noises and interruptions of therapy. A colleague who shared the office with me complained a few days later that the music was just driving him crazy. I softly chuckled to myself and talked to him about the value of interrupted learning.

No Wasted Energy

Dr. Erickson was a proponent of the scientific and philosophic rule of Occam's razor, "multiplicity ought not to be posited without necessity."[1] From the very beginning I was shocked by his crisp responses. He said everything concisely, so that in no way was I able to hang on to ward off any insecurities within me.

He answered his telephone calls to others in the same manner. They didn't last over thirty seconds and he did so right in the middle of the teaching sessions. He asked callers, "What do you want?" "What is your educational background?" and possibly one or two other comments before hanging up. That in itself can be of value to many practicing psychotherapists who abuse themselves and their energy during their sessions as well as when answering telephone calls. Therapists who permit patients to drain them will be hard pressed to teach their patients not to abuse themselves. In addition, therapists who do not foster patients' assumption of responsibility by responding responsibly, may eventually burn themselves out.

I find there are many times when I am confronted with such decisions. Patients who call and want to hang on after I have given them all they need; patients who take a long time writing their checks at the end of the session; those who attempt to make an unnecessary problem out of scheduling; those who always have that one last question after the time is up; and those whose basic message to the therapist is that they must be treated as special. One of the basics involved in doing therapy with these patients is to treat them just like everybody else. I have such people write their checks at the beginning of the session and deal with scheduling at that time. I tell them to bring up their question at the beginning of the next session, etc.

Yet, there are people I have treated in the film industry who were famous people, and who had these same traits and needed to feel special, but who sensed that this was their problem and actually appreciated my treating them ordinarily even though a large part of them found it distasteful while it was happening.

The Essence of the Work

Dr. Erickson's work transcended much of the technical wizardry that he was noted for. It is as if he realized that if he didn't get to the heart of the matter in his teaching, the world might not be able to recreate the essence of one of the greatest therapeutic minds it has yet to know. Although Dr. Erickson enjoyed doing one demonstration per visit, in a feisty and challenging way, he talked about people making hypnosis much too mysterious. He told people all they needed to do was have the patient focus on an object, tell them about the vast learnings that are part of their unconscious minds, talk to them about how it was to learn the alphabet–distinguishing an "a" from a "b" from a "d," and how difficult that was to learn, and how our unconscious minds are full of many other learnings that were difficult for us to learn, things we *didn't even know that we knew.* He would say, tell the patient his heart rate has changed, his respiration rate has changed, his blood pressure has changed and his muscle tone has changed, talk about the patient's arms becoming heavier and heavier, as they get more and more relaxed– then begin telling stories via indirect suggestion. He demystified the hypnosis process so that people would realize it is something they could continue to use throughout their lives. For example, the second time I wanted to learn hypnosis he said, "By the very fact you have asked the question already shows you are half in trance, and that you can go as deeply as you wish, for however long you wish, and come out whenever you wish." I hadn't realized I had the power to do all that at that stage of my career.

Dr. Erickson more often than not referred to his sessions as teaching sessions, where he used no formal hypnosis. He just experienced the people present, looked at them, asked them to write down some brief statistics about themselves–name, educational background, marital status, and occupation–and then began telling stories. This is THE ESSENCE OF THE WORK. HE TAUGHT PEOPLE ABOUT LIFE BY DIVERTING PATIENTS' CONSCIOUS MINDS, TALKING TO THEM FROM THE CORE OF HIS EXISTENCE TO THE CORE OF THEIRS, FULLY TRUSTING THAT EACH PATIENT'S UNCONSCIOUS MIND WOULD TAKE FROM THE EXPERIENCE WHAT IT NEEDED AT THAT TIME AND NO MORE. HE HAD A FULL ACCEPTANCE OF PEOPLE AND THEIR BEHAVIOR

AND THIS WAS OFTEN SHOWN TO THEM IN HIS RESPONSES QUITE SOON AFTER THEY BEGAN WORKING. For example, his acceptance of the man who said his wife had the problem and his working with them in that way–talking to her and not the man, when telling the stories. The man later told me that if Dr. Erickson had not done this he would have lost him, but the fact that he did do it gave him a sense of all-rightness at the gut level and permitted him to grow from that point.

What Therapists Need to Know and Practice

1. *Diagnostic acumen.* Dr. Erickson had an ability to zero in to the person and to his own unconscious mind, and that is how he diagnostically knew what stories to tell–not that it's strategic. Thus, by whatever therapy or other means people can trust their unconscious minds, they are more likely to be able to tell the right story at the right time. The more they practice the more they will be able to continue to tell consecutively stories that have indirect suggestions that make therapy relevant. The ability to make very fine detailed discriminations is helpful, and a therapist might, to practice, go to a botanical garden and learn to distinguish a variety of different kinds of plants, anything that will sharpen the immediacy of the therapist's ability to discriminate even the most minute details.

2. *Developing a curious mind.* Dr. Erickson told us how he would read a book by Thomas Mann, and another by Hemingway, *good books*–and read the last chapter first. He would then attempt to figure out what happened in the preceding chapter and read the entire book in this fashion. Practicing exercises of this kind will help therapists to view things from as many directions as possible.

3. *Communicating with your unconscious mind.* Through therapy, meditation, hypnosis, or other ways that you may find appropriate, come to trust your unconscious mind to be able to just let it flow while you work. This is quite different than waiting for the other person to respond, and then reacting passively to the situation.

4. *Practice your storytelling.* As the issues come into your unconscious mind when working with a patient, little by little the appropriate stories will also come into your mind. The more you practice, the better you will get at indirect suggestion, providing you are trusting your unconscious process.

5. *Talk to people from your heart.* Talk about your experience of you and them in a way that will touch them in a meaningful way. If you do not do this, what you say is likely to be unconnected words that have no relevance for the patient or for yourself.

COMMENTARY ON MY WORK WITH DR. ERICKSON

Experiencing training, teaching, advising, and hypnotherapy with Dr. Erickson was the most meaningful and unusual experience of my life. I was a dedicated student of Dr. Erickson and his work, yet, no matter how many times we were in contact over a two and one half year period, he did things that left me in total chaos. He was the master of surprise. Not all were of a pleasant nature, although some were. But on a deeper level I learned to have a sense of joy at being surprised even when the surprise stung.

He did his most effective therapy with me through letters. I would send him what I thought to be a casual letter discussing the current course of events in my working with hypnosis, and he might not respond, or he might send along a friendly note, or on a few occasions say and do something that was so out of line with what I thought I had sent him, that I just didn't know what to make of it. His letters would take me on long searches in which insights and actions would occur that would be major breakthroughs in my life. When he responded was uncanny. His dynamite came when the chips were down; when my back was pressed right against the wall. Oftentimes I did not even know this was the case. His letter would precede an event that, if I had not done my homework as a result of his letter, could have been responsible for major negative turns in my life. For example, what brought me to realization about a false sense of guilt, a false sense of power and a false assumption of responsibility in my work was a reply by Dr. Erickson to what I felt was a casual letter.

Dear Dr. Bergantino:

Your letter of October 1 was most appalling, because of its total disregard and disrespect for William of Occam.

Until you give evidence of respect for the law of parsimony, I suggest you discontinue your correspondence with me and your study with me.

Sincerely yours,

MILTON H. ERICKSON, M.D.

Dr. Erickson was very aware of the fact that I was dedicated to my work with him, and that I felt that working with him was most important to me. Needless to say, he sure knew how to get my attention. I couldn't think of anything worse than being thrown out of training with him. And who the hell was William of Occam? I went to the library and began to research William of Occam. Further the letter I had sent to Dr. Erickson was about five pages long. I was also getting the idea about the "razor's edge," of William of Occam, that I should write shorter letters that were more to the point. After much deliberation I wrote back:

> Dear Dr. Erickson:
>
> Your letter caused much turmoil. It was doubly difficult to deal with while recovering from an appendix operation. However, this letter is submitted to give evidence of my respect for the law of parsimony in the hope that no hours will become one, two, three, four, five or six as previously scheduled in November.
>
> What initially appeared to me to be a slight difference in perspective is now seen as a major change in personality—the dealing with a tragic flaw that left me with a false need to feel powerful—a false sense of responsibility—and a false assumption of guilt. The change I am now embarking upon will make a critical difference in my work. Patients will feel my respect for them as well as a fuller sense of self-accomplishment. When getting

into the area of "magic" it is critical for therapists and hypnotists to realize that they really aren't doing any magic at all–and that they only provide an environment where patients can heal themselves through whatever means their own unconscious minds make available to them. This is in accord with William of Ockham who postulated that we only know individuals and the rest are constructions of our mind. Multiplicity ought not to be posited without necessity.

Please respond as soon as possible in two respects: 1) Whether you are willing to work with me as previously scheduled. 2) This is what I do see. Is there anything I missed?

Thank you for your letter.
Sincerely,

Dr. Erickson responded:

Dear Dr. Bergantino:

I was pleased to receive your letter and note that you have reached a realistic appraisal.

You may attend the teaching sessions as scheduled. I am, however, finding it more and more difficult to allot time for individual consultations and I intend during the forthcoming year to discontinue this entirely. Therefore, I would not be able to give you five or six hours. I will, however, do my best to give you one to three hours although I cannot promise.

When I went to Phoenix to work with him, Dr. Erickson began by acknowledging the reddish purple shirt that I was wearing. To my amazement, after his letter, without any explanations whatsoever, I did not receive any individual time over the three day period.

However, Dr. Erickson began the session by looking me right in the eye, and saying "You wouldn't believe the psychiatrists and psychologists I train. They all have amnesia." He repeated the same thing again. I then realized that I went back to ask him the same questions I asked him on my first two trips to Phoenix, and that my letter to him had already answered the questions. Dr. Erickson had that challenging twinkle in his eye. Here it was I had gone through hell to get back in his training, only for my unconscious mind in reaction to what he was saying and doing, knowing that was my last visit and my training was over. I was shocked! He then began the session by looking around to the rest of the group in a challenging way, saying "I take no responsibility for blindness." He paused and repeated, "I take no responsibility for blindness." With such a challenge, conscious or unconscious, I knew damn well I wasn't going to forget anything I already knew but continued to block out due to my own rigidity. It should be mentioned that on this particular trip Dr. Erickson's health was unusually poor, and he also had to cut short the group sessions a bit. Whatever his reasons for not giving me individual time, which I do not know for sure, as I never knew anything for sure with him, it certainly did hit my need to be treated special. The message was clear in my mind that I needed to accept becoming one of a group and give up my grandiose position.

During the group session Dr. Erickson dealt with all the issues I had raised in the piece of paper I handed him at the beginning of the session. In other words, I got everything I wanted by going to see him in a group setting. Yet, I was in doubt. Was he talking to me during the group session? Was he just telling stories and my unconscious mind made what it needed to make out of the situation? Was he making sure I got what I needed while cutting into my need to be treated special? Why was he so formally impersonal, while at an unconscious level he felt like he was being very personal to me in the group setting? Was any of this reality? Was I imagining the entire thing? In any case I left the two-day session feeling very satisfied with my experience and very dissatisfied with not knowing any of the answers to these questions, and not really being sure if I was being personally slighted or not. Each time I worked with him or corresponded with him it was like being in the twilight zone. It is still hard to believe that I could be that unsure of so much at a conscious level. This method forced me to trust my unconscious as the only means in which I could respond at all.

On one occasion I was feeling very personal toward Dr. Erickson and addressed my letter, "Dear Milton." He wrote back the most formal of his letters, "Dear Dr. Bergantino." He made it clear that our relationship had a basic professional aspect to it and that he in no way planned to dilute his authority.

All the questions from my prior visit kept churning in my mind for months. A close friend and I wanted to go to another of his training sessions, so I dropped him a note. There was a longer period of delay than usual before he answered. This in itself caused further search. I kept remembering the story he told me the first time in which one of his patients could "stay in his back yard as long as he needed." I knew I didn't need the back yard any longer, but I wanted to go. In other words I had turned the tragic corner in my life and I was consistently experiencing and acting in positive ways.

A few weeks passed and one night it came to me. I couldn't wait for morning, as my unconscious became very clear and powerful about what I needed to write to Dr. Erickson.

Dear Dr. Erickson:

I trust you know that I do not have amnesia. In fact, my experiences with you are as deeply imbedded as was Cain's experiences with the Old Kung Fu Master.

My experience with you the last time was as unusual as all the rest. While at the conscious level I was disappointed that I didn't get to work with you individually for one to three hours, I felt that I got *everything* I came for. Further, I, at the unconscious level felt you said goodbye to me. ("I like to get new patients. I like to see them for awhile. Then I like them to leave and to refer me other new patients.")

I realize that you delivered the ultimate dynamite prior to that session. My errors tend to run in the direction of obsession, so all I really need to do whenever I feel any difficulty doing hypnotherapy, or personally, is see if I am assuming any false sense of power, false sense of responsibility, or false sense of guilt. It's an ABC method to clarity.

So I do not have a need to see you in February, although I have a want to see you in February. When I did not hear from you I began to examine my want. I love to see you be outrageous. I feel that I could listen to your stories forever and still be fascinated. Your ability to call your shots never fails to surprise me. Of course, when I thought about it I realized that you have taught me how to do all this. I just haven't practiced enough. The method is in developing a *curious mind*, making my *prediction*, and then *testing my hypothesis*. Even Ted Williams didn't *hit .406* until he had a lot of *batting practice*.

On the personal side there are even more important reasons why I am writing this difficult letter. While I am ready to come into my own, there is a part of me that wants to remain a perpetual student. To hang on.

I have one helluva time with separation. I could easily become your lifetime student, but then I might have missed the most important part of the lesson–how to become an adult who is willing to assume responsibility for his life. So I will continue to study your work, as I am doing in the pain section of one of your books, but I will not make myself your lifetime student. I guess this is how a person would feel at the end of a five to seven year intensive psychoanalytic experience.

You were correct when you said you could charge five hundred dollars an hour if you wanted to. My entire life has turned about since knowing you. Things have never been better. Even the off days are pretty good. I feel that I have the strength to deal with whatever comes.

So how does one say goodbye to the person who has provided the most significant impact in that person's life? I am embarrassed that I can think of nothing more than a simple–thank you.

Sincerely,
Len Bergantino, Ed.D., Ph.D.

Saying goodbye was most difficult for me. Three weeks later I received a note from Dr. Erickson.

Dear Len:

I received your letter of July 22, but before I had answered it I received the letter you sent by certified mail on August 11.

I wish to say that I appreciate the content of this letter and I hope that in the future we can meet casually.

Sincerely yours,
Milton

As I was uncertain as to what he meant by "casually," in his last communication to me he said, "I meant to imply that our meeting would be on a friendly basis and not directed to a specific goal of teaching and learning or advising."

I include this commentary, not to suggest that Dr. Erickson wanted to be my friend, but to comment upon an evolutionary process in my therapy with him. While his offer to meet on a friendly basis came as a surprise to me, given the previous formality of our relationship, perhaps at the deepest levels I needed such affirmation from someone whom I considered to have impeccable judgment in order to heal the most deep-seated wounds and insecurities about my own humanity that existed within me. While I certainly never questioned the sincerity of his words, I also understood that he had a way of sensing precisely which personal needs were most in need of fulfillment in his patients. Perhaps this was part of the cure for the remnants of my narcissism. Perhaps it was but a simple statement of his position. In any case, once again he left my unconscious mind with the surprise of not knowing for sure.

Further, while most of what has been written about Dr. Erickson describes him as exemplifying technical wizardry in his therapy that may never again be seen or experienced, I mean to show through the context of his letters that what I believe he was most concerned about was the development of a human being. And it was in that context that I experienced Milton Erickson (and he gave all that he was, which was more than I could have ever imagined) in much deeper and more profound ways than merely his technical wizardry which often appeared to be at the levels of magic. My suspicion is that much of what patients cooperated with at the unconscious level, that appeared to be magic, was in response to a deeply moving human being.

Our casual meeting never came to pass as a result of Milton's death. Throughout our relationship I experienced his responses to be impeccable at the most subtle levels. His mind had a kind of clarity that one is fortunate to encounter in a lifetime. HIS ABILITY TO WORK IN TERMS OF THE SHIFTING SANDS AS OPPOSED TO THE SOLID ROCK OF TRUTH perhaps made him the most unusual therapist, ever. He could reach people that others found to be hopeless. He could utilize whatever they used against themselves, and help them use it for themselves.

On a personal level I felt touched by Milton. For I have never met such a person, who, fighting incredible degrees of sickness (polio, gout, arthritis, myasthenia gravis), waning energy, and great demands upon his time, still never let me down. Whether by letter, hypnotherapy, or his teaching sessions, he found ways to free a rigidity of mind that was so well cemented that it might never have been penetrated enough to turn the tragic corner in my life. For this I am forever grateful. I trusted him implicitly.

Looking at what he did from a strategic viewpoint, it was absolutely ruthless as well as outrageous. My fear was abandonment. He used the threat of abandonment as a way to motivate primal levels of change. But even when I was stung by him, I felt pleased that he cared enough about me to surprise me in those ways. It is rare that I get surprised to such an extent in either direction, and his responses allowed me to tolerate, and even look forward to surprises throughout the course of my most intimate relationships. In fact, my joy with Milton was that he could continue to surprise me. A great deal of my sadness, although less and less so since working with Milton, was in either not being able to surprise myself or in not being able to be surprised. While his method was outrageous, I never felt that anything he ever said or did with me was anything but respectful.

Milton was a very generous man. When asked about his fee, he would tell people to pay him what they could in terms of what they felt the experience was worth to them. And if they couldn't afford anything, he said that was alright, too. In his sparkling, mischievious way, he told one of my friends, "If I were paid on the basis of the results of my work this weekend, I would be a very rich man."

The degree of courage he had in dealing with his illnesses, while sad, was inspirational. I couldn't help but feel that if he could use self-hypnosis to help him survive each day with tremendous pain, my job ought to be relatively easy. He had been confined to a wheelchair for more than a decade.

With Milton's death, I felt a great personal sense of loss, as I know that it is very rare indeed to meet a man with such great substance tempered with that degree of liberated wisdom. At the deepest levels, I loved Milton.

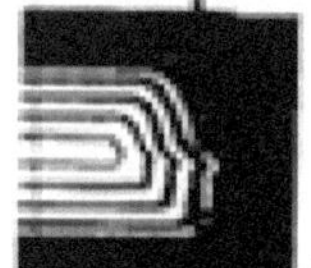

THE MILTON H. ERICKSON FOUNDATION, INC.

3606 North 24th Street • Phoenix, Arizona 85016-6500 • USA
Telephone: (602) 956-6196 •   Fax: (602) 956-0519
e-mail: office@erickson-foundation.org
http://www.erickson-foundation.org

February 16, 2008

To Whom This May Concern:

I am the daughter of Milton H. Erickson M.D., and a member of the Board of Directors of the Milton Erickson Foundation.

Prior to and during the 1970's, Dr. Erickson held weeklong professional teaching seminars in the home office. The content of the seminars included basic and advanced techniques of clinical hypnosis and uncommon therapy. The teaching involved didactic, metaphorical and experiential methodology.

Dr. Leo Berganitno first participated in this educational opportunity on September 11, 1977, returning several times for more in depth study with Dr. Erickson. Dr. Berganitno breadth of knowledge is remarkable in that he has studied under numerous world-renowned psychotherapists. Dr Erickson remarked to him that he "respected your dedication to the work". The mutual respect that Dr. Erickson and Dr. Berganitno held for each other was reflected in the friendship that continued until Dr Erickson's death in 1980, and has continued with Dr. Erickson's widow, Elizabeth Erickson, now 92 years old.

Sincerely

Roxanna Erickson Klein

About Milton Hyland Erickson

My professional life may be divided into BME (Before Milton Erickson) and AME (After Milton Erickson). I read the original Jay Haley version of *Uncommon Therapy: The Psychiatric Techniques of Milton H. Erickson, M.D.* by Norton Press 1973). I was so taken with the miraculous work that I wanted to see if Dr. Erickson was still living and I might go to Phoenix, Arizona, to study with him. So I called information and they had one Milton H. Erickson, M.D., with two addresses, one on 7th and one on 12th. He was known for his confusion technique, "Into every person's life should come a little confusion and a little enlightenment." It started with the two addresses for one person. I had never encountered that before, nor what he did in session. I called and said "I'm looking for a Dr. Milton H. Erickson, M.D." He said "y y y e e s s s." Already I was taken off balance. I told him I wanted to study with him but I wanted to read Haley's *Advanced Techniques* book first *Advanced Techniques of Hypnosis and Therapy: Selected Papers of Milton H. Erickson* edited by Jay Haley, Pearson, Allyn, & Bacon, 1967). He said "That will be fine," and immediately hung up. I got a quarter of the way through the book, and without direct experience realized that I was at a stuck point, so I called him back and said with some trepidation,

"I want to come and see you the weekend of September 11th [1977]." Dr. Erickson said "Come, you will get what you want" with such certainty that I was again taken off balance, as I was not sure what I wanted.

Erickson told stories for between four and six hours at a time at a very slow pace that Margaret Mead told him she had only heard in a rare African tribe relatively free of disease. Oddly enough this was the same pace of Wilfred Bion, the great British psychoanalyst. After 1 1/2 hours, patients gave up resisting and customarily gained access to their unconscious minds where therapists and patients alike had been consciously controlled and customarily made commentaries about what they were aware of. After working with Erickson, the unconscious mind which you came to trust implicitly gave you flashes that were like red neon signs showing your moment-to-moment course of living. Essentially, it was hard to get lost after Erickson.

Erickson saw me individually, after another of his six-hour sessions, and said, "What can I do for you young man?" I said, "Dr. Erickson, you are the foremost psychotherapist in the world! When I get out of here I want to be as good as you are!" (This was the kind of comment that had many people who had trained me wanting to crush my skull, and is also a point that sons hardly ever resolve with their fathers.) Erickson matter of factly said, with no bones to pick, as if he didn't care one way or the other, "Where do you think you stand now?" Very bulldog-like, I challenged him saying "The top of the average." He said, "Why don't you be the best top of the average you can be then. You will never be Milton Erickson." This freed me up to be whatever I could become, and seven years later while doing live demonstrations in Australia my work was described as "a kind of mental precision that electrified the Australian therapeutic community and had lasting therapeutic impact."

Erickson worked with a woman named Barbara in front of the training group. He loved to take on negaters or those severely resistant. He asked her if she wanted to be hypnotized. She said "yes." Twenty minutes later he asked her if she thought she was hypnotized and she said "no." He leaned over from his wheelchair and flipped her right arm upward and there it stood. Then he looked over at me and said, "Old Dr. Bergantino over there, he believes in magic. He doesn't know all I do is pay attention to details." I spent the remaining three years with him learning to pay attention to "minimal cues" that would let me call my shots as best I could, which resulted in my success in Australia.

One of Erickson's better students was a clinical social

worker named Stephen Lankton from Florida. The last time I saw Erickson, he began by saying "I understand that young Steve Lankton is prematurely mourning my death. Well I want you to tell young Steve Lankton that dying is absolutely the last thing I plan to do." Erickson had the spirit of a Viking in terms of fighting for life force and it was contagious. Oftentimes when I feel like throwing in the towel in some situation in my life, I remember that session and carry on with "vigor."

Lastly, Erickson made a point to get your attention right off the bat by "opening the set" as it is described. I was one of five, the only clinical psychologist in a group with four psychiatrists who were dedicated enough to come from Europe to train with him. He began by saying "You wouldn't believe these psychologists and psychiatrists I train. They all have amnesia. I've got to tell them a first time, and then a second time, and then a third time."

He turned the brightest of clinicians around in the first few

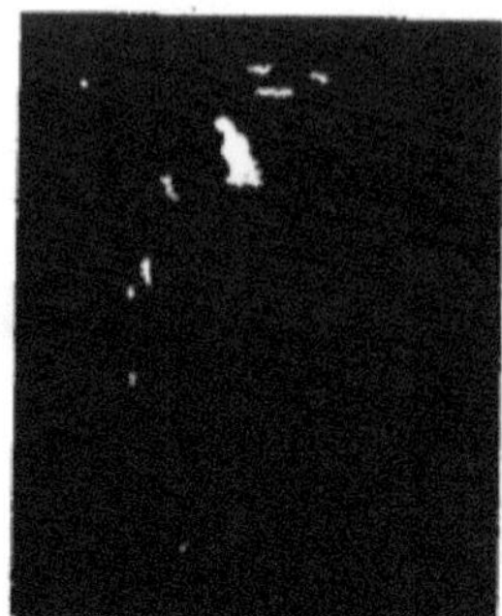

minutes. One day there was a clinical psychologist who had a name that sounded German, and Erickson did this detailed search (seemingly nonsensical to me at the time) for the roots in his name. After a bit we discover Swedish roots in his name. As soon as Erickson finds this out, he says "So you are Swedish. Heh! Well I am Norwegian" and goes into a tale about "One Norwegian chasing one hundred Swedes through the weeds." Then he began the session's work, after having established who the teacher was and who the student was.

With me, he did it this way: "S you're a clinical psychologist, heh Me: "Yes." Erickson: "I'll bet you don't even know why I am wearin purple." Me: "I guess it's just part of Dr. Erickson's style." Erickson: "Heh! I'm color blind. It's the onl color I can see!"

Erickson is known for brief therapy, but he got results becaus he had extraordinary dedication. There was one patient at Wayne State Hospital who spoke only in word salads. Erickson went to the hospital's park bench where the patient spoke three hours of word salad, and Erickson took down every word; then he went home and wrote out a word salad of his own which he took back to the park bench and read to the patient. He did this for two straight weeks, reading his own word salad to the patient each time. After two weeks, the patient said, "Hey Erickson, why don't w go down to your office and talk."

LEN BERGANTINO, a Clinical Psychologist licensed in California, Arizona, and Hawaii, and Diplomate in Family Psychology, American Board of Professional Psychology, is currently willing to work with families in their homes or telephonically 310/207-9397.

Humanizing A Creek

Steven Dubovsky

An occasional respite in a park, preferably near a creek, can absolutely be a soothing experience from the daily responsibilities and trials of life. Momentarily, pause, let one's mind blend with the flow of the creek while gazing at the serenity of a perfectly shaped bubble lethargically wandering on the surface of the water. The bubble might remain a single entity or bond together with other bubbles, creating a kaleidoscope of shapes and color reflections through the rays of the sun. A bubble's fleeting presence is an integral part of a creek's soliloquy, so to speak, as it is meandering through a park, a forest, paying homage to the absolute beauty of nature, her enchanting mysteries, her imposing grandeur.

A creek, en route to uniting with a larger body of water—lake or river or ocean, besides irrigating and beautifying the landscape, also enhances the life of many a human being coming to its banks seeking a tranquil refuge to rest, admire, commune; or in the case of a fellow "cousin" animal, quenching its thirst and satiating its hunger from the bountiful vegetation flourishing on a creek' banks.

February 11, 2010

Guest Editorial

Get Informed
By: Koinie Manuel

As of press time, Prime Minister of the Honorable Dean Barrow was addressing the country in his State of the nation address. During his speech, Honorable Barrow is touching on issues that affect our day to day life, our bread and butter and our future. It was being aired live through the frequency of Love FM. Media and parliamentarians gathered at the Radisson Fort George Hotel to listen to the Prime Minister's presentation.

As we listened, Honorable Barrow spoke of issues on tourism and future projects which may be implemented on the island. He spoke of police issues which have been affecting Belizeans across the nation and the fact that soon, we may have more human resources joining the force. Such an important speech and live coverage, did you listen to it?

Speeches such as the one presented by Honorable Dean Barrow shape up our country and shed light into our economy. At most times, these issues make headline news, whether it be print, television or radio. However, as Belizeans these issues were discussed prior to media houses submitting articles on the subject.

On the island, Her Worship Mayor Elsa Paz offers similar presentations, which we have had the privilege of attending. At these meetings, the attendees can be counted; what does this say about our in-

landers can know how much money was generated through taxes, through donations and how much was spent for infrastructure, streets and education, etc. During the meeting, the opportunity is given for a question and answer session where residents can either voice their concerns or clarify issues which might not have been too clear.

Consultations for developments are also carried out in the same manner. Before a development is set to begin construction, the Government requires the investor to submit an Environmental Impact Assessment (EIA) and then carry out public consultations. These meetings are advertised and the general public is invited to attend. During the meeting, the proposed plan is laid out and again, residents are given the opportunity to ask questions or voice their concerns.

Throughout these meetings, attendance is low, why? These are issues that affect our community, our island, our Belize. These meetings do not happen every day or every week, they happen once in a while. Taking the time to sit through these meetings provides us with important information, information that lets us know what direction we are heading into. With the world in the state that it is now, and the issues plaguing our country it is imperative that we all, as Belizeans, take more interest in these sort of meetings and speeches. By taking a role and being informed,

Letters to the Editor

The San Pedro Sun welcomes letters from its readers. Letters cannot be libelous or slanderous and must be signed, with a return address or telephone number and mailed to The San Pedro Sun, P.O. Box 35, San Pedro Town, Ambergris Caye, Belize. Letters are not the views of The San Pedro Sun. The San Pedro Sun reserves the right to edit and shorten letters. Please do not exceed 300 words when submitting letters.

Dear Editor,

I Love San Pedro

I was here for two days in April 2008 and knew I had to come back. What I love about San Pedro:

1. You fly in from Belize City on a 12 seat – Tropic or Maya Air – and land two streets away from the Main Road.
2. If you travel light you just carry your bags across two streets and are at a hotel.
3. You do not have to rent a car and get a golf cart.
4. I stayed at Ruby's Hotel and both times which is at the begining of the cobblestoned Barrier Reef Drive. You walk out the back door and you are on the beach. You walk out the front door and you are at the begining of a pleasant walk.
5. The airport here has a sign that says something to the effect that nobody is a stranger in San Pedro. The people are naturally friendly to visitors.
6. Most of all I feel good here. I walk out the door of Ruby's Hotel around 7:15 a. m. and usually I see three or four people I know on the empty cobblestone street ahead of me.
7. It gives one the feeling of "It's good to be alive every day!"
8. It is pleasant to walk the cobble lined streets unencumbered by masses of bodies as you would find in many big cities.
9. The weather is warm and balmy with some wind and not too hot but you don't get chilled either.

IN OTHER WORDS SAN PEDRO IS LIKE A LITTLE SLICE OF HEAVEN ON EARTH!

/s/ Dr. Len Bergantino
Los Angeles, CA U.S.A.

Dear Editor,

I have been asked the question way back in early 2009 and continue to be

ize is precariously bordering near chaos with all these senseless murders and assaults with no end seemingly in

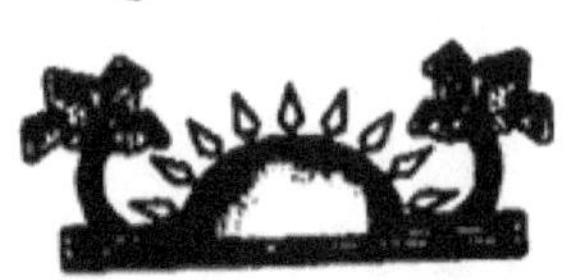

THE SAN PEDRO SUN

P.O. Box 35
San Pedro Town
Ambergris Caye
Belize
Central America
(501) 226-2070
(501) 226-2905
tamara@sanpedrosun.com
www.sanpedrosun.com

March 19, 2019

Whom It May Concern,

As the owner and editor of The San Pedro Sun I give re-print permission for a Letter to the Editor that was submitted and printed by The San Pedro Sun on February 11, 2010.

The letter, titled "I Love San Pedro" was submitted by Dr. Len Bergantino.

Feel free to contact me should you require further information.

Regards,
Tamara Sniffin

Owner/Editor
The San Pedro Sun

The Board of Psychology (State of California)'s Decision to do Away with The Oral Part of the Exam for Psychology Licensure: A Dissenting Opinion

— Len Bergantino

Psychology has moved from a profession of personal growth on the part of the clinician, which could be put into one's private practice on Monday morning, to one of legal deadness. It is now a care and caution that make the fullness of being of the clinician in enhancing the patient's ability to become, a legal impossibility. The nonclinicians who run Boards of Psychology and state Psychological Associations and psychologists themselves have capitulated in their own castration. Now there isn't even a penis left to envy in the practice of psychology. I have seen the death of a profession I once loved and now have nothing in common with.

I think the State of California Board of Psychology's decision to do away with the oral examination is wrong on several counts:

1) It shows extreme cowardice on their parts when they have put each and every psychologist (admittedly with their own complicity in the project) at risk since the mid-1980s.

2) Having an oral examination is the only way to get a fair look at an examinee's clinical abilities.

3) Even if the Board of Psychology is sued by a disgruntled person who flunks the oral examination, the Board would probably win. (Dr. Steven Frankel in his course on law and ethics describes Board of Psychology bulldozing tactics as not having to adhere to law at all.)

4) The written examination has no validity for evaluating actual clinical practice. It primarily measures the ability to pass that kind of test and knowledge of some academic content of psychology.

The Board of Psychology's actions, along with lawyers looking for a new field in which to make money, and with the complicity of psychologists whose clinical acumen and lack of courage are suspect, have decimated the private practice of clinical psychology. Because practitioners can no longer be on the cutting edge of clinical practices nor have an interest in developing that ability, the profession has become one in which those kinds of services can no longer be rendered to patients, and therefore clinicians with courage can no longer function nor make a good living doing so.

Psychologists continue to publish articles about new areas, which they will not be able to practice, nor make a dime on. They go to continuing education classes (36 units a year) like good students and take courses of no use to private practice or to making a living. Many psychologists are making $75 an hour, which I made in 1975, and they are happy to get it. I write this because there has been a great deal about hard times and psychologists not being able to make money. But if you can offer quality of service and a *quality of response,* you can make money. For all intents and purposes, the Board of Psychology and the psycholegal system have made quality *verboten!*

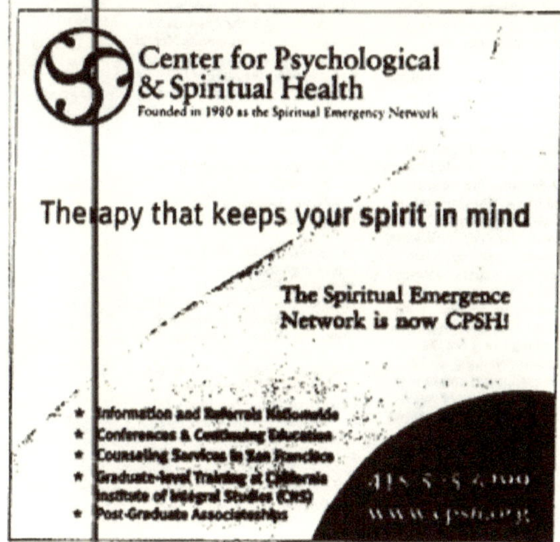

Given that the California Board has participated in the death of psychology and asked psychologists to bear the brunt of fear by which they continue to castrate themselves, it is now a "totally bad faith decision" to do away with an oral examination. It is the only way one can determine if someone has any clinical abilities whatever. The decision deals a final blow to a profession that will attempt to sell the words *clinical psychologist* to the public when all they have are people who are able to pass academic examinations.

Wilfred Bion, the great British psychoanalyst, once said: "The entire psychoanalytic library is good for about the first hour and one half of an analysis. After that you have to know what to say to the patient." The Board's decision to do away with the oral examination will ensure that psychologists are no longer able to determine firsthand who knows what to say to a patient.

Their fear is unfounded in the following respect:

1) They actually do hold clout over the way administrative law is set up.

2) If three independent clinicians meet with an examinee and two flunk him, even if there are countertransference difficulties that preclude a purely objective examination, there is still the rule-of-thumb presumption that if someone doesn't pass the smell test of two out of three, then they ought to get some help, try again, or perhaps go into administration.

3) Written tests measure the ability to take tests and to go to school. (Dr. William B. Michael, USC Professor of Statistics, and writer of SAT and GRE exams, has stated emphatically that the tests don't even measure academic ability but only the ability to take those exams.)

4) There is the "halo effect" regarding graduate school clinical supervisors' recommendations, which says: "You are my supervisee. I have chosen you. Therefore you are worthy."

5) Tuition paid by students may make the university or professional school reluctant to judge a student as not having clinical skills when they may have good grades. But they have decided anyway to try to save themselves a few lawsuits by basing licensure upon an examination that does not look at the ability to do clinical work.

CLINICAL INTERVIEW EXAMPLE

Twenty-eight years ago, I worked as a clinical psychologist in a community mental health center in South Central Los Angeles, which was predominantly African American. An African American psychiatrist and an African American social worker had already interviewed a prospective Caucasian psychologist for a position and wanted to hire him.

He had a resume about twelve pages long, which stated that he had a law degree from the University of Michigan, a degree in clinical psychology, a great number of publications, etc.

My primary interest was how he would survive with the street population he would serve. Did he know what to say? Would he know what to do clinically? He came in and said to me, "Do you want to ask me about my resume?" I said, "I can read." He said, "Well, what do you want to ask me?" I said, "Nothing." His anxiety continued to rise. Then he said, "You have to ask me about my resume." I said, "No, I don't." He said, "Well, what are you going to ask me about then?" I said, "Nothing, all I'm interested in is what you have to say to patients, and what you do with them, and so far you haven't showed me shit!"

While this was confrontive, and may even seem harsh, it gives the fellow a chance to show me anything if he has anything to show, and believe me the patients attempted to rough me up a lot worse than that. He said, "I am going to get Dr. _________ (the psychiatrist)." I said, "If you need help with the interview, I strongly urge you to get him!" The man ran out of the office. And he did not come back with the psychiatrist. That told me he would not know what to say to clients in this neighborhood, nor what to do with them. If I was asked, he was clinically a "no-hire." I could not have known this from reading anything he submitted. It took a clinical interview.

After lunch, the psychiatrist said, "What did you do to Dr. _________, you really freaked him out?" I told him exactly what I said, and he said to me, "If you said and did that to me, I would have hit you in the head with a two by four." And I said, "If you had hit me in the head with a two by four, I would have hired you!"

He hired the man, and I soon after went into private practice. One day I read in the *Los Angeles Times* that that Community Mental Health Clinic was on probation and being fined by the State of California for hiring and having in their employment a fraudulent man who had never had any schooling or training in clinical psychology, law, or anything else for that matter.

Now that happened when the clinical exam was still in!

LEN BERGANTINO, ED.D., ABPP, retired from the private practice of clinical psychology after 30 years. He has authored 75 publications and the book Psychotherapy, Insight and Style: The Existential Moment (Boston: Allyn & Bacon, 1981). He gave workshops at the international level, the focus being "Keeping the Space Open While Doing Therapy So That Experience Is Not Destroyed By Education." Three major influences were the training he received from Milton Erickson, M.D., Carl Whitaker, M.D. and his exposure to Wilfred Bion, M.R.C.S. and his analysands who trained him in Bion's methods.

> *The entire psychoanalytic library is good for about the first hour and one half of an analysis. After that you have to know what to say to the patient.*
> *— Wilfred Bion*
> *(1897–1979)*

Cosmetically Speaking

Coasting along on my bicycle, rounded a gentle curve on the Sanibel [Island] "multiple-use path." That's the official and proper name for the paved mini-street that serves walkers, runners, baby strollers, dog-jockeys, and, of course, bikers. I braked to a stop in order to dismount and get a drink of water at the "multiple-use fountain." That's the one with three user-friendly bubblers—one mounted chest-high, the next waist-high, and the the last ground level for pets. Seeing a shady spot to park my bike and cool down, I stepped off the path into the welcoming shade of what I thought was a thicked branched tree. On closer examination of the leafy bulk, I discovered the hidden trunk and root-ball of a huge Australian pine that Hurricane Charlie had blown over in August of 2004.

The trunk and branches had been cut up and trucked away soon after the storm, but the 15-ft. diameter mound was left lying there. As time went by, Mother Nature lavishly decorated the little mountain with native greenery. The sight reminded me of the haunting image of a Mayan ruin draped with lush jungle vegetation. It seems that not only does nature abhor a vacuum, but nature loves to redecorate—to disguise the unsightly by adorning it with living "bling."

Human beings have the same urge to refashion what lies around them. Outside, we yearn to landscape the lot and trim the tree. Inside, we love to redesign the living spaces, remodel the rooms, and rearrange the furniture. Then, when it comes to our bodies we are the only species to have created the science of cosmetology and the economy of cosmetics.

After all, the word *cosmetic* comes from the Greek root verb *cosmeo*, which literally means "to order." A well-mannered citizen was often described by the adjective *cosmeo*. Philosophers and teachers observed the logical processes of nature and called the world a *cosmos*.

To notice, search for, record, and cooperate with order is what we do. To want to reorganize and rearrange is who we are. It is a mark of our human worth and dignity, or some would say our callig, to create order and harmony around and within us from the vast spaces of the universe to the nearer places around us, culminating with the most personal boundaries of our being—how we look and how we dress.

It is good to be a cosmetician—to be skilled in bringing order to our chaos and beauty out of disarray. Cosmetics is the motive, the means, and the marvel of making music and art; it is the driving force behind science and technology; it is the lure for personal growth; it is is the promise of healing for body, mind, and spirit; it is the hope for man's recovery from mean feelings and alienation.

RANDALL H. NIEHOFF recently retired after 41 years of parish ministry. This is excerpted from the column Gulf Coast Zeitgeist in *Times of the Islands* magazine, *17*(4), June/July 2012, p. 18.

Braer Rabbit, the Avenging Angel

Trained by Milton Erickson from 1977–1980, I learned to tell stories therapeutically for hours on end at a very slow pace (see article on Erickson on p. 15 of this *AHP Perspective* issue). James S. Grotstein, M.D., a training analyst known for his book *Projective Identification*, and his book *Do I Dare Disturb the Universe?* about Wilfred R. Bion, the great British psychoanalyst, wrote that my storytelling was "reverse analysis." Erickson said I had "pinpoint accuracy" when I tell stories from my unconscious mind to the unconscious mind of the client or the group at large.

In 1977 Charlie Kpvowitz, M.D., internist to the stars, referred a man to me who was second in command at a major television network and who had already had analysis. He came to me because he was highly stressed from what I sensed to be a politeness that prevented him from demanding what he needed to function at his job in a more stress-free manner.

He began seeing me once a week for fifty minutes. I wrote themes for the session in my unconscious mind for five minutes and then told stories for the remaining time at the "Ericksonian" extremely slow pace based on the themes I identified at the beginning of our session.

The fifth week he walked in and said "You are not going to believe what happened. I walked into the President's meeting with executives and after ten minutes slammed my fist down on the table as hard as I could yelling out 'Braer Rabbit!' Everybody thought I was completely nuts and that I had lost it. And I got everything I needed at the meeting."

After this experience, he was so pleased with the results that he started seeing me four days a week for this slow-paced storytelling.

He went on to become President of two major

movie studios He was able to therefore to have a copy of the movie *Song of the South* made for me, as it is no longer available to the public. Naturally it featured my first therapist, Braer Rabbit! He often referred to me as his avenging angel.

LEN BERGANTINO, Ph.D., Ed.D., ABPP, a Clinical Psychologist licensed in California, Arizona, and Hawaii, does family therapy, 310/207-9397. He is the author of the book *Insight and Style: The Existential Moment*.

High School Graduation Talk

You only live once . . . you only go through this adolescence at one point in your life. By the time we reach the end of our high school careers, we have been through literally a lifetime of school, and many of our memories are school-related. At points school may have gone by in the blink of an eye, while other days it seemed to be the longest seven hours of our lives. Adversity truly stared us in the face at moments, but we all remained resolute and gave adversity a nasty glare back. We burned the midnight oil studying for the countless tests (at least some of us did), we tried to stay awake through those first-period classes, and we even had fun once in a while. None of it would have been possible without the the consistent dedication we displayed throughout our high school careers. What my lacrosse coach Pete Kervin said before every season, "Every action you do and every decision you make will affect everything that you do in the future," is relevant to us today. . . . for every action there is a repercussion based upon that action. . . . The repercussions for our efforts were the successes and satisfaction of being able to partake in the grand scheme of things. The act of receiving a diploma has proven the character that developed in each and every one of you. Through all the adversity and almost drastic change that has occurred in the past four years, one thing is truly evident: Moral character and pride are but two that were strengthened and will be further developed as we go on.

A bang for your buck. This is what I thought of when I first started to write my speech. I'm the last one today to speak at one of the biggest moments of your lives, so I thought it had to be something good. I fell upon significant advice from Steve Jobs that I urge you to consider. "If today were the last day of my life, would I want to do what I am about to do today?" When the answer to that one question was "no," then something was wrong and changed. I won't guarantee the success that Steve Jobs had, but I can guarantee that if you ask yourself this every morning you will gain much in little time. That question goes back to the motto *Carpe Diem*, Seize the Day. With both Jobs' question and the attitude of the motto in mind, the chance of success (or maybe death for those thrill seekers) increases. I've seen it with my own eyes: the state records and titles, the academics, club participation. Success will continue on into the future as long as you pursue it. If you join the military and decide to serve your country, success will come when you rise to the next rank. If you enter the workforce, it will lead to that promotion down the road. If you seek higher education, it will be graduating from college with flying colors. If you seek a higher education and decide it's not for you, you might be the next Steve Jobs. . . . In any path you seek, I wish you the best in your ventures, no matter what the pursuit (well, as long as they are in the legal confines of society). I'm sure happiness will find a way into all our lives if we bear in mind and remember the motto: You only live once.

Despite all our differences, we have at least two things in common: 1) we all have the potential for success, and 2) we were and always will be Huntingtown Hurricanes. I'm proud to congratulate the Class of 2012 and am honored to be part of it. Thank you.

MAURICE MANUEL STANLEY HARRIS, a recent graduate of Huntingtown (Maryland) High School, is Past AHP President Stan Krippner's grandson.

EXISTENTIAL MOMENTS IN CLINICAL HYPNOSIS

In terms of hypnosis, existential moments may be viewed as those moments in which a person is so deeply relaxed that he or she is once again in touch with the way he or she felt before being strung up in knots as a way of surviving in the world. In addition to this very relaxed and sometime euphoric meditative state, there are increased levels of concentration, and suggestion to patients takes hold much quicker; also, patients may be able to drift off and let their unconscious flow easily.

My introduction to hypnosis was with Dr. Erickson, and the preceding section was written between my first two training sessions with him, which were six months apart. However, much happened during that six months that was responsible for major changes in my life. Many of these changes centered around the use of hypnosis, self-hypnosis, and the accumulation of existential moments.

About the time I returned to Los Angeles after my first visit to Dr. Erickson, I was reading *Type A Behavior and Your Heart*. I realized that I had the following traits:

> a tendency to utter the last few words of a sentence far more rapidly than opening words; move, walk and eat rapidly; impatience with others at the rate of speed most events take place; irritated when a car in lane ahead went at pace I considered too slow; polyphasic thought, striving to think or do two or more things simultaneously; bringing the theme of any conversation around to the subjects that interest me, and if not successful, pretend to listen while absorbed in my own thoughts; feeling guilty when relaxing; schedule more and more in less and less time; believe that my success has been due to ability to get things done faster and faster than others and afraid to stop doing things at this speed; not making time to become the things worth being because I was preoccupied with the things worth having.[3]

Working with Dr. Erickson gave me the opportunity for many experiences which helped me take charge of my life by taking control of the above personality traits and going from a Type A personality to the opposite Type B personality. His method of hypnosis helped me make the connection in my unconscious mind that clinical hypnosis via the storytelling approach was an excellent way to work with both young and old Type A behavior personalities. It is known that clinical hypnosis has been used to control high blood pressure (hypertension), one of the primary causes of coronary artery disease. But it has not been recognized that by telling indirect stories at a very steady and slow, almost monotonous pace, these suggestions would begin to set into the unconscious minds of Type A personalities who might otherwise not be open to direct suggestion.

The following is an example of how I used indirect storytelling with a very slow and steady pace, followed by having the patient tell me a story with the same pace. The man was a severe heart attack patient who was well-entrenched in his self-defeating behaviors, and could not help himself even though his brushes with death sent him to the hospital. The patient, a man in his mid-sixties, had had two prior heart attacks and several tachycardia attacks (rapid heart beat that would continue to pound for as long as ten hours on one occasion) and was suffering from recurring tachycardia attacks during the night. His heart rate was stable during the day, however. One of the cardiologists asked him if he had any bad dreams. He acknowledged that he would constantly dream of fighting but he could never see the faces of the people and the battle would never end. I visited him shortly after he talked with the cardiologist. He relayed the story to me, telling me the cardiologist told him that it was his dreams that got his tachycardia going at night. The man felt helpless to do anything, yet he was pleading for help. I began talking to him about his inner conflict in a gentle but direct fashion. Although on one hand he was pleading for help, on the other he kept switching the subject. He kept telling me that all his problems were physical problems and that I did not understand his physical problems. I was getting nowhere fast. I retreated and began telling him a story about a former patient of mine named Joe (actually in this instance I made this story up spontaneously because I never had a patient named Joe who was in the situation I described. I made it up by watching the patient's behavior.). I said, "Joe would complain about a certain problem but just before he got to solve the problem he would change the subject. He was so afraid of feelings that he didn't even know that he was afraid of, that he was too afraid not to change the subject. The tragic part about Joe was that Joe didn't even know that he could feel good, or that he could satisfy himself, or that he could get what he wanted." About this time, the patient began to laugh. We had connected through my use of indirect storytelling when this patient had been unreachable through more direct methods–a common trait among Type A personalities. The storytelling resulted in an existential moment that turned the session around. I then asked him if he could remember a happy feeling when he was a little boy. I knew that if I could tap into a happy feeling and highlight it, the problem might be solved. He wasn't going to make it that easy. He said that he was a Jew who grew up in Nazi Germany, and that he could not remember one happy feeling during his entire childhood. At this point I thought I would take whatever I could get so I asked him if he could remember one happy feeling at any time during his life. He said he could–his wedding day. I began to make suggestions about relaxing and had him talk about the details of his wedding day. At first he was very vague. He was accustomed to severely underplaying the happy experiences in his life. I kept asking him for more and more details about every joyous moment and sensations of his wedding day. As he continued to talk a very peaceful feeling increasingly came over his face. He drifted off into a peaceful sleep and slept well the entire evening–and without a tachycardia.

The value of the indirect storytelling approach can further be seen when we look at what Friedman and Rosenman say about Type A personalities.

> For every five men who exhibit unquestioned Type A behavior, perhaps four will deny or underplay the intensity of the syndrome. The Type A person will particularly deny the existence of this pattern in himself if it carries the slightest pejorative connotations. It must be remembered that Type A subjects do not easily admit–even to themselves–the effect of any defect or emotional stigma. Certainly the most difficult Type A man of all to convince about his possession of this behavior pattern is that one who not only suffers from a sense of time urgency but also from free-floating hostility.[4]

The use of indirect suggestion via the storytelling approach while the patient is in hypnotic relaxation makes this entire population of patients more amenable to treatment because their egos are not being challenged and their defenses are not being directly assaulted. At the same time they are satisfying themselves via deep relaxation so they have no other reason to be immediately hostile. The storytelling method, in addition to being valuable with the older patient who has already suffered from a heart attack, is also valuable for the striving, competitive younger patient–ages thirty five and up.

While my first exposure to clinical hypnosis was an uncommon one, I felt a need to become acquainted with the more direct approaches to hypnosis and so I took a sixty-hour course between my first and second visits with Dr. Erickson.

A very fascinating experience took place. One of the trainers, who had explained Dr. Carl Simington's treatment of cancer patients through the use of visual imagery as an adjunctive method of treatment along with proper medical care, said that just before he was to fly to Texas to work with Dr. Simington he was suffering from an extremely bad sore throat and cold. His secretary told him that if he was going to learn how to cure cancer patients, the least he could do was get rid of his own sore throat and cold. He took her challenge seriously. He was working–doing therapy and hypnosis from eight a.m. to four p.m. and had ten-minute breaks between each session. He used each of these ten-minute breaks to hypnotize himself, while imagining that his white blood cells were engulfed in a warm soothing fluid, and that this fluid was bathing all the sore and raw areas in his throat and nose. By four p.m. his sore throat and cold were gone. He said he used this method of self-hypnosis whenever he felt a cold or sore throat coming on, and as a result he had avoided any colds or sore throats for three years. I was fascinated!

This trainer went on talking about working with pain patients. He told of how people could have pins stuck through their hands without feeling the pain in demonstrations. I was all set to volunteer when the other trainer told a story about a man who had been hypnotized, had a pin stuck through his hand, and claimed he felt no pain. However, the hypnotist asked him to engage in automatic writing with his free hand. (Automatic writing is uncensored expression that comes from the unconscious mind.) The man wrote, "Ouch, you son of a bitch!" At this point I decided not to volunteer to have a pin stuck through my hand, but said that I did have a problem that was bothering me. The following is a good example of visual imagery in hypnosis to create physical well-being.

My right eye had felt strained several times each day ever since I was thirteen years old. Eye doctors said my eyes were in perfect health, and my glasses were of the right correction. The trainer asked me what eye doctors had told me before he agreed to use hypnosis. He spent about twenty minutes telling me in a very soft and soothing voice that THE WHITE BLOOD CELLS WERE IN A WARM FLUID AND WERE BATHING THE RAW IRRITATED AREAS, AND THE RAW RED AREAS WERE BECOMING PINKER AND HEALTHIER, and that my eye was feeling more and more soothed. At the end of twenty minutes my eyes felt as if they were set in a different place in my head. They felt so soothed I couldn't believe it. An existential moment for sure. I remembered where my eyes were now set as opposed to where they were formerly setting. After the tension was removed I had a much softer look in my eyes. I was able to keep my eyes in this new position, and haven't had eye strain in nearly a year since that twenty-minute session. I have also had a great deal of success in cutting off colds and sore throats before they develop fully.

I was gaining a real sense of self-confidence and began to use self-hypnosis for a variety of physical ailments. I had seborrhea for about fifteen years and when it got bad I would have a red spot right in the middle of my forehead that looked grotesque. I hypnotized myself for four hours, imagining the white blood cells were focused on this one little area, before going to sleep one evening. When I woke up in the morning the red spot was gone. This condition had not been treated successfully through conventional medical procedures and recommended medicated shampoos. Of course, I may have had lasting results with both my eyes and the seborrhea because my entire pace of living had changed from Type A to Type B.

On one occasion I made the mistake of trying to see if my car radiator needed water when the car was hot. The cap blew off and my entire arm was burned. I was also late for a patient I had to see so I quickly stopped at the drugstore and bought an ointment recommended by the pharmacist, although he said the burns would take a week or two to go. When I got to the office I put my arm on a pillow and hypnotized myself while doing therapy and hypnosis with patients. My arm became colder and colder, more numb and more numb, and at the end of four hours all the burn marks were gone.

Again, I was astonished that I could produce these existential and healing moments as a result of hypnotizing myself.

I also found that patients who had an addictive nature–marijuana, alcohol, cigarettes–could be taught to produce a euphoria through hypnosis done at a very slow pace for about an hour. One young lady said "This feels just like a lude." I asked what a lude was. She said, a quaalude. I told her it would save her a lot of money to produce her own euphoria through self-hypnosis. Being a practical woman, she agreed, and proceeded to live accordingly.

About this time I began to get a different kind of referral. One physician called and told me that he had a patient whose vagina was very tight and hurt every time she had sex, and that her fiancee was threatening not to marry her if she did not get this problem fixed. The physician wasn't particularly interested in any intrapsychic conflicts she had about sex, or in the communication difficulties she had in her interpersonal relationship with her fiancee. He wasn't even interested in my using hypnosis to help her relax her vaginal muscles. He wanted me to help her develop anesthesia through hypnosis so she wouldn't have any pain in her vagina during sex–and that was that. I felt that the long-term effect of such anesthesia would be to permanently reduce or eliminate sexual sensation and sexual gratification of a physical nature. In addition, I felt there were probably many psychotherapeutic reasons why the woman was using this painful situation to avoid sex. I did not take the referral. However, I did feel that I probably needed to learn more about developing anesthesia through hypnosis and I heard that Dr. William S. Kroger was very good at doing that. I contacted him for some supervisory sessions.

CLINICAL HYPNOSIS, WITH WILLIAM S. KROGER, M.D.

Dr. William S. Kroger is author and co-author of many books, papers and articles in the field of hypnosis. He is a pioneer in psychosomatic medicine, psychosexual problems and hypnotherapy. He is founder of the Institute for Comprehensive Medicine in Beverly Hills, California and a co-founder of the American Society of Clinical Hypnosis, the Academy of Psychosomatic Medicine, and the Society for Clinical and Experimental Hypnosis.

Dr. Kroger had an unusual kind of practice. Beverly Hills was the kind of place where most of the physicians saw psychoanalysis as a method of choice and were making their referrals accordingly. However, after certain patients would fail in psychoanalysis, or in other forms of therapy, they would be sent to Dr. Kroger with a heavy expectation on the part of both patient and physician that he would cure them. I couldn't help but be curious about how he practiced hypnosis. His method was mostly to use direct suggestion, but was very unique with its focus on the development and control over the five senses through the use of visual imagery. Dr. Kroger felt that when people could reignite their senses and take control over these senses through visual imagery, they could take charge over the troublesome aspects of their lives. The images are used "as an adjunctive method for decreasing anxiety, and developing self-control and hypnotic concentration."[5]

I, and several colleagues to whom I have recommended Drs. Kroger and Fezzler's book, have used visual imagery via direct suggestion with patients who feel they need to grasp something right away. Indirect storytelling sometimes is too frustrating for a desperate and heavily-controlled conscious-minded person (as opposed to someone who is at least willing to let their unconscious flow a little bit). Therapists and hypnotists need a place to enter the patient's world, and visual scenes are often an appropriate and pleasant way to do this.

I am going to present one scene verbatim from the book by Drs. Kroger and Fezzler, to give the reader a feel about how fully this imagery is developed.

Image I

The first image is usually given in the second session after the subject has had one week to practice self-hypnosis. Its focus is on the recall of five basic senses emphasizing tactile feelings of warmth and cold, visual colors, the basic taste and smell of salt, and rhythmic sound. The therapist paints the picture as follows:

Beach Scene

You are walking along the beach; it is mid-July. It is very, very warm. It is five o'clock in the afternoon. The sun has not yet begun to set but it is getting low on the horizon. The sun is a golden blazing yellow, the sky a brilliant blue, the sand a dazzling glistening white in the sunlight. Feel the cold, wet, firm, hard-packed sand beneath your feet. . . . Taste and smell the salt in the air. There is a residue of salt deposited on your lips from the ocean spray. You can taste it if you lick your lips. Hear the beating of the waves, the rhythmic lapping to and fro, back and forth of the water against the shore. Hear the far-off cry of a distant gull as you continue to walk. . . .

Suddenly you come to a sand dune, a mound of pure white sand. . . . Covering the mound are bright yellow buttercups, deep pink moss roses. You sit down on its crest and look out to sea. The sea is like a mirror of silver reflecting the sun's rays, a mass of pure white light, and you are gazing intently into this light. As you continue to stare into the sun's reflection off the water, you begin to see flecks of violet, darting spots of purple intermingled with the silver. Everywhere there is silver and violet. There is a violet line along the horizon . . . a violet halo around the flowers. Now the sun is beginning to set. With each movement, with each motion of the sun into the sea you become deeper and deeper relaxed. (It is important to pair physical sensations such as breathing with elements in the image so that the imaginal elements will cue relaxation.) The sky is turning crimson, scarlet, pink, amber, gold, orange as the sun sets . . . you are engulfed in a deep purple twilight, a velvety blue haze . . . you look up to the night sky. It is a brilliant starry night. The beating of the waves, the smell and taste of the salt, the sea, the sky, . . . and you feel yourself carried upward and outward into space, one with the universe. . . . I am now going to count to 3. At the count of 3, you will open your eyes, you will feel completely refreshed, totally relaxed: 1, 2, 3. (The subject is always brought out of hypnosis by reciting the above three lines.)

The last two lines in this image should produce a feeling of detachment and often dissociation.[6]

There are twenty-five such scenes of varying length and purpose which will provide a useful guide in helping those wanting to improve their visual imagery skills. During the process and at the end of each of these scenes, patients experience a peace with self that may be considered another type of existential moment.

I can recall when I first experienced visual imagery with Dr. Kroger, how difficult and how slow the images began to form. Yet, after practice, I felt much richer in my imagery. I felt as if I had been able to open myself up to another world in letting my images flow along as rapidly as Dr. Kroger was speaking them. In my opinion, richer imagery is directly related to the seeking of a more fulfilling life that will be congruent with the expanded imagery.

I often heard Dr. Kroger tell patients that after they have practiced the beach scene at home thirty or forty times (he usually makes a tape for them), they will be able to go into a deep hypnotic state, achieving the same degree of deep relaxation, by just thinking the words "beach scene."

Another concern I had was doing arm levitations with patients who were more invested in scalp hunting than in their own well being. In my readings it was clear that if the hypnotist failed, it would be a setback in the treatment process. Dr. Kroger had a fool-proof system for dealing with such patients.

He said verbatim, in a tape-recorded session:

Hypnosis is not mystical and you don't go under anything. It is a very alert state of awareness while you are experiencing deeper and deeper relaxation. You will learn to take greater and greater control over your five senses, over simple and elementary feeling states by suggestions you give yourself; heaviness, lightness, tightness, stiffness, limpness, and other sensations like wetness and dryness and others involving taste and smell and touch, you will be able to understand and put these combinations together for whatever purpose you want to achieve.

Look at a spot. Your lids are getting very very heavy and that is the first sensation you are taking control over, not because you have to but because you really want to feel these other sensations and get them under control. Your lids are sticking tighter and tighter together as you are becoming deeper and deeper relaxed. Imagine a nice warm bath. Feel the warm water, breathing slower, deeper, more regular, if you want to go still deeper, and want to learn how to control your smoking and eating habits. I want you to learn how to control the flexing of one part of your body first, as much as you wish to, or as little as you wish to, raise your right arm or your left arm, and you can extend this control to any part of your body. I want you to listen very carefully: you will raise your right arm or your left arm two inches at a time, pause for a second or two and suggest to yourself, "I will become deeper and deeper relaxed"–it will get lighter and lighter and it will become light as a feather–light as a sponge. You are allowing yourself to go into this relaxed state, more aware. If you want to go deeper, the stiffer your arm and your fingers will get. I know you want to cooperate. Now if you want to go still deeper, I want you to suggest to yourself another sensation of limpness. Say to yourself, my arm is getting limper and limper, dropping two inches at a time until your arm drops with a thud to the couch; you are able to relax and have begun taking control over your five senses.[7]

The patient would not feel threatened about losing control, and Dr. Kroger's presenting them with choices–left arm or right arm, "as much or as little as you want, because you really want to feel these sensations–not because you have to," insured patient cooperation throughout the session. I had seen other hypnotists induce arm levitation by saying something like, "You will notice your arm beginning to move, it is gradually becoming lighter and lighter." Sometimes it didn't move, and the hypnotist would have to do a fast change of direction and say, "It is becoming heavier and heavier" in order to save face. Dr. Kroger's method continually puts responsibility with the patient and is geared to their own wants. It is an excellent way to work with what is voluntary when patients are not willing to have an experience that is involuntary.

The Impact of Automatic Writing: Breakthroughs into Existential Moments

One of my trainers sensed I would sometimes get stuck, and not knowing what was going through my unconscious mind, would pressure myself to figure things out consciously. Once he grabbed his pad and began to write, directly from his unconscious mind. The unconscious writing said:

> be patient, be patient, lay aside fear. Love and peace can be yours, but let the love come to you. Loving and being at peace will come as you lay aside fear. No need to grab for it, it can come with ease as you let it come. Yes, a lot easier said than done. But a good do of this kind must wake a conscious awareness first. You can do it unconsciously while you are aware of the need consciously. Relax and let it happen by itself. You are giving a lot, and can go a lot further if you do not try to keep books on it.

> Many levels of operation are here being given a loving and appropriate inner examination. Do you ask to know it all as a conscious awareness? Not possible! Be more trusting of the wisdom of the inner knowledge and the love you are a part of will carry you to your life opportunity. May we open to you an awareness of your own ability to do this? Lay aside fear and let the hand be lovingly free.

I picked up the pen and pad and wrote,

> I am really divided as to which hand I should be writing
> with. It is becoming clearer now that I can switch and
> have two different kinds of experiences that are both
> rewarding. If I let both sides of the straddler develop,
> although I am sometimes wasted in terms of energy
> depletion, I am confident at the unconscious level that
> such pursuits will lead to the development of a unity I
> might not have otherwise known.

My trainer wrote, "Both are a part of that unity! Who you are is all of the parts you know and those you are not yet aware of."

To say the least I was surprised about what popped out of my unconscious mind. The issue of being a straddler had been lurking around without my conscious awareness for several months, and all of a sudden my unconscious mind gave resolution to my frustration in trying to make a choice of one side or the other. My unconscious mind affirmed the necessity of my straddling behavior at this time in my life. I was at ease.

However, two weeks later I came for my appointment feeling depleted of energy and I began to do automatic writing–

> I want to space out. I feel disappointed about a feeling of
> depleted energy. I feel as if my body was about to break
> out of its encapsulation on a more sustained basis and
> now I have decided to postpone becoming one with my
> energies. Your automatic writing is easier to swallow
> consciously than unconsciously. A whole different trust
> level is involved. One thing this automatic writing is
> doing is slowing me down enough to go with whatever
> flows through my unconscious. I am not sure I can do
> it as a lifestyle. How the hell does one resolve the issue
> of exuberant life–spirit–body energy–and a terror about
> just letting that happen? You gave me the how and I am
> stilling asking the question. Remnants of fear are very
> slow in leaving.

The trainer wrote,

Many are the ways of approaching a goal. You are at liberty at all times to choose. A good deal of old and outworn fear has been given away, but you are still caught up in a pattern of trying to go your way under conscious control more than is justified by the results obtained.

No way can the conscious mind control the inner mind, a part of you which can go the whole distance. By giving the inner self a freer hand, you can find a better balance. Bouts of doubt and uncertainty are the result of trying to control consciously more than is right or possible. Bouts of calm and peace are the result of learning to trust the inner self to know what to do, to say, to put into action. Bouts of wise and competent artistic production also are the result of such letting the inner self have a free hand. You are reading now a result.

Each day you are laying aside a bit more of the fear. Who you are, at a down deep inner level is quite aware of the needs of the conscious self, and is doing a good job. You are laying aside gradually the felt need to control things consciously, which you will give up as soon as you feel safe enough. Who you are at a down deep level automatically does these things at the right speed. You can trust that inner self, but you need to test out old pain and fear being gone in a slow enough way to feel comfortable. Who you are at a deep level is very protective of you while you learn!

Each time the trainer or myself picked up the pen I found myself to be pleasantly surprised at what I felt was a more profound way in which to view life than I had been accustomed to. So I began to experiment with automatic writing in my practice.

Automatic writing had several benefits for me when doing therapy/hypnosis.

1. It gave me a growing sense of confidence and trust in the flow of my own unconscious processes in responding to patients. Although I had always been intuitive and responsive via my unconscious, I was now responding at a much deeper level. After a few months this level of depth transferred to my verbal therapy with patients.
2. Whenever I feel stuck in a therapy session, or a patient feels stuck, I can pick up the pen and know that what comes out will be trustworthy. Patients also know what comes out from me and them will be trustworthy when doing automatic writing.
3. Patients and myself tend to view automatic writing as a detached observer whose accuracy is impeccable, thus, the power of suggestion that might be defended against by the conscious mind is usually more readily accepted. It is not as if I am giving the suggestion, but as if the suggestion comes from something much more trustworthy–my unconscious mind–and the unconscious minds of patients themselves.

The following are some of the ways in which I used automatic writing with patients. In each case there was an impact that was surprising to both the patient and myself. I began to realize that a way to continually be surprised and enriched was to trust and go with my unconscious response. Also, I felt that my continued use of new methods kept patients' conscious defenses off balance, making it easier for me to provide an experience for them at the unconscious level.

Case of Jerry–Sex, Guilt

Jerry was a very bright patient with whom I could take liberties because he was both pretty together and had a good sense of humor. Jerry was speaking of his sexual problems with his wife, but I realized from the way he went about asking for guidance he was also laying a burden of responsibility upon me. I felt a bit fearful with this kind of pressure and became blocked in the therapy session. I picked up the pad and began to write, "Guidance is forthcoming–Go fuck yourself! Guidance is forthcoming. Fornication is an experience that one should not do without because it is only when satisfaction wreaks and creaks through the limbs and codpiece that one is connected to the outside world." I handed him the paper. He laughed like hell and wrote, "How true!" As the session went on he began to talk about guilt in his relationship with his wife. Again I began to write, "Guilt is something people feel when they do what they do over and over again and resent getting caught. In your case guilt is good for the soul. Your guilt is the other side of your sociopathic behavior. You should probably be whipped daily and even that wouldn't make amends." An existential moment. At this point he wrote, "I'd like to fuck everybody out of everything they've got!" This is the first time Jerry acknowledged that all of him was not the amiable fellow he presented himself to be. Furthermore, part of him was blind to people who had the same tendencies and he kept getting "screwed out of everything he had," which presented a series of financial crises throughout the course of therapy.

I wrote, "Guilt will only subside when your response to people becomes more founded in your compassion and good will as opposed to your ambitious desires." He wrote, "I do a lot when I don't feel threatened, but when I fear I will lose or be disapproved of I start manipulating and my approach becomes stressed–i.e., not spontaneous, i.e., dead." I wrote, "The problem with which you grapple is that you are the one who is disapproving–and well you should. You are disapproving of adapted child on the one side and sociopath on the other. It is only the more human side of you that will draw an approval that feels real to you."

Case of Joe–Obsessive, Depressive, No Fun!

I was getting stuck in Joe's flurry of words, so I broke the pattern by beginning to write. "You look happier and more spontaneous when you let yourself play. It becomes you." Joe wrote, "I fully agree and can feel that difference when I am playing." However, at this point we were still engaged in words when my unconscious mind provided the fun, rather than making it a task for Joe. I wrote, "I'll bet you can't stand up and sit down at the same time." He was taken aback when he wrote "Can you?" I wrote, "I'm the therapist. You have to answer my questions first."

Joe responded with, "Give me a high chair!" An existential moment in which we both had a good belly laugh!

In summary, clinical hypnosis in its various forms has been very useful in helping patients deal with hypertension, pain that is not clearly related to organic causes, and in some cases pain that is directly related to organic causes. Automatic writing is but another way to reach existential moments. While on paper it may appear to be imprecise language that may or may not have meaning, during the context of hypnotherapy it often provides an important key to that patient becoming free.

Perhaps the best way to end the chapter on hypnosis is to tell one last Erickson story. "I remember someone asking Dr. Erickson what he thought the effect of one hypnotherapy session might be. Dr. Erickson said, 'You only had to be born once!, didn't you!'"

ENDNOTES

1   Encyclopedia Britannica, Chicago: William Benton, Publisher, 1965, Vol. 16, p. 858.

2   Ibid.

3   Meyer Friedman and Ray Rosenman, Type A Behavior and Your Heart, Greenwich, Conn.: Fawcett Crest Book reprinted by arrangement with Alfred A. Knopf, 1974, pp. 100-101.

4   Ibid., p. 206.

5   William Kroger and William Fezzler, Hypnosis and Behavior Modification: Imagery Conditioning Philadelphia: J. B. Lippincott Co., 1976, p. 103.

6   Ibid.

7   William Kroger, A Tape Recorded Session. Beverly Hills, Calif., 1978.

REFERENCES

Encyclopaedia Britannica. William Benton Publisher, vol. 16, 1965.

Erickson, Milton H., and Rossi, Ernest L. *Hypnotherapy: An Exploratory Casebook.* New York: Irvington Publishers, 1979.

Erickson, Milton H.; Rossi, Ernest L.; and Rossi, Sheila I. *Hypnotic Realities.* New York: Irvington Publishers, 1976.

Erickson, Milton H. *The Nature of Hypnosis and Suggestion. The Collected Papers of Milton H. Erickson on Hypnosis Vol. I.* Edited by Ernest L. Rossi. New York: Irvington Publishers, 1980.

Erickson, Milton H. *Hypnotic Alteration of Sensory, Perceptual and Psychophysical Processes. The Collected Papers of Milton H. Erickson on Hypnosis, Vol. II.* Edited by Ernest L. Rossi. New York: Irvington Publishers, Inc., 1980.

Erickson, Milton H. *Hypnotic Investigation of Psychodynamic Processes. The Collected Papers of Milton H. Erickson on Hypnosis, Vol. III.* Edited by Ernest L. Rossi. New York: Irvington Publishers, Inc., 1980.

Erickson, Milton H. *Innovative Hypnotherapy. The Collected Papers of Milton H. Erickson on Hypnosis, Vol. IV.* Edited by Ernest L. Rossi. New York: Irvington Publishers, Inc., 1980.

Erickson, Milton H. *Advanced Techniques of Hypnosis and Therapy: Selected Papers of Milton H. Erickson, M.D.* Edited by Jay Haley. New York: Grune & Stratton, Inc., 1967.

Erickson, Milton H. *A Teaching Seminar with Milton H. Erickson.* Edited by Jeffrey Zeig. New York: Brunner/Mazel, Publishers, 1980.

Friedman, Meyer, and Rosenman, Ray. *Type A Behavior and Your Heart.* Greenwich, Conn.: Fawcett Crest Book, reprinted by arrangement with Alfred A. Knopf, 1974.

Haley, Jay. *Uncommon Therapy: The Psychiatric Techniques of Milton H. Erickson, M.D.* New York: W. W. Norton, 1973.

Kroger, William S. *Clinical and Experimental Hypnosis.* Second Edition. Philadelphia: J. P. Lippincott Company, 1977.

Kroger, William, and Fezzler, William. *Hypnosis and Behavior Modification: Imagery Conditioning.* Philadelphia: J. B. Lippincott Company, 1976.

Regarding the books of Milton H. Erickson. I recommend beginning with *Uncommon Therapy* as it gives an action oriented account of Dr. Erickson's unique way of doing therapy and a feel for what the man was all about. Then, to begin to delve into his hypnotic work start with *Hypnotic Realities* (accompanied with tape). *Hypnotherapy* and *Advanced Techniques* I have read a couple of times. It was rough going and I did not remember very much. However, in these two books Erickson deals with a variety of difficult cases that sooner or later may get referred to you. At that time, go back and read the specific section that deals with that kind of problem. While each patient and situation is unique, I find that the processes Dr. Erickson described in dealing with a particular problem in some way come together in my unconscious mind so that

I can formulate a unique treatment plan for my patient. This method helps me to work with patients I might otherwise have very little idea of how to treat. Many of the other books are newer, but can be used in the same way. Erickson's work can be used as a lifetime project in this way.

10

Direct Confrontation: The Treatment of Schizophrenia, with Jack Rosberg, M.A.

JACK ROSBERG IS a clinical psychologist in the Los Angeles area. He is director of the Anne Sippi Clinic. Jack has been involved in the treatment of schizophrenia for over twenty-five years, and has lectured widely throughout the United States regarding the method of treatment he has developed called "direct confrontation," since his earlier two years of training with Dr. John Rosen.

Introduction

When I was discussing impact and style in doing therapy, Dr. Martin Grotjahn told me that he met Dr. John Rosen at his farm in Pennsylvania. He described Rosen's treatment of a schizophrenic adolescent girl.

The girl kept telling Rosen that she saw communists on the upper floor and they were talking about her. Rosen insisted there were no communists on the upper floor of his house, but the girl persisted. Finally, he grabbed her by the hand, saying, "All right. I will go up there with you and we will see if there are communists. I know there aren't any and if there aren't any I am going to throw you down the flight of stairs." Martin said the girl thought about it and said she realized there were no communists on the upper floor, and began to talk to Rosen in a normal manner.

What I realized regarding impact and style in doing therapy were:

1. Rosen shocked the girl back to reality through the use of strong language with the threat of physical violence.
2. Even though she was schizophrenic, many schizophrenics have character disorders, and SUCH A SHOCKING METHOD COULD BE USED TO CUT AWAY CHARACTER DISORDERS, in addition to bringing delusional systems (e.g., the delusional claim that there were communists on the upper floor) back to reality in a potent way.

I BEGAN TO SEE HOW THE USE OF VIOLENT AND PROVOCATIVE LANGUAGE COULD BE USEFUL, even with character disorder patients who were not schizophrenic, and who were not suffering from delusional systems. IT MIGHT PROVIDE A METHOD TO STOP THE CHARACTER DISORDER BEHAVIOR WHEN ALL ELSE FAILS, OR EVEN SOONER.

While I have not had the opportunity to come into personal contact with Rosen, I had contact with Jack Rosberg, a clinical psychologist who studied with Rosen. It is of this approach in doing psychotherapy that I shall write about. While Jack primarily treats schizophrenics, I feel that there are times and places during the context of more traditional therapy that such techniques may be useful. They may also be useful for those who may use direct confrontation as an adjunctive method of treatment even though their approach to treating schizophrenia may be quite different.

Further, the approach provides a primal kind of emotional contact that may be necessary to reach patients who have hardened themselves to normal human touching, and through the character disorder, continue to pollute their interpersonal environment so badly that they become tragic loners. The use of direct confrontation may help them stop a negative behavior so that fruitful human contact can then take place.

While seeing Jack Rosberg work on videotape and hearing him present his way of viewing therapy I felt that direct confrontation, as practiced by Jack, is an intuitive, creative, and effective therapy. Jack has an uncanny way of confronting using unusual and sometimes bizarre responses that really capture the moment (an existential moment) and reach the unreachable. Jack treats a patient population which is characteristically chronic, and which psychotherapists across the board have not had a great deal of success in treating. Jack describes his work by saying "it's intuitive." It just comes through him as it may come through others if they can listen to themselves and have the courage to respond when dealing with a patient population whose characteristics are so well-ingrained. While Rosen's method was called "direct analysis," Jack refers to his method as "direct confrontation."

Jack confronts patients with their craziness during the first session. In fact, he does so during the first encounter. He defers interpretation. In the intensity of his interactions he annihilates patient's defenses and invites deep cathartic experiences. Rosberg has moved from the analytic to a more eclectic position, focusing on the here-and-now.

Jack states,

> I confront the person with the fact he's nuts. It's important that he knows he's nuts, that he has a distorted view of the world, and acting on this view, he makes misjudgments and says weird things. The idea, of course, is abhorrent to him; and the harder I push, the more he resists. But the patient isn't fragile. The defenses are extraordinarily powerful. You can't penetrate them by reality or psychoanalytically-oriented therapy with the use of interpretation. By participating in the patient's delusional system, becoming a part of his nightmare, the therapist weakens the psychotic defenses to the point, eventually, where the patient becomes accessible to psychotherapy.[1]

Jack feels that therapists must be dramatic to capture the attention of schizophrenics. He feels it is important to show them you are not weak, but that you are a strong figure with whom they can identify. He says these patients are terrified, and therefore, do not need a therapist who is also terrified.

It is important to appreciate the high level of caring that is involved. Jack cares enough to put everything he has into his work with people who many therapists might write off as being hopeless cases. There is a tremendous expenditure of energy. It appears from a process point of view that Jack tries to break the internal parental symbiotic connection between the patient and the patient's introjected parents, by forming a new tie to the therapist. However, to hold them in the therapy, the tie must be strong, and he puts out constant energy until they begin to talk in a more sane way. If you, as a therapist, find this is too demanding, and it may well be, then it would not be wise to begin to work in this way. For it was Jack's caring about these people that transcended all of what he said and did. It was only with such caring that his stroking, poking, aggressive, and loving ways encouraged patients to relate to him.

It is important to preface the work with Jack's capacity for caring because if one reads the content of what he is saying without experiencing the process, the literal meaning of the words spoken may appear to be anything but caring. And in no way is this chapter intended to be a license for non-therapeutic violence on the part of therapists.

Direct Confrontation: The Treatment of Schizophrenia

During his twenty-five years in practice, Jack has developed and refined direct confrontation which is designed to make quick contact with the most seriously regressed schizophrenic patients.

Jack's approach is both effective and stylistic. It is also quite unusual because of the kind of confrontations he makes and the degree of force, and what may even appear to be violence, involved in his responses. Jack deals with patients who are both delusional and contained within themselves and who are unwilling to make contact. Further, they often block contact through violence or threats of violence toward the therapist. Jack feels that he has a real battle on his hands when working with a chronic schizophrenic with a well-organized and systematized delusional system. However, he feels that if the therapist can *cut away the character disorder, the schizophrenia will go away.* This is what his responses via direct confrontation are intended to do. He feels the difficulty of the case, in terms of acute vs. chronic in addition to being contingent on the character disorder, is also affected by the schizophrenic delusions and the number of times the patient has had the episode. The greater number of times, the tougher the case.

Jack is a no-holds-barred therapist. He says, "You need to find something that works for you." He commented that many of these patients act in rotten, hostile, and abusive ways. He feels that such character problems must be confronted so these patients will be made aware they can't get away with it. I feel this is a crucial issue, because most of these patients have lived such hardened lives, and have such cold spots inside, that it is difficult, if not impossible, to reach them with even the most compassionate responses while they are hammering away at the therapist. Getting them to stop the craziness may then become the first order of business so they will respect both themselves and you. He feels that, particularly in this kind of work, it is crucial that therapists "have the freedom to be spontaneous." He further states that "spontaneity gets to the delusional system. Therapists have to be a little crazy. Schizophrenics are geniuses at their craft. They expect regular psychotherapy questions. I never do that. I get involved instead."

One example Jack used when talking about spontaneity was about a Jewish girl who thought she had intercourse with the Holy Spirit and that she was pregnant. Jack asked, "Did he have a big dong?" The woman was stunned, but proceeded on with her delusion. Jack asked, "Did he come in you?" The woman then became angry at Jack's unwillingness to play by the unspoken set of rules for the professions of psychotherapy. She said, "Doctors are not supposed to talk that way." And she began to talk to Jack without her delusional system.

Jack made it perfectly clear that therapists who want to treat this kind of patient cannot be more interested in the politics of their profession (e.g., community standards) than they are in responding to patients in whatever way to get the job done. He felt this was particularly important because everything schizophrenics do is designed to push people, and therapists in particular, out of their lives. Jack went on to say that there are about two million people in this country suffering from schizophrenia, but that the treatment of the problem somehow gets lost in the interprofessional battles of psychiatrists fighting psychiatrists, and psychologists fighting social workers. He feels that these groups then become more invested in their professional images rather than being willing to risk the kinds of responses necessary to reach such a difficult population. He said, "If you fight too much, if you bend your efforts along political lines, if you try to think along medical lines in terms of training in diagnosing, you may not have the time or courage to do the treatment of schizophrenia." Jack went on to say that regardless of what discipline people come from among the therapeutic professions, they can work out the problem successfully. Then he exclaimed, "If you don't want to work with it, for God's sake, don't work with it!" "Do something else! I hate to see the copout continuing in the field!"

Jack went on to say: "To treat schizophrenics therapists must be involved with them emotionally. You can't be outside the periphery of their disorder. You have got to be part of it in some way. It doesn't mean you have to be that crazy, but you have to be somewhat loose and spontaneous."

Jack reassured the group that even though therapists may have a battle on their hands when dealing with well-organized delusional systems of chronic schizophrenics, it doesn't mean these patients are hopeless. They are treatable.

He feels it is important to catch their attention. Otherwise you could easily be fooled into thinking they hear you, when they do not. When giving examples of how he sometimes catches their attention, he yelled words in what to me felt to be a loud, shocking, and somewhat frightening voice. I could see why patients would be afraid to continue being crazy. He felt this worked for him, and again urged that what we needed to do was find something that worked for us, no matter how bizarre it may appear on the surface.

Jack commented that Jay Haley said a direct intervention therapist is someone who does a lot of talking. Jack suggested,

> Don't let the patient talk. I do a lot of talking and sometimes patients get very angry at me because I am not listening to them. I tell them very directly and candidly that when they start to make sense I will listen to them and in the meanwhile they should listen to me because I make more sense than them.

> In hospitals they TLC (tender loving care) people into chronicity. What should you do if a patient comes up

and kicks you in the balls? Should you say, "Hey, you must be angry?" Is that how you would deal with that? Not me. Not me. If they do that to me, I will express my anger. I will not be benign to ruthless, hostile and assaultive people. I will yell like hell at them.

When talking with Jack at a later time I asked him if physical violence was ever a part of the treatment process. He said that it was not, and that when he uses strong language for shock purposes there is rarely any physical outburst by patients. However, on the occasions where such an outburst might occur, the only physical intervention would be to restrain the patient. He cautioned this as being particularly important when using direct confrontation and assured "no one will get hurt that way."

Jack described his work with Anne Sippi, a schizophrenic patient who had been a patient at a small private psychiatric hospital at the time Jack met her. She was delusional. She heard voices and carried on conversations with dead people from her past. She was self-mutilating in addition to being assaultive. She was kept in restraints 70 percent of the time.

Anne's vocabulary had shrunk to a few words, and she would not make eye contact. Jack grabbed her by the chin and held her head in a fixed position in order to gain her attention. Jack feels that in terms of economy of time forcing a patient to listen to the therapist can be valuable. He then told Anne, *"I understand you kick people, bite people and tear their hair out. That's perfectly fine with me because that's exactly what I do."* Jack said that he does not like violence and he will not permit patients to violate him. "I thoroughly respect, encourage, and recommend patients' rights, but there is such a thing as therapists' rights, too. We have to live." Jack's shocking comment to her prevented any violent outburst on her part. He felt it was critical to be spontaneous with her in that way. In a few weeks she was out of the closed unit and into the open unit.

Jack commented that therapists might say,

"Hey, you are scaring me, but you are not going to chase me away because I am here to stay." And you have to be committed with them in that sense. If you are inconsistent they will pick up on this and they've got you. They will win that tremendous battle that you and they are fighting. It is war. And you fight, and you fight, and you fight, and you keep fighting, and then they start getting better. Can a schizophrenic recover fully from his illness? Sure.

If you are doing therapy with them, and you are nudging them, you have to expect a reaction. So they hit somebody, or they throw a chair or something like that. The traditional setting will give them 300 mg. of thorazine and those patients will run away from dealing with themselves and they will be safe again. That is, they will have their position protected again. When we have somebody acting out usually we have some indication that something is happening. Patients run away. They hide from us. They hide underneath the bed sometimes. We have to drag them out of the closets. This is because something is happening and it should not be misconstrued as regression in any sense of the word.

Jack believes that psychotherapy alone is not enough. He feels that patient management is a large part of the treatment process. "A fifty minute hour isn't enough. What do you do with the rest of the day, twenty-three hours a day, seven days a week? There has to be a program. There has to be structure. There has to be activation. There has to be intellectual stimulation."

Jack feels that thearpists must have dealt with the *sufferer in themselves* and their *own anger* and *aggression to treat schizophrenics*. It takes that kind of honesty and a certain degree of strength.

The following are portions of dialogue that I imagine are both unusual and possibly somewhat shocking to therapists who are unfamiliar with Dr. John Rosen's work. Each of Jack's comments were made at an extreme and shocking intensity of volume that produced in me a reaction of attentive fear. There will not be any particular continuity to the comments, as I am only describing the freedom Jack gives himself to respond with what goes through him. For the most part during the first part of the session the patient tried to keep his head down and ignore Jack. The edited video tape that was shown to us was cut from three and one-half hours to manageable proportions for the purpose of Jack's presentation. What was seen was a dramatic emergence of this patient from a severe schizophrenic condition. Jack makes contact quickly, using his knowledge of the moment as his diagnostic tool. Jack continually uses the element of surprise.

Now for some of the dialogue. Jack begins:

Jack	Stand at attention! Stand at attention! Stand up! Salute! Stand at attention!
Patient	I'm burning the United States flag! (His actions symbolize his "go to hell" attitude toward everyone else.)
Jack	That's OK. Stand at attention while you are burning the United States flag! (Jack's responses acknowledged that it was all right to be angry, but that Jack was present as a person and that the patient was going to have to pay attention to Jack while learning to respect both himself and Jack.)

Jack felt that the patient was asking him to make an intervention. The patient customarily spoke in the gibberish of the schizophrenic. Jack felt that it was important that he talk in the language of the patient. Meanwhile, the patient's response indicated a position of "I'm not going to give you anything until you can break the code." When the code has been broken patients typically feel they have been cared about in a way that makes hiding pointless. At this point they gain self-control and Jack gains control of the session. Jack describes his method as that of getting involved in the patient's delusional structure.

Patient	(Puts a paper cup in his mouth and begins to eat it and ask for some marijuana. The patient had a history of living at a board and care home in California where he used to eat out of garbage cans.)

Jack	This is just like shit! Here, have some shit! Eat it! Eat the shit!
Patient	(To another girl in the group) You came from a savage primitive planet beast. (Another patient tells Jack that this patient gives him a headache when he acts crazy.)
Jack	You give him a HEADACHE!
Patient	I was born retarded.
Jack	No. No. You're acting crazy, but you are not a bad crazy man.
Patient	The Chinese came.
Jack	(At this point it was about time to end the session) Goodbye. We'll see you. (Jack wanted him to leave)
Patient	(Walking out into the hall; he did not want the session to be over) You want me to break it? (As he said this he smashed a chair against the wall out in the hall. Jack became more aggressive in dealing with the patient's aggressiveness)
Jack	Hey . . . COME HERE . . . YOU COME HERE . . .
Patient	Okay . . .
Jack	YOU COME HERE . . . YOU GET YOUR ASS BACK HERE . . . LISTEN YOU SON OF A BITCH . . . TURN AROUND . . . ARE YOU EVER GOING TO BE VIOLENT? HUH? ARE YOU? I'LL BREAK YOU . . . I'LL BREAK YOU . . . DO YOU UNDERSTAND THAT? . . . Now you walk quietly back to your unit. I'm going to stamp out

	your head. Do you understand that? Your head! DO YOU UNDERSTAND THAT?
Patient	Kill me.
Jack	I'll kill your craziness.
Patient	Kill me.
Jack	I'll destroy your craziness . . . I'LL GET INTO YOUR BRAIN AND I'LL KILL IT.
Patient	Kill me.
Jack	Now you may go.
Patient	Kill me. I need the poison.
Jack	You need the poison?
Patient	Kill me, I need the poison.
Jack	I'll give you the poison. Go . . .
Patient	Give me the poison . . .
Jack	LEAVE . . .
Patient	That little red fox (?)
Jack	LEAVE . . . . Get out of here . . . go . . . go, go . . . you may leave. (The patient walks out and then returns.) Go, crazy man! Go, crazy man!
Patient	Help me, man . . . .
Jack	What chu want me to do?
Patient	I told you . . . I got to have the weed . . . (marijuana)

Jack	Give me your hand.
Patient	Let me have the weed, man.
Jack	No.
Patient	I got to have the weed.
Jack	You can't BE CRAZY ANYMORE . . . . YOU CAN'T BE CRAZY ANYMORE . . . .
Patient	GOT TO HAVE WEED . . . .
Jack	YOU CAN'T BE CRAZY ANYMORE . . . .
Patient	Got to have weed . . . .
Jack	You CAN'T BE CRAZY ANYMORE. . . .
Patient	Got to have weed . . . .
Jack	YOU CAN'T BE CRAZY . . . YOU CAN'T BE CRAZY . . . .
Patient	(All the time here is trying to interrupt Jack, with the same phrase) . . . I got to have weed . . . .
Jack	YOU CAN'T BE CRAZY . . . . CAN'T???? . . . CAN'T . . . CAN'T . . . CAN'T . . . CAN'T . . . CAN'T . . . CAN'T . . .
Patient	WEED.
Jack	NO. You act crazy and I won't like you . . . .
Patient	Weed . . . .
Jack	NO . . . .

Patient   Again Joe insists on having weed . . . .

Jack   NO. NO. NO. NO. NO. NO. NO. NO. NO. NO. NO. NO. NO MORE . . . . NO MORE. NO MORE. NO MORE WEED, NO MORE CHINA . . . . NO more ghosts . . . NOTHING . . . . NO WINE . . . . NO BLACK BELT . . . .

Patient   I'll remember that.

Jack   You will remember that.

Patient   I'll remember that the rest of my life.

Jack   Yes you WILL . . . . NO MORE WEED, NO MORE WEED . . . . DO YOU UNDERSTAND THAT . . . . NO MORE WEED . . . NO MORE . . . NO MORE . . . NO MORE WEED . . . NO MORE . . . DO YOU UNDERSTAND THAT? NO MORE CHINA . . . NO MORE CRAZINESS . . .

Jack   NO MORE . . . NO MORE . . . No more . . .

Patient   I have to . . .

Jack   NO MORE . . . I DON'T CARE . . . NO MORE . . . .

Patient   I have to . . . .

Jack   NO MORE . . . OUT WITH IT . . . OUT WITH THE CRAZINESS . . . . OUT WITH IT . . . STOP IT . . . STOP IT . . . STOP IT . . . Now look at me . . . . I want you to act like a sane 22 year old black man with a good right MIND I do not want you to hide any . . . more . . . do you understand that?

Joe   I'm going back to my Chinese connections.

Jack   I SAID NO MORE . . . WITH THAT . . . now shall
            I say it again . . . ? I want you to act like a bright
            twenty-two year old black man . . . . Do you hear
            me . . . ? Do you hear me . . . ? Do you hear me . . . ?
            Do you hear me . . . ? Do you hear me . . . ? Do you
            hear me . . . ? no craziness . . . no more . . .

Patient   They only teach me self-defense.

Jack   NO MORE . . . no more craziness . . . Do you
            understand me? . . . DOWN . . . DEAD . . . .
            BURIED . . . . FINISHED . . . . and you will live.

Patient   Kill me . . . .

Jack   I want you to live . . . . I'm going to kill that insanity
            in your head . . . .

Patient   Kill me . . . .

Jack   The insanity I will kill . . . I will kill the insanity . . . .

Patient   Kill me . . . .

Jack   The insanity I will kill . . .

Patient   Kill me.

Jack   The insanity I will kill . . . I'll kill it . . . .

Patient   Kill me . . . .

Jack   I'LL KILL THE INSANITY . . . .

Patient   Bite me . . . .

Jack   No. That's crazy . . .

Patient   Bite me . . . .

Jack   That's crazy . . . .

Patient I'll die . . . . (Jack bites the patient)

Jack   Die?

Patient I'll die for real . . . .

Jack   All right . . . .

(The bite was effective and symbolic. The patient was asking Jack to get very close. The action was so strong it allowed the patient to come out of it for a bit. And for the first time he speaks sanely as he says:)

Patient Fuck you all damn whites . . . . Fuck . . . Fuck . . . . Take it . . . . It's yours . . . . You want the ress of me . . . . You want the ress of me . . .

Jack   I want your craziness . . . . the craziness I want . . . . THAT'S WHAT I WANT. I'LL BITE YOU AGAIN . . . I BITE YOU AGAIN. I'LL BITE YOU AGAIN . . . IT'S A DOUBLE DEATH . . . AAAGHHHH . . . . Sit.

Patient Search me . . . search me . . . . search me . . . . search me . . . search me . . . go ahead . . . search me, take my clothes off . . . Do anything you want . . . .

Jack   THAT'S CRAZY . . . . THAT'S CRAZY . . . . I SAID NO MORE CRAZINESS . . . . DO YOU UNDERSTAND THAT . . . . NO MORE . . . . I SAID NO MORE CRAZINESS . . . . NO MORE . . . . Come here . . . to me . . . Let me take the craziness out of your head . . . squeeze it out of your ears . . . . PULL IT OUT OF YOUR NOSE . . . . Do you understand me? . . . You can't be crazy anymore . . . . You can't be crazy anymore. You can't be crazy anymore . . . YOU CAN'T BE CRAZY ANYMORE.

Patient   Take it.

Jack   That's one piece of craziness . . . . I . . . stamp on it . . . . (Jack begins to smash his foot into the floor over and over.)

Patient   Take it . . . .

Jack   Kill it . . . . Kill the craziness . . . . Kill it . . . . Kill it . . . . Kill it . . . . Kill the craziness . . . . Kill the craziness . . . . Kill . . . . Kill . . . . Kill the craziness in your head . . . . Stamp on it . . . . Stamp . . . . STAMP . . . . STAMP . . . . MORE . . . . It's all gone . . . . That's part of it all gone . . . .

The patient was a very provocative patient who would not stop. Jack took the patient off guard by responding to him directly. He was playing off of what was given in the here and now. The patient was the stimulus and Jack's responses are to gain control of the session.

IF I WERE THE PATIENT I MIGHT BE TERRIFIED OF BEING CRAZY IN JACK'S PRESENCE. I WOULD CERTAINLY BEGIN TO WONDER IF THE THERAPIST WASN'T CRAZIER THAN ME, AND POSSIBLY MORE ASSAULTIVE (JACK'S TONE IS OFTEN VIOLENT, ALTHOUGH HIS ACTIONS ARE NOT). Such aversive stimuli was used in the face of the patient's irrationality to encourage the patient to speak rationally.

The patient was wearing beads around his neck to indicate that he was an African warrior. Jack was stamping his foot on the floor to symbolically destroy that piece of craziness. When Jack said, "I'll kill the craziness," he was responding to schizophrenics' depersonalization of themselves. Schizophrenics often say something else told them to do it. Jack was depersonalizing that aspect (the craziness) of himself, so as to respond in kind by speaking in the patient's language. They are crazy and that's the craziness–as though some foreign body has gotten into them. Jack's approach makes them want to integrate themselves. The craziness boundary can be kicked out of them in this way. Once the craziness was kicked out Jack got to the real issue, the patient's anger about what he felt to be unjust treatment of himself as a black man and blacks over generations.

Jack	Clicking fingers . . . uhuh . . . uhu . . . melodiously . . . . . ahhh. My soul brother . . . . my soul brother . . . my daahlin . . . my daaling . . . my soul brother . . . . my sweetheart . . . . my crazy black beauty . . . . what would you do if you had 29750092172 . . .
Patient	You asking me a question?
Jack	Yes.
Patient	I'd blow up the world . . . .
Jack	VERY GOOD . . . . . . EXCELLENT . . . . Now you know what the right number is, don't you?
Patient	Yeah.

Session Two

A second session begins four days later on a much more rational basis. What is remarkable is the degree of progression in the patient in such a short time. The following session took place in a group with two other patients involved in the dialogue. I will refer to them as P2 and P3, while the first patient be referred to as Patient:

P2	Whether or not you are going to continue to work with him and help him and protect him, and he wants to do things that are going to make you feel like you should, continue to be nice to him. Huh? All those things are going around in your mind right now.
Jack	Right. Is he correct? OK, that's good. As long as you recognize it, I'm going to continue to work with you.

Patient   OK? And I have no trouble being nice to you because you are a very, very likable person. Do you hear me? And it's OK, as far as I'm concerned, if you think it's going to be helpful to you, to clean yourself out, go ahead and do it. You know.

Jack   It certainly can't hurt you. But that's not the solution. OK, the solution is to realize that again, that you lived in a world of fantasy for a long, long time, you've gotten used to it, you've come out of the world of fantasy, and you are living in a world of reality and it's going to take a little time to get used to that, too. But you don't have to do it all by yourself. There will be other people around you, and especially me, who will help you understand how to do it. Still scared, huh? Trust yourself?

Patient   Uhuh.

Jack   Trust me.

Patient   Uhuh.

Jack   Good, gimme a hug.

Jack   Ahh, give me a good one . . . . . . AHHHHHH. YEAH, that's a real good one, boy, I'll tell you. I like to see you smile. (Laughter in background) Yeah, well we'll work it out OK, it's going to take time, you know. You have certainly developed very quickly and that's scary too, OK?

Patient   Uhuh.

Jack   But I'm going to see you frequently and have long talks with you, all right? And I'm not going to write on paper. I'm just going to talk to you like man to man and man to son. All right? And I'm not going

	to run away, and I'm not going to turn my back on you, OK? You'll see, you'll see. OK, that's good. All right?
Patient	Is that the end of the rap session?
Jack	Pardon?
Patient	Is that the end of the rap session?
Jack	Do you want to talk some more?
Patient	Uhuh.
Jack	About what?
Patient	Blacks–girls in our country.
Jack	OK, go ahead . . . .
Patient	They used to sell something for the girls. UH, cosmetics . . . .
Jack	What else do you want to talk about?
Patient	I used to be a carpenter.
Jack	I know that. You know, I have the feeling that you just want to keep talking, which is fine, because you're afraid that if you stop talking you will lose me. You're not going to. Again, I think that you don't want me to work with anyone else but you? Right?
Patient	That's up to you.

Jack   No. I'll work with other people. I think that you want me to be completely devoted to you. I am very much devoted to you, OK?

Patient   Uhuh.

Jack   And maybe it kind of annoys you when I speak to other people too, does it?

Patient   I like to have this between me and you, that's all. Nobody else.

P3   Does it bother you if I'm sitting behind, I'm just behind you and I'll move, if you'll feel better. Would you? Truthfully, I'll move back over there, in the other chair, would it?

Patient   I'm talking to him.

P3   All right.

Jack   You want us to have private talks, from now on, huh?

Patient   Uhuh.

Jack   OK, that's good, we'll do that. All right. Just me and you and nobody else . . . . . agreed? OK.

Patient   Can I stay here?

Jack   Yes, you certainly can, I want you. OK.

Patient   How ya doin'

Jack   OK. That's nice . . . . . . yeh I care for you a lot. And you care for me a lot, you feel good when you feel that way don't you?

Patient   I feel . . . . I feel better when I'm around a man that has as much education

Jack   Uhuh . . . . . that's stimulating to you, isn't it?

Patient   Uhuh.

Jack   Makes you think better.

Someone in Room And just in the same way, you can get that same education that he has in your head.

P3   That's what you want to do, is go back to school.

Someone in Room You can go back, get a trade and do something, where you don't have to depend on somebody, when you can be your own man.

Jack   Well, that will come about. He wants to go to school and he will. We'll work that out. OK, Joe, why don't you just sit here.

Summary

Direct confrontation is a method that can be quite successful in the hands of a caring therapist, who has *street savvy* for how to use it. It has the potential to reach a population that has, for the most part, been given up on. This is a rather large population of about two million in the United States, and there are not nearly enough therapists trained or interested in dealing with this population.

It is hoped that what I have written will keep the initial work and thoughts of Rosen alive and open to further research, and that some of the newer methods that have come as a result of Jack Rosberg, who was stimulated by Rosen's work, will have a wider audience.

In addition to Rosberg's *caring capacity*, his *attitude of hopefulness* for cure is most important. He told a story that early on in his career he was referred a patient and the patient became well. Rosberg later found out the patient had endogenous depression, and that such an illness was incurable. He said that he would rather use his intuition in helping him cure patients before being influenced by hopeless predictions about the treatment which may effect its outcome.

It can also be seen that many powerful existential moments took place between Jack and the patient, who might otherwise have been thought to be unreachable if it were not for Jack's strong use of direct confrontation.

ENDNOTES

[1] My wife at the time Snader, "A Part of the Nightmare," Human Behavior (July 1977), p. 42.

All other quotations by Jack were taken from a seminar entitled "Psychotherapy and Schizophrenia," sponsored by The Anne Sippi Clinic for the Treatment of Schizophrenia. The presentation was given in Beverly Hills, Calif., on November 3, 1979.

REFERENCES

Rosen, John. *Direct Analysis, Selected Papers.* New York: Grune & Stratton, 1953.

Rosen, John. *Direct Psychoanalytic Psychiatry.* New York: Grune & Stratton, 1953.

Rosen, John. *Selected Papers on Direct Psychoanalysis, Vol. II.* Grune & Stratton, 1953.

Snader, My wife at the time. "A Part of the Nightmare." *Human Behavior* (July 1977), p. 42.

These related books by Dr. Rosen are available in a single volume form. That is, I am not sure if they are still in print, but were put in a single volume form.

11

<u>DR. LEN BERGANTINO, A. B. P. P.</u>

THE GODFATHER OF CLINICAL PSYCHOLOGY

It is rare you would have a book based on psychotherapy interventions I made when I was 37 years old as well as ones at close to the end of my doing professional psychotherapy. This spans a gap from 1968 when I was a doctoral student at The University of Southern California and a time when I was forced by a recession that wiped out 40% of my annuities to work as an independent contractor in a California State prison working with murderers almost exclusively. This was different than my Beverly Hills private practice and also included my having to deal with the institution of the prison system.

I found it fascinating to work with murderers almost exclusively in that they need to be dealt with at a primitive level that goes far beyond what most private practitioners were either trained or therefore able to do. I set a State of California record in that 93% of them came out for sessions when most clinicians could not get 70% weekly psychotherapy sessions.

As I was a quick learner I ALWAYS TOLD INMATES EXACTLY WHAT I WOULD DO AND WHAT I WOULD NOT DO, IN THAT I WOULD NOT DO ANYTHING TO GET ME FIRED BECAUSE I NEEDED THE MONEY. ONE MULTI MURDERER SAID, "OH, YOU ARE A HOLY MAN! YOU CAN DO SOME GOOD AROUND HERE!

AS DR. CARL WHITAKER, MD, TRAINED ME TO DO PSYCHOTHERAPY BY TELEPHONE I ATTEMPTED TO DEVELOP A TELEPHONIC PRIVATE PRACTICE OF MURDERERS, BUT THERE JUST WERE NOT ENOUGH MURDERERS WILLING TO CALL IN DESPITE THE UNIQUENESS OF MY ADVERTISING WHICH I HAVE ENCLOSED. IN THIS CHAPTER. However, with the increase of gun related murders, it is hopeful the reader will be a file to expand on the lessons in Chapter Eleven.

Psychotherapy in a California State Prison: The Real Story

About five years ago, I was employed as an independent contractor by a California State prison. A law had been passed that 70% of all inmates had to be seen one time per week in psychotherapy, and a Special Master was appointed to see that this took place or the prison might be shut down.

THE MAIN PROBLEM

Administrative staff would not support the psychologists in the face of the correctional officers who found this new rule an undue burden.

WORKING CONDITIONS WITH AD SEG POPULATIONS

In Administrative Segregation (ad seg), the Hole where all the murderers and severe cases were housed, the working conditions were the following. For me to see an inmate, two correctional officers would have to go to an inmate's cell, put him in chains, and escort him over to a cage where the handcuffs and chains were then taken off for what the Administration said had to be only a "5-minute psychotherapy" session. However, under these conditions, the Administration was not meeting its quota of 70% inmate participation, because inmates did not want to be dragged around in chains for a 5-minute session, and correctional officers did not want to bring them to the cage for therapy, chaining and unchaining them at their cell and at the therapy cage and escorting them.

In addition, correctional officers discouraged them from coming out, and the Administration did not back the psychologist. Further, the correctional officers had the strongest union in the state, and the Administration was afraid to go against them. Also, the Administration requested that the psychologist go from cell to cell with a bulletproof vest and a plastic face mask (to prevent knife injuries or acid on the face), and that he personally recruit each inmate to "come out" for psychotherapy sessions.

Articles about working in a prison as a psychologist leave out this background information, because there is a rule that anything published by anyone working in a prison has to be approved by the warden. I am writing this now because I no longer work in the prison system.

In my private practice in Beverly Hills, seeing private patients 5 days a week for between 3 and 7 years, I didn't get to use some of my specific skills as much as I did in the prison. These included those skills from my training with Milton H. Erickson, M.D., and Carl Whitaker, M.D., two pioneers who helped me create a style of work that I referred to as "existential shift", where I had a chance to "make a difference" in a person's life each and every time I saw them, no matter how short a time period it was. Without this technique, you might not enjoy working with ad seg populations (comprising mostly murderers). On the other hand, if you do have the ability to do brief therapy and make a difference in a short time, this population challenges every bit of creativity a therapist could bring to bear, and for that reason this was the most interesting job I ever had.

Up until the time the prison and I parted ways, 93% of the inmates came out of their cells on a weekly basis, which was a record, since most therapists couldn't get the required 70%.

HOW I GOT INMATES INTO THERAPY

Doing Favors

I tried to figure out what the inmate wanted most: Someone who was a straight shooter who would not lie to them. So if they asked me to do something for them and I could do it without getting fired, I told them I would and did it in the time promised. If I could not do it or it presented a risk to my livelihood, I merely stated:
"You could get me fired! It's out of the question!" So the inmate knew where he stood with me from the beginning. They tolerated a "No" just fine, as long as it was not a lie "yes" that meant "no".

Asking for Favors

An inmate would say: "Why should I come out to see you for 5 minutes and be dragged down in chains and put in a cage?" (This particular inmate lived in darkness all day and all night, never taking down a towel that blocked a window where any sunlight might go in, and he was supposed to have been one of the worst multiple murderers.) I said: "Because I need a favor. If I don't get 70% of you guys to come out every week, they are going to fire me!" The inmate said: "You are a holy man. You can make a difference around here. I will come out." His words kind of shocked me in that he scoped out the situation in about 30 seconds. By my telling the truth and not having any "hidden agendas", these murderers were not murderous toward me, were trustworthy, and did not threaten me at all.

Playing Fair

I maintained a nonjudgmental attitude despite the crime the inmate was in for. For example, if someone was in for life (having committed one or two murders—one fellow had two life sentences plus 80 years and he was only thirty years old), most people would judge them and treat them badly, while they were asking the psychologist to treat them for suicidal depression. I maintained the following attitude: I did not sentence them. The courts had sentenced them to life imprisonment, and I was ordered to "lift their spirits so they would not commit suicide." So I basically treated them as a tabula rasa, as if I knew nothing of their history, nor did I really care what they were in for as that had little to do with what I was hired for, which was to lift their spirits, prevent suicide, and prevent the prison from being closed down by the Special Master. So I treated them like I would anyone else, and worked with what they voluntarily presented to me that they saw as a problem. It was clear they were not going to escape, as rifle sharpshooters were in the towers, and they would never get past their chains anyway.

So picture yourself in a cell for the rest of your life. Want to commit suicide? See the problem? How does the therapist reinforce the desire to live and keep their spirits up when they have nothing to live for except the next garbage-like meal being served to them?

MOMENTS THAT STAND OUT

Suicide Escape

One of the bosses of the correctional officers, a good guy, said: "You better see Mr. Smith in Cell #x as he tried to kill himself last night." They brought the man to the cage, and he was drooling saliva, and had his head down looking totally dispirited. He had tattoos all over his body and rings coming out of his nose, belly button, ears, etc. He was a big, bulky, tough guy you would not want pissed off at you. I looked at him and said in the most scolding way I could: "What the fuck are you still doing here?!" That pulled him out of his stupor, as it was totally unexpected, and he said: "What do you mean?" I said: "I thought you would have escaped by now!" He beamed from ear to ear, not that he was going to escape, but that I had enough confidence in him that he could escape from an impossible situation. That was his five minutes; and one comment was all that was needed that day.

Note: You might wonder about mentioning the word escape in ad seg. But there was no way to escape, and my job was to lift spirits.

Group Therapy

I was doing group psychotherapy, which meant there were six cages lined up with one inmate in each in a semicircle, and they sent down about five guys with machine guns to watch the group. I was sitting in a chair that could roll between the cages to wherever I could do the best work at the moment.

One little African American guy seemed to have little or no contact with reality that day, and he shouted wildly at me "What are you, one of those correctional officers?" Meantime, I was taking notes (mandatory), and said: "Would you excuse me for a moment? I will get to you next." When I finished the notes, I said: "What the fuck makes you think I am one of them?" (I was really pissed off when I said it, as if to say "Can't you see straight?"). The inmate looked up at five Darth Vader looking characters and said: "I don't trust them!" I looked away from the inmate in his cage and at the guards and leaned over to him and whispered through the cage: "I don't trust the sons of bitches either!" He trusted me implicitly after that, and that one sentence set the groundwork for the therapy to begin. I "joined his psyche" "as if I were one of the prisoners" and I spoke to tough guys "as a tough guy".

When I had my own radio show in the early 1990s entitled "Psychotherapy Live", a call-in show, my promoter Audrey Franklyn (who was Ella Fitzgerald's promoter throughout her life) used to pitch me as "a cross between Sigmund Freud and Sylvester Stallone"! She would say: "He's brilliant but he talks like Rocky." Two Ericksonian principles are "utilization of what the client provides you and utilization of your own personality characteristics in treating them." Thus, as I grew up as a street kid in Waterbury, Connecticut, I talked to them like the street kid in me.

Physical Escape

There was a very bright Italian who was a cellmate of a very loyal German. They had both been trustees, but decided to arrange an escape because of what the Italian described as poor medical treatment that he could only get taken care of on the outside. So they arranged an elaborate escape, where they were to have someone pick them up and drive them to the Mexican border, where they had phony passports made up, and would then take a flight to a country without extradition. Great, plan, right? Wrong! They depended on someone to pick them up in the center of town and that person never showed, so there they were in their prison suits waiting for six hours, where they were captured and put back in prison, only now instead of being trustees watering the flowers, they were in ad seg for years to come.

There were team meetings where every so often a psychologist, a psychiatrist who prescribed prison meds, and a correctional officer would meet and confer with the prisoner about the plan for the next three months. These meetings were bullshit because the prisoner was going back to his cell for the next eighty years, but these meetings (quarterly I think) were part of the overall plan of therapy.

No Rehab in Prison

There is no rehabilitation program in the three prisons in which I worked. So during a team meeting for one of the two who had escaped, I said: "I recommend a rehab program for this inmate that he be sent to chauffeur school." The inmate was rolling under the table laughing, while the psychiatrist and the correctional officer thought I had made a mistake and didn't understand the prison system, as there was no rehab unit. And there certainly would not have been a chauffeur school if there had been a rehab unit.

I used to have both those cellmates brought down together (the Italian and the German) for therapy, and the one the team meeting had been for said: "What was that bullshit about chauffeur school?" I said: "You stupid bastards, the next time you break out, drive your own car!" They laughed and laughed. Of course, they knew there would never be a next time because they were now in ad seg with the murderers until the end of their sentences, to which had been added another five years for the attempted escape.

My first week working in the prison was devoted to training, which required the reading of the 125-page think manual and then a meeting with the warden. Hardly anyone read the manual, but I found it interesting. At the end of the introductory week, the warden said: "Well, did you learn anything?" I said: "Yes! I learned how to run a big business." The warden was furious and said: "Why do you say that?" I said: "Because you run the only place of business I have ever seen with a 93% recidivism rate." That means 93% of inmates released on parole get sent back to California State Prisons.

To my knowledge I am the only psychologist in the history of the State of California who was in charge of a plea bargain (to release John Marks (Marks I and Marks II, 1368 Law regarding mental illness and prisoners). He had appellate work that was brilliant from Bob Gerstein, and he had a court-appointment attorney who was a panel attorney and friendly with all the judges in Pomona, none of whom wanted Marks on the street. I sent out two mailings to about 2,000 criminal lawyers and attorneys throughout the State of California pro bono, and got attorneys Tom Mesereau (noted for winning the Michael Jackson case) and Stan Rozanski to do a few pro bono motions for Marks. Despite that legal work, Mr. Gil Garcetti invited me to facilitate the meeting with his top two D.A.s. Sunstedt and Mueller, and I was able to facilitate Marks' release based on the legal work Marks had done himself and that of appellate attorney Bob Gerstein). Sunstedt was furious and said: "What the hell gives you the right to be in this meeting?" I said: "I'm the only one Marks will talk to!"

In any case, the "release" was not all it was cracked up to be. Marks had been in for about 15 years, and at about 4 a.m. he was released with a pair of overalls, a blue dungaree shirt, and $13. Attorney Stan Rozanski gave him room and board for a while. Mesereau bought him a suit.

I introduced him to all the members of the California Supreme Court on the one night that all but Stanley Mosk attended the Italian American Lawyers annual event. Lucas (Chief Justice) said: "I've never met anyone I have ruled on before." Arabian told Marks his motions were brilliant and invited him to meet him in San Francisco for lunch. Arabian was a regular guy so to speak.

Marks encountered a few problems. Every job he had, when they found out he was a released felon, they fired him. He had severe diabetes and could not afford proper medical treatment. So after 15 years in prison and no rehab treatment, recidivism is what you get.

Marks, who was born John Balbo, was a structural genius and figured a way to get himself back into prison by having his relatives call the police for a nonviolent crime—possession of a weapon—which in his case was a third strike. So while he liked his freedom, freedom without having rehab to train you for a job and without money for even the barest necessities puts a person in a tough spot, and another prison doesn't look as bad as it did before.

Another first for a psychologist was when Judge Gibson in Victorville in 1997, presiding over the John Balbo trial, let me sit at the trial table with Balbo (in propia persona) along with the court-appointed investigator (who Balbo thought was better than having no legs at all). Balbo did not want a court-appointed attorney, and no attorney I or he could think of would take the case for the small sum of money that was paid for three-strike case.

It was after Johnny Cochran and the O. J. Simpson case, so the sheriffs made fun of us calling us "The Dream Team". In any case, for reasons far beyond the scope of this article, we lost, and Balbo, formerly Marks, got a third strike, and has been an appreciative pen pal ever since.

The bottom line message is that we need to install rehab into the prisons so when a guy gets released he can go get a job, make some money honestly and a life for himself. Anything else is bullshit.

My Five-Year-Old's Power

I have a brain-damaged son named Alexander, who when he was five or six years old used to talk to John Marks when he called the house from LA County Jail. Alex, developmentally delayed at birth, used to watch a lot of action films, which made him feel powerful, and he was enamored with Schwarzenegger as the Terminator. So one night, Alex tells Marks: "Hey, John, I'm coming down to bust you out of that place! I've got the dynamite, and I'll have the car running waiting for you." Then we didn't hear from Marks for a long time. I said: "Where the hell have you been?" He said: "In solitary confinement." I said: "Why?" He said: "The prison people listened to Alex and they thought he was for real, that he was going to break me out of here." And we laughed, and my son felt very powerful that at least someone took him seriously. The thing is that Alex speaks with floppy muscle tone, and you could barely understand his pronunciation.

Medical Care "Favors"

I complained to my supervisor about the work of a particular medical doctor and his lack of follow-through with inmates, and my supervisor had one comment: "After awhile everybody gets beaten down who works here." In terms of the kinds of favors I would do for inmates, they were things that should have been done anyway—but weren't because of prison red tape. Let's look at two examples.

An inmate told me that he did not urinate for a week and wanted to be sent to the infirmary to have a catheter inserted in his penis and the urine extracted, which sounded like a relatively unpleasant situation. I ordered him down to the infirmary. Two days later I stopped by his cell to see how he was, and he said: "The medic (a correctional officer) overruled you and cancelled the order." I was pissed. I took it up with the medic. He said: "The prisoner is lying to you." I said: "Why in hell would he lie about having a catheter shoved up his penis?" He said: "Because he is a prisoner and all prisoners lie." But they hardly ever lied to me because I never lied to them. I overruled him, and the medical doctor who performed the procedure said the patient had so much urine in his body "it was going to start to float out his ears." I told the medic the result, and he said: "Look Bergantino. I've got about 200 inmates a day to service and what you do screws me up; I have to fill out papers. It takes so much time. Cut the shit!"

I got an inmate moved up on the dental chart because I was friendly with the dentist. The inmate was screaming with pain and the waiting list was 1,500 inmates with appointments ahead of him, which would take about six months. I got him in in two weeks and the tooth was pulled. He looked at me like I was Santa Claus. Imagine having unbearable nerve pain and having to eat with it and live with it for six months.

In other words, my favors were no danger to the prison and in fact boosted morale and gave the inmates the feeling, that in addition to the psychotherapy work, it was worth their effort to come out of their cells to see me once a week.

My Mafia Image

Bergantino is of Italian descent, so a lot of the prisoners would yell from their cells when I came in the building: "Hey, Bergantino, are you with the Mafia?" I never answered them for the therapeutic reason of technical neutrality, and the less they knew about me the better; as well as going with Erickson's advice of "utilizing the patient's resistance, and my own personality characteristics"—the work might go better if they thought I was with the Mafia.

While the inmates and I got on pretty well and for the most part I trusted that they would not harm me, I did not have this feeling about all the correctional officers, all of whom were armed, and who kept telling me I worked too many hours and that I should be out of there by 3 p.m. I worked four ten-hour shifts Monday through Thursday. About six months after I no longer worked at the prison, there was a bust and several correctional officers were under arrest for bringing in illegal drugs to the prison. The correctional officers also hadn't been too sure if I was with the Mafia or not and I liked it that way.

Stand Down
Around 1993, Attorney Tom Mesereau brought me to Phil Paolino who had a gym on Fairfax for white-collar boxing. For about one and a half years I did 15 rounds five days a week of training. There was a three-minute bell per round. Five rounds were spent jumping rope. Five rounds were punching a light bag, three punching the heavy bag, and two sparring in the ring or hitting the mitts of a trainer.

Phil, trained by former champ Archie Moore, liked to see people get hit, and so one afternoon he said to me: "Len, I got a call from Tom Mesereau at 2 a.m. I said: 'Tom, what do you want? It's two o'clock in the morning.' Mesereau said: 'Phil, I don't want to get hit! I don't want to get hit!' I said: 'Tom, this is boxing. In boxing, people get hit.'" Phil spent most of his time with a heavyweight who had 18-inch arms, and when he hit the heavy bags with either hand, smoke would come out. I pretty much stayed out of his way as he took the entire floor when he worked the heavy bags. One Saturday I went in and Phil said: "Len, I have a sparring match for you" (and it was this guy who looked like Evander Holyfield). I said:

'Phil, I have a stomachache today, I think I'll go home early." Phil said: "You chickenshit bastard, get in the ring! It's only a sparring match." I got in the ring and the bell went off and I hit the guy with a left jab and he fell backward on his butt with his hands and feet up in the air, like he was in stirrups. I realized instantaneously that it was rigged and a big joke but I acted like I didn't know it was a joke and I helped him off the canvas apologizing for hurting him in a sparring match, and telling him my problem throughout my life was in not knowing my own strength, and I walked out apologizing for hurting him while they were all laughing like hell.

The reason that anecdote came to mind was that I heard two correctional officers telling an inmate "Don't go down to see Bergantino! That son of a bitch is crazier than you are!" So in front of 100 cells, 200 inmates, I called them both out at the same time. I said: "C'mon, let me see what you got!" And I backed them down in front of the inmates. I was pretty sure they were not crazy enough to beat a psychologist in a State prison, and that such a move would go beyond even the power of the Union to protect them. One of them later said to me: "You are lucky you are an old man." (They were 20 years younger than I. I was about 60 at the time.) I looked the guy right in the eye and said: "You are lucky I am an old man." For a few days after that the inmates would rattle their cups on the small window bars and yell, "We want Bergantino." They saw me stand up for myself, and for them, which they could not do for fear of abuse.

A Request to Reduce Violent Thoughts
"Hey, doc, can you help me? When most people get pissed off at someone they want to punch them or beat them up in a fistfight [something I could identify with given what I had to deal with walking to grammar school in Waterbury]; but me, my first thought goes to chainsaws, axes, AK47s, dynamite, etc. Can you help me reduce these violent thoughts to a more normal level?" Frankly, this was not the kind of question I had encountered in psychotherapy and I took it up with my supervisor who was also stumped on any intervention that might be helpful.

This inmate had committed multiple murders and was only 30 years old. He was one of the ones who used to yell out of his cell window anytime I was in the building, "Hey, Bergantino, are you with the Mafia?" So at least part of him thought I was a thug (from Erickson I had learned to utilize my own personality characteristics, and from Whitaker I learned how to use the craziness of the inmate or patient in invading his or her unconscious mind to gain an existential shift in the problem).

So one day he was in the cage waiting for a paralegal who would come around once every two weeks (and had a caseload of 2,000 inmates). While he was waiting, something just occurred to me on the spot and I blurted out: "Hey, Joe, when I am pissed off at somebody I throw them down three flights of stairs. When you are pissed off at somebody, you kill them. That's why you are in here and I am out here."

After that, everytime I came into the building, he would yell out, "Hey, Bergantino, three flights of stairs!" I realized that while three flights of stairs might be awful, it actually reduced his level of violence from thoughts of chainsaws.

I had combined the Ericksonian storytelling method based on an intervention made by John Rosen, M.D., a creative genius in cutting out character disorders, in his work with a 13-year-old girl who claimed there were Chinese communists on the third floor of her farmhouse in Doylestown, Pennsylvania (the story was told to me by Martin Grotjahn, M.D., a psychoanalyst observing Rosen's work at the time).

Conclusion
While the methods of Erickson and Whitaker and Rosen were certainly helpful in my prison work, the key ingredient was that I was not a phony.

LEN BERANTINO, ED.D., ABPP, is in the private practice of clinical psychology specializing in telephone psychotherapy or supervision. He is a diplomate of the American Board of Professional Psychology and a licensed psychologist in the states of Arizona, California, and Hawaii, and he can work with those who call from one of those three states or internationally (1)310-207-9397. He resides in West Los Angeles, California. In addition to being trained by Milton Erickson, M.D., and Carl Whitaker, M.D., and other world-renowned therapists, he has authored 80 publications and the book Psychotherapy Insight and Style: The Existential Moment, 1981, Allyn & Bacon.

From:	Voices Business Manager <voicesaap@gmail.com>
Sent:	Tuesday, May 7, 2019 11:33 AM
To:	usa1164@fedex.com
Subject:	[EXTERNAL] Dr. Lenbeurgentino

Hi!

You have permission to use your article as you see fit in your own publications. We would love to know when the book is published!

Lisa

Lisa Kays
Voices Business Manager
VoicesAAP@gmail.com
230 Washington Ave, Ext Suite 101, Albany, NY 12203

Twitter & Instagram: @VoicesAAP
Facebook

Voices is unique, nourishing, and transformative. Reading it changes lives.

Click here to subscribe!

Psychotherapy in a State Prison: Some True Stories

Len Bergantino

A FEW YEARS AGO I WAS EMPLOYED AS AN independent contractor to provide psychotherapy to inmates in a California state prison. A law had been passed requiring seventy per cent of inmates to be seen one time per week in psychotherapy, and a special master was appointed to see that this took place; otherwise the prison was in jeopardy of shutting down.

In order for a psychologist to see a prisoner in Administrative Segregation (aka "Ad Seg" or "The Hole"), where all the murderers and severe cases were housed, two correctional officers would have to put the prisoner in chains and escort him to a cage, where the handcuffs and chains were taken off for what the law stated had to be "five minute psychotherapy sessions." The prison was not meeting its quota because inmates did not want to be dragged around in chains for a brief session in a cage, and correctional officers did not want to do all the

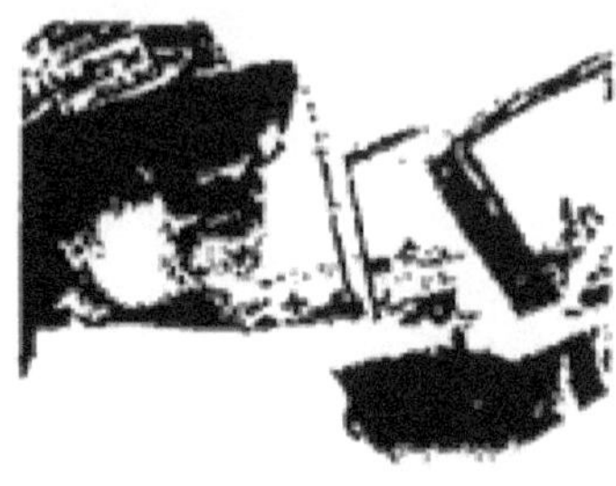

LEN BERGANTINO, EdD, is a licensed clinical psychologist in the state of California, where he currently practices Gestalt therapy. He received his doctorate from the University of Southern California and is a Diplomate in family therapy of the American Board of Professional Psychology. He has been in private practice for most of his professional life. Dr. Bergantino was trained in family therapy by Carl Whitaker (1981–1985) and by Walter Kempler (1977–1983). He is a graduate of Erv and Miriam Polster's three-year program at the Gestalt Training Center San Diego (1976–1979).

required escort work. Prisoners refused to come out, and correctional officers did whatever they could to discourage them. Yet we psychologists had to get seventy percent of them to sessions or get fired.

In addition, psychologists were expected to go from cell to cell wearing a bulletproof vest and a plastic mask (to prevent being knifed or having acid thrown on their faces) and personally recruit each inmate to "come out" for psychotherapy sessions each week. Incidentally, articles about working as a psychologist in a prison usually leave out this background because anything that is published has to be approved by the warden.

In my private practice as a psychoanalyst in Beverly Hills, I saw patients five days a week, and they were in treatment for between three and seven years. However, with these patients I never got to use the particular skill I had learned in my training with Milton H. Erickson and Carl Whitaker. These two pioneers had helped me create a style of work that I refer to as an "existential shift" where I had a chance to make a difference in a person's life each and every time I saw them, no matter how brief our time. Without this skill I would not have enjoyed working with an Ad Seg population mostly comprised of murderers. On the other hand, having the ability to do brief therapy and make a difference in a short time challenged me to bring every bit of my creativity to bear. This made it the most interesting and compelling job I ever had.

Most of the psychologists employed in the prison did not meet their 70 per cent quota, but I managed to get 93 per cent of the inmates out of their cells on a weekly basis.

My policies were to be honest with the inmates, to treat them with an attitude of fairness, and to keep my word. Unlike other prison officials, I always tried to be a straight shooter, someone who would not lie to them. I tried to figure out what the inmate wanted most. If they asked me to do something for them, and I could do it without getting fired, I did it in the time I promised. If I could not do it because it presented a risk to my livelihood, I merely said, "You would get me fired. It's out of the question." I found that inmates tolerated a "no" just fine as long as I did not lie or say "yes" when I really meant "no."

Another important part of my success was to maintain a nonjudgemental attitude and treat the inmates as fairly as I would treat any other human being. Most people these men dealt with on a day to day basis judged them to be scum and treated them accordingly. They felt free to deny the inmates their basic rights—e.g. for medical care. Paradoxically, the prison created an atmosphere of helplessness and hopelessness while asking psychologists to treat prisoners for suicidal depression. I maintained the following attitude: I did not sentence inmates, the courts had already sentenced them to life imprisonment. My orders were to "lift their spirits so that they would not commit suicide."

I went in to sessions as if I knew nothing of their history nor did I care what they were in for. I was hired to "lift their spirits" and prevent the prison from being closed down by the special master. So I treated them with basic human dignity and worked with issues they voluntarily presented to me. It was clear that they were not going to escape—the prison was guarded by rifle sharpshooters in towers, and anyway they would never get out of their chains. If you picture yourself in a cell for the rest of your life (one 30-year old man was serving two life sentences plus eighty years) looking forward only to the next garbage-like meal, you get a sense of these men's spirit and the challenges for any psychotherapist.

CREATING AN EXISTENTIAL SHIFT

In addition to my early training with Carl Whittaker and Milton Erickson, my work with Walter Kempler and Jim Simkin helped me gain confidence that I could, when I chose, shoot an authentic comment out of a cannon and trust that the resulting force would facilitate change in certain unique situations. The work I did with inmates called for that confidence in the power of truth-telling, the power of one single statement to make a situation work. This kind of maneuver was like the times during my college years, when an all night card game would come down to one ride-it-all moment. My partner would spin a card in the air, betting the entire pot, and call out "NBNBC!" ("No balls, no blue chips!")

Here's an example of the existential shift that one of those comments can cre-
ate. One inmate who never spoke to anyone asked me, "Why should I come out
to meet you for five minutes to be dragged down in chains and put in a cage?"
He said there was nothing in it for him and it would basically mess up his whole
day. This inmate lived in darkness all day and all night, never taking a towel from
blocking the window where any sunlight might go in. He was reputedly the worst
of the multiple murderers.

I answered him like a con: "Because I need a favor." (This is something any
inmate could understand.) "If I don't get 70 per cent of you guys to come out
every week they are going to fire me, and I need the money."

I was shocked at his response. He said, "All right, I will come out. You are a
holy man! You can make a difference around here." My comment had changed the
terms on which we were negotiating with each other. Instead of pulling rank and
insisting that he needed my expertise, I put him in the position of helping me.

Because I told the truth and had no hidden agendas, these murderers were
not murderous toward me. In fact I found them quite trustworthy. Ironically,
my trouble came from the correctional officers, who did not want the hassle of
bringing 93 per cent of them out each week. And since the correctional officers
have a very powerful union, the prison administration was reluctant to support
someone in my position.

Another time, I was doing group psychotherapy, which meant there were six
cages lined up in a semi-circle, with one inmate in each. There were five guards
with machine guns watching the group therapy and listening to what I said to the
patients. I sat in a chair that could roll between the cages to wherever I could do
my best work at the moment.

There was one African American fellow who seemed to have little or no con-
tact with reality that particular day, and he shouted wildly at me, "What are
you, one of those correctional officers?" I was taking notes (a mandatory part
of the job) and I said, "Would you excuse me for a moment? I will get to you
next." When I finished the notes I turned to him and said "WHAT THE FUCK
MAKES YOU THINK I AM ONE OF THEM?" (Really pissed off, as if to say
"can't you see straight?") The inmate looked up at five Darth Vader-like characters
and said, "I don't trust them." I looked away from the inmate at the five Darth
Vaders, leaned over to him and whispered through the cage, "I don't trust the
sons a bitches myself."

He trusted me implicitly after that, and this one sentence set the groundwork
for the therapy to begin. I had joined his psyche, as if I were one of the prisoners.
Also, I spoke to this tough guy as a tough guy—as if I had happened to sneak
by the guards to come in and work in the prison. I did not do this because I was
putting on an act. It is an authentic part of who I am, having grown up as a tough
Italian kid in Waterbury, Connecticut.

On one occasion a boss of correctional officers, one of the good guys, came
to me saying, "You better see Mr. Smith in cell 99, as he tried to kill himself last
night." They brought the man to the cage, his head down, drooling saliva, look-

ing totally dispirited. The guy had tattoos all over his body and rings coming out of his nose, belly button and ears. He was a big bulky tough guy you would not want pissed off at you. I looked at him and said in the most scolding way I could, "What the FUCK are you still doing here?" That pulled him out of the stupor, "What do you mean?" he asked. I said, "I thought you would have escaped by now!" Now, there was no chance to escape from prison. He was in administrative segregation and there were two guards escorting him to sessions in chains. But the fact that I placed such a vote of confidence in him turned him around in a split second. He laughed and laughed and was no longer in a suicidal mood. He beamed from ear to ear.

No one who cared what the prison administration thought about ideas of escape would have said what I did to that guy. But I saw my job as lifting his spirits and that is what I did. I saw that as *authentic trickery*, causing him to shift his perspective on himself from being a worthless piece of garbage who is ready for suicide to a self-confident person worthy of thinking about escape. All I needed was five minutes. Actually one comment was the psychotherapy that day.

When I had a radio call-in show in the early '90s called "Psychotherapy Live," my promoter used to pitch me as a "cross between Sigmund Freud and Sylvester Stallone." "He's brilliant," she used to say, "but he talks like Rocky." The way I talk is natural to me, and I put it to good use in the prison setting. One of Milton Erickson's principles of treatment was "utilization of what the client provides you." To that I added utilization of my own personality characteristics. I used the street kid in me to talk to my prison clients, and checked my Ph.D. self at the door.

DRIVING LESSONS

There were two cell mates, one a very bright Italian-American and one a very loyal German-American. They were both trustees (i.e. privileged inmates) but they decided to arrange an escape because the Italian needed outside medical treatment. Their escape plan involved a third party who was going to drive them to the Mexican border. They had phony passports made up and were booked on a flight to a country without extradition. Great plan—except their pick-up person never showed. So they waited in the center of town, in their prison suits, for six hours until they were captured and put back in prison. And now, instead of being trustees watering the flowers outside their cell, they were in Ad Seg for years to come.

In the three prisons where I worked there was no rehabilitation program. There was, however, a thing called a team meeting where every three months a psychologist, a prescribing psychiatrist and a correctional officer would meet with the prisoner and confer about the plan for the next three months. These meetings were total nonsense because the prisoner was going back to his cell for the next eighty years. That was the plan.

During the team meeting for one of the captured escapees I said, "I recommend a rehab program for this inmate that he be sent to chauffeur school." The inmate was rolling under the table laughing, while the psychiatrist and the correctional officer thought I had made a mistake and did not understand the prison system. There was no rehab unit. And if there had been a rehab unit there certainly would have been no chauffeur school.

I used to have the two former cell-mates brought down together. The next time I met with these two one of them asked, "What was that bullshit about chauffeur school?" I said, "You stupid bastards, the next time you break out, drive your own car!" They laughed and laughed. Of course, I knew there would never be a next time because they were now in Ad Seg with the murderers until the end of their sentences, with another five years added on for attempted escape.

DOING FAVORS

I mentioned that part of my approach to dealing with my prison patients was to figure out what they wanted and, when possible, do them favors. The kind of favors I did for inmates were things that should have been routine but weren't because of prison red tape. Here are two examples.

An inmate told me he had not urinated in a week. He wanted to be sent to the infirmary to be catheterized. I wrote an order that he be sent to the infirmary and two days later stopped by his cell to see how he was. He said, "The Medic (a correctional officer) overruled you and cancelled the order." I took it up with the Medic, who said, "The prisoner is lying to you." I responded, "Now, why the hell would he lie to me about having a catheter shoved up his penis, a treatment that is going to have him screaming with pain and hanging from the ceiling?" The Medic said, "Because all prisoners lie." I overruled the Medic. The doctor who then treated the prisoner said he had so much urine in his body it was "going to start to float out of his ears." When I told that result to the Medic he said "Look, Bergantino, I've got about two hundred inmates a day to service and what you do screws me up. I have to fill out papers. It takes too much time."

Another favor I did was to get an inmate moved up on the dental chart, since I was friendly with the dentist. The inmate was screaming with pain, and the prison waiting list had fifteen hundred inmates ahead of him—a wait of six months. I got him in in two weeks and the tooth was pulled. After that he looked at me like I was Santa Claus.

The favors I did were no danger to the prison and in fact boosted morale and gave inmates the feeling that, in addition to my psychotherapy work, it was worth their effort to come out of their cells to see me one time per week.

A USEFUL CONNECTION

Here are two ways I put into practice the principle of using your own characteristics to aid the therapy. My surname is Italian, so a lot of the prisoners would yell from their cells when I came into the building, "Hey, Bergantino, are you with the Mafia?" I never answered them, for the therapeutic reason of technical neutrality. The less they knew about me the better. In addition, I figured the work might go better if they thought I was with the Mafia, so it suited me not to answer the question.

The inmates and I got on pretty well, and for the most part I trusted they would not harm me. However I did not have this feeling about the correctional officers, all of whom were armed. They kept telling me I worked too many hours and that I should be out of there by 3 P.M. My schedule was to work four ten hour shifts, Monday through Thursday. About six months after I left my job at the prison, I read that there had been a bust and several correctional officers were under arrest for bringing illegal drugs into the prison. I was not totally surprised. They weren't too sure if I was with the Mafia or not, and I liked it that way.

During the time I worked at the prison, I used to train at a local gym for white collar boxing. I enjoyed using my fists, which I first learned to do on the way to school every day in Waterbury. One day I heard two correctional officers telling one of my inmates, 93 percent of whom were now coming out for their psychotherapy sessions with me, "Don't go to see Bergantino! That son of a bitch is crazier than you are!" So I called both officers out at the same time, in front of a hundred cells, two hundred inmates. "Come on," I said, "Let me see what you got!" And I backed them down in front of the two hundred inmates. I was pretty confident they were not crazy enough to beat up a psychologist in a State prison, that such a move would go beyond even the power of the Union to protect them. One of them later said to me "You are lucky you are an old man!" (I was about sixty at the time and they were twenty years younger than me.) I looked the guy right in the eye and said, "*You are lucky I am an old man!*"

For a few days after that confrontation the inmates would rattle their cups on the small window bars and yell, "We want Bergantino!" They loved me for standing up to the kind of abuse that was meted out to them on a daily basis. They were in no position to challenge the correctional officers the way I had done, but they respected me for doing it.

A LEGITIMATE PSYCHOTHERAPY REQUEST.

"Hey Doc, can you help me? When most people get pissed off at someone they want to punch them or beat them up in a fist fight. But me, my first thoughts go to chain saws, axes, AK47s, dynamite, stuff like that. Can you help me reduce these violent thoughts to a more normal level?"

This was not the kind of question I had ever encountered in outpatient psychotherapy, and I took it up with my supervisor who was also stumped on any intervention that might be helpful. This patient had committed multiple murders and was only 30 years old. He was one of the guys who used to yell out of his cell window, "Hey, Bergantino, are you with the Mafia?" So at least part of him thought, doctor or no doctor, I was a thug.

One day, when this patient was in the cage waiting to meet with a paralegal, an idea occurred to me. I blurted out, "Hey Miguel, when I am pissed off at somebody I throw them down three flights of stairs and break every bone in their body. When you are pissed off at somebody, you kill them. That's why you are in there and I am out here!"

He laughed like crazy and, for months, anytime I was within shouting distance he would break out laughing and yell, "Hey, Bergantino! Three flights of stairs!" This was an existential shift in that the humor and how funny it struck him depotentiated many of his own more violent thoughts. It was an example of what Carl Whitaker used to recommend—i.e. using the patient's own craziness to invade their consciousness in order to create an existential shift. My statement to him was within the limits of my own threshold for violence—something I might actually consider doing if pushed to my limits—therefor I was not lying to him. You lie to a guy like that once and you lose credibility with him forever. Although "three flights of stairs" might be at the outer limit of what I would ever do, it was authentic to my own primitive truth, and I considered the intervention a successful, authentic piece of trickery. Although throwing somebody down three flights of stairs might be terrible, I had actually reduced Miguel's level of violent fantasizing from chain saw murders to three flights of stairs.

Both Martin Grotjahn and Carl Whitaker used to tell me about the work of John Rosen, a psychiatrist best known for his book *Direct Psychoanalytic Psychiatry*. He was a genius in using confrontation and reality to "cut out the character disorder" in character disordered patients—and you find a lot of those in prison. I believe that what I did with Miguel and some of my other prison clients borrowed something from Rosen's way of thinking. When I wrote my own book about my psychotherapy methods, Carl Whitaker wrote a preface in which he used the work "trickery" to describe my style—and I have come to understand that there is a true part of my character that is a trickster. This is an aspect of the real me that I use in my treatment of difficult cases.

CONCLUSION

While the methods of Erickson and Whitaker were very helpful to me in doing psychotherapy in the state prisons, the most important ingredient in my success is that I was not a phony. I was operating from the truth of my identity as both the former street kid from Waterbury, Connecticut and as the trained psychotherapist.

A rule of thumb is that if you are afraid of working with these kinds of patients, don't do it. Pay attention to your fear. For some reason, I was always pretty skillful at working with these kinds of patients on a primitive level, even before I was well-trained. In my second job at a VA outpatient clinic in 1972, I was asked to take over a group for a psychiatrist who was leaving the clinic. There was a large African American fellow in the group who came each week with a huge machete strapped to his leg. The psychiatrist told me that not much happened in the group because all the group members were afraid of him.

When I came in and was introduced by the psychiatrist, I stood near the door so that if I had to run out in a hurry I could be the first one out. I looked at the man with the machete and said, "Hey you! You are going to get rid of that machete right now! And if you don't I am going to throw your ass out of this group and cut your disability payments!" He looked at me and said, "Man, with you here I don't need the machete. I wish you were with me in Vietnam." His response was totally unexpected and relieved everyone. Although I was not conscious of it at the time, the bit about cutting his disability payments was a threat designed to "cut out the character disorder" and to appeal to the part of him that appreciated reality.

What drew me to the work in the prison? First, I needed the money after losing a significant amount of my annuity during the recession of 2000-2002. Second, although most of my working life had been devoted to longterm intensive psychotherapy, I had been trained in briefer treatment methods. I felt challenged to see if I could actually be effective in a situation where I would have just five minutes or, on a good day, maybe twenty minutes, and would be able to put the "trickster" part of my personality to work in the service of improving people's mental health.

So, what if you are not a tough guy? How would you manage to work in a prison environment? Walter Kempler taught me that it was important for the therapist to show him or herself, warts and all, in order to give the patient something to rub up against. In other words, be yourself with as little bullshit as possible. This requires that you do your own hard work in order to know your primitive self well enough to be honest and to make your statements forthright.

REFERENCES

Bergantino, L. (1981) *Psychotherapy Insight and Style: The Existential Moment*. Boston: Allyn & Bacon.

Rosen, J. (1962) *Direct Psychoanalytic Psychiatry*. New York and London: Grune & Stratton.

Len Bergantino

Brief Psychotherapy—Family Therapy and the Pursuit of Excellence in a World that Only Tolerates the Illusion of Safety!

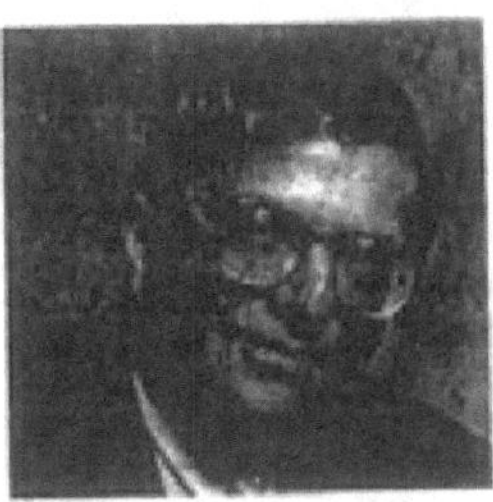

Len Bergantino, Ed.D., ABPP is in the private practice of clinical psychology in West Los Angeles. His book, *Psychotherapy Insight & Style: The Existential Moment* is being republished as a Master Classic by Jason Aronson Publishers under a new title: *Making an Impact in Therapy: How Master Clinicians Intervene*. He has trained psychotherapists and family therapists internationally. At this time in his professional life, he enjoys doing family therapy and brief psychotherapy by invading the unconscious with the patient's own craziness to create existential shifts.

Brief psychotherapy can be deep, short-term, meaningful, and impactful! Brief therapy has customarily been thought of as less than, not as deep as, not the treatment of choice if one could afford a more in-depth treatment, and superficial to the point of not having any lasting deep results. Brief therapy is primarily thought to be either the short-term psychodynamic work taught by Davanloo and his followers or the cognitive-behavioral work initiated by Albert Ellis and later expounded upon by Aaron Beck and his followers.

My experience in having been trained in brief therapy was somewhat different in that it was both more primitive and more primal, and lifelong shifts were created in me from which I could never return to the way I was. In other words, whether I was a cooperative patient or trainee or not, certain things were done to me and I came out different, like it or not!

Perhaps the day of the guru has passed because of the psycholegal flavor of super safety for the presumed protection of the consumer from so-called untried and untested methods; yet what this actually robs the consumer of is the creative genius of those therapists who have the courage and capacity to break new ground in situations that for the most part currently remain hopeless.

Of those gurus, perhaps the last of a breed who taught me were Milton H. Erickson, Carl Whitaker, and Walter Kempler. I suppose what I came out with is a synthesis of what I learned from them, a reformulation in my own way at the level of the primitive unconscious.

Most therapists follow the patient's conscious lead with the material they present and say or do things that are experienced by the patient as relatively understandable and safe. Not so with Erickson, Whitaker, and Kempler. They did things that were not easily understood by the patient and might even be thought to be ruthless. That is, at the levels at which they worked what I came to learn was that while a great deal of psychotherapy was spoken with many many words, those words did not necessarily change the patient to someone who was a tolerable human being to live with or be with, or the kind of behaviors they engaged in that added to their intolerability. I found that most patients were so frightened of change that they were morally collusive and corrupt with themselves and others. They could not or would not voluntarily stand the chaos and anxiety of not knowing which was necessary for primitive movement and change. Thus, I had three mentors from whom the message I received was, then, "JUST DO IT TO THEM!"

I will give you a flavor of each with a story or two, saving Whitaker for last. When I naturally do what I do best, my colleagues tell me I work like Carl Whitaker. I said to one, "It's a good thing he was born first!"

I have long been impressed by Erickson's work (Haley, 1973). What stood out for me was the ruthlessness of approach and getting a complete turnaround in one session!

When I went to Phoenix to be trained by Erickson, therapists would come from all over the world to be trained by him. He would tell stories as a way of accessing the unconscious potentials of patients. I will tell one such story about what I saw him do. A 26-year-old former patient of his, whom I will call Sarah, called up while the training session was ongoing. She said it was an emergency, that she couldn't sleep and had been up all night coughing with an asthma attack. Erickson asked her to come right over.

He asked her if she wanted to be hypnotized. She did. She went into a very peaceful trance state for about 20 minutes. When she came out of trance she said, "But Dr. Erickson, how is this hypnosis going to help me stop coughing and sleep at night?" Erickson looked at her intently and said, "Take it from an authoritarian old man like me that you have very kissable lips."

Sarah just beamed. It was as if someone had reached in and given her a warm heart massage. The tension came off her forehead. However, Erickson knew the conscious resistance was always lurking there and did his best to use his creativity to bypass the resistance. Sure enough, as she got up to leave and walked toward the door she turned and said, "But Dr. Erickson, how is that going to help me stop coughing and sleep tonight?"

Erickson, who had polio, was in a wheelchair, had paralyzed lips and a dislocated tongue, began to sing, "AND THE LIP BONE IS CONNECTED TO THE CHEEK BONE, AND THE CHEEK BONE IS CONNECTED TO THE NECK BONE, AND THE NECK BONE IS CONNECTED TO THE CHEST BONE." HE TURNED AROUND TO THE GROUP WITH SUPREME CONFIDENCE (NOT CARING IN THE LEAST IF ANYONE THOUGHT HE WAS GRANDIOSE, BUT ONLY TO MAKE A LASTING IMPACT THAT WOULD RELIEVE THIS WOMAN'S SUFFERING) AND SAID AUTHORITATIVELY, "I KNOW THAT SARAH IS GOING TO SLEEP VERY VERY WELL TONIGHT" (AGAIN, IT WAS NOT SAID DIRECTLY TO HER). THEN SARAH SAID, "CAN ONE SESSION MAKE A DIFFERENCE?" ERICKSON REPLIED, "YOU

ONLY HAD TO BE BORN ONCE, DIDN'T YOU!" AND WITH THE CONFI-
DENCE BOTH IN HIMSELF AND THE OUTCOME, SHE FELT RELIEVED
AND DEPARTED.

I began to see that every time out of the starting gate Erickson would try to
attain a solution that very session! I learned that he had supreme confidence in
himself because of the painstaking details he took. I learned that if I paid my
dues by paying attention to "minimal cues" I, too, could significantly increase
my abilities to reach people successfully in much briefer periods of time.

Erickson never said anything to me "directly" (vs. indirect), but trusted my
own unconscious would come up with the answers I needed as a result of my
experience with the minimal cues he assessed when working with me. On one
occasion I said to him, "Dr. Erickson, your stories have pinpoint accuracy." He
said, "I'm just an old man who tells stories. It's your unconscious mind that has
the pinpoint accuracy!" The more I came to trust that statement was true and act
on it, the more it was true.

Then there was Walter Kempler. Most of the work I saw him do was with
couples and some with families. Watching him work reminded me of Zeus.
Kempler had an intensity, a fury, a passion, a correct sense of where the life force
was, and what other family members either did or needed to do to bring value to
another person's life, that was remarkable! He was ruthless. Where most thera-
pists would leave patients alone with what might be referred to as "belt line
respect," if Kempler felt one suffered from what he diagnosed as a "rotten per-
sonality disorder," he would work with a force that had one partner go for the
place in which both had destroyed the relationship and life. He would show the
person whom he assessed had the best chance of movement. "What the job was"
was to provide value to their partner's life in a way that their partner might at a
later time be able to provide value to his or her life (the person giving first).

The other unusual thing was that one had the impression that Kempler had a
taxicab meter. He would turn it on. He would charge a healthy fee, as he knew
his "one of a kind abilities" (even though psychologists and psychiatrists are not
supposed to think or say things like that), and he would stop two or three hours
later. You had probably spent $600 by then. However, when you were done, you
were done! You had a resolution!

So, in one three-hour session, major impact was made at the deepest levels of
life force! Perhaps, the very recalcitrant would go back for a second or third time,
with several weeks in between, but certainly no more frequently than that. So
the entire therapy was between two and nine hours and there was a resolution of
major import each time he worked.

An example: I was in a weekend couples workshop where Kempler was the
leader. There was a 270-pound physician whose life, weight, and life force were
out of control. I knew he had had excellent psychotherapy training and personal
growth work over a period of years without touching his basic self-destructive
pathology. He came to the couples workshop with a thin woman with whom he
had a serious relationship that had hit an impasse. Kempler started off the work-

shop by looking at her, and with the intensity of Attila the Hun, saying, "It's your job to stop him!" It appeared that most of the people in the group didn't understand what Kempler meant, but the woman did. When he felt someone's life force was at stake he did not concern himself with how what he did was perceived by others. He only concerned himself with making the impact required to save life!

Part of the kind of problem in today's vast psycholitigation world is that therapists have become too timid and too frightened of being misperceived by patients who will sue them; and thus, they don't go for the home run ball in terms of making the greatest impact in saving lives or enhancing life force. We as a society have psycholitigated professional impotence, except for a very few that are willing to consider the theme of psychotherapy as a revolution. Wilhelm Reich said, "If you can't do politics, you can't do psychoanalysis," and as a whole it appears we may have lost the battle of doing potent therapy.

The woman Kempler was working with said, in a way that surprised me in strength as she looked like a weak mousy type, but was challenging Kempler with equal intensity, "Every time he goes near the refrigerator I tell him to stop!" Not missing a beat Kempler came right back, "You don't need to say anything to him! You only make him feel guilty! Just smash the food all over his clothes! That will stop him!"

Without ever using these words in his teaching I deduced, "Oh, so that is what EFFECTIVE ACTION is with character disordered people." With such people words or more normal therapies I have found to be nearly a total waste of time.

Perhaps the thing I liked best about Kempler was his fire in contrast to a profession of colleagues I for the most part experienced as placid and timid by comparison, and certainly nowhere near as impactful in such a short time, or even a long time.

From Kempler's writing (Kempler, 1973) I have selected some quotes I think are most applicable to a brief therapy that is to reach patients at a deep level.

> The task of therapy is to arouse (remind) forgotten desires; to fire up abandoned conflict, and to keep all combatants at the front until everyone wins. In the wake of such victories, new and old struggles will awaken and be guided similarly. When the family catches on to the therapeutic process, therapy is ended. (p. 70)

> Regardless of the number of family members and irrespective of the many things happening at once, the therapist, with himself as the starting point, selects as the other point the greatest obstacle to resolving that current conflict, and engages it. If he can't find it, his own lostness becomes the other point for a brief engagement, either alone or with the help of the family. (p. 70)

> Such changes are not easily achieved. One must go through the rigors of hell each revealing inch of the way, experiencing the loss of treasured traits and valued virtues as though it were death itself. There are no volunteers. Everyone who goes is forced, either by an already existing unbearable pain inside himself, or by family, i.e., a significant other with whom he cannot live and cannot live-without. And, as a rule, without a family to inspire the task, unbearable pain within is dealt with largely by denial, desensitization, and social achievement. (p. 78)

While describing one of my cases, Kempler once severely chastised me for "not curing the patient in one session!" Actually, I had neither the thought nor knew I had the capacity to do so until he mentioned it. He saw, and approached me with a fury for denying that ability in myself.

And then there is Carl Whitaker, a strange and gifted bird indeed. I remember the first time I heard him speak to a group of 700-plus psychiatrists, psychologists, and social workers in Los Angeles. He began by telling a story about a father and his son. The story went like this: "Dad, I'm going over the hill to get me a wife. . . . Good, Son, when will you be back? . . . A couple of days, Dad. . . . Good, Son, I'll look forward to seeing you then." The son comes back in a couple of days. The father says, "Well, where is she, Son? . . . The son says, "Dad, I found her but she was a virgin." The father says, "Son, you did the right thing. If she's not good enough for her own family she is not good enough for us." About 700 therapists were left there with their mouths hanging open in total shock, as this was out of their "left brain" way of viewing things and the world.

Whitaker refers to what he does as "Experiential-Symbolic Family Therapy." He rarely if ever explains anything in a left brain ordinary conversational English way of rational thinking and speaking. He, and I too, find such banter to be not very effective and worst of all boring to the interpreter, making psychotherapy a joyless venture. The fun of it is when you pick up the craziness of the patient or family, and you put it back to them while responding from your own unconscious with the craziness projected. It can be new and refreshing to the therapist. In this way the therapist can provide an enlivened experience and stay fresh. It must be remembered that if the therapist dies in session through the illusion of safety, so does the patient. Whitaker has done more than most in giving us an example of having the courage to work with chaos and anxiety in the midst of professional litigators of today.

The goal of this experiential-symbolic way of working, which certainly has an existential flavor, is to create more chaos and anxiety in the patient's guts than they came in with. It is opening up the space and forcing the patient to tolerate this chaos and anxiety. It is forcing them to deal with the absurdity and craziness of what they do and what they project that is curative! This therapeutic use of the unexpected permits having greater individual freedom and a capacity to live more freely in a family. All members of the family can come to "normalize" what was previously thought to be taboo and abnormal.

Whether it was Erickson telling Sarah she had very kissable lips, or Whitaker "invading the unconscious" with his story that helps normal humans get in touch with their own incestual fantasies, having and taking the therapeutic freedom to fully respond to patients is critical to having the greatest opportunity to move them and to create an "existential shift." Yet, each of those comments could be misunderstood by a literal patient and a literal investigator of the attorney general's office who has not been trained in knowing about such methods, and might very well consider the psychotherapist to be in violation of the community standards of practice, as well as committing gross negligence with possible overtones of sexual enticement. Yet, these comments by Erickson and Whitaker clearly were not that.

I picked the Whitaker example to demonstrate another outrageous example, because what I am proposing is a brief therapy treatment modality I know to be highly effective and highly charged, making lasting impact which patients can benefit from. In fact, I do not see contraindications. *Over the years I have found patients are more resilient than therapists give them credit for.* What I have found is that if patients feel a particular interpretation is useless to them or untimely they hardly make anything of it and tend to dismiss it. This means that nearly all patients have the possibility of benefiting from this brief and forced psychotherapy at an in-depth level that deals with both the conscious and unconscious. It means that very few, if any, will be or can be injured by the impactful "invasion of the unconscious" in a way that puts the patient's own madness back to them so the possibility of rapid therapeutic movement always exists.

However, let me make a very significant point so therapists do not commit professional suicide while "invading the unconscious" or engaging in "ruthless behavior intervention." Both Erickson and Whitaker had a way of utilizing the patient's anger against them to evoke and create therapeutic movement. This was a way to gain effective change with rebellious, paranoid, and sometimes paranoid schizophrenic patients, or those who had those tendencies. The problem was that the patients would be angry at Whitaker and Erickson, and would remain angry at them throughout their lives. This was an accepted price the doctor paid for healing his patient. The problem in today's day and age is the environment now encourages the poor little dear or so-called victim of such invasion of the unconscious or ruthless behavioral intervention to go to Boards of Medical Quality Assurance and Boards of Psychology with complaints where the therapist could easily appear "crazy." This could easily cost $150,000 for the therapist to fight out of pocket. Thus, we have a society that says it demands excellence while it ensures impotence in the professionals it hires.

In the therapies done and shown to me by Whitaker, Erickson, and Kempler, there was no or little emphasis or necessity for dealing with the transference or working through of a relationship as is customarily thought about in long-term psychotherapy or psychoanalysis. It was not a concern of Erickson, Whitaker, or Kempler. Erickson said in two of the training sessions I attended, "I like to see patients for awhile, then I like to get rid of them. Then I like them to refer me new patients." At one time when he thought I was settling in to a long-term psychotherapy relationship with him, he began the training session by looking around at all of us and saying, "You wouldn't believe all these psychiatrists and psychologists I see! They all have amnesia!" One sort of had the feeling he was saying, "Look, I gave it to you the first time, and I gave it to you the second time, and if you don't get it by the third time, you're a dope and I am wasting my time and yours by falsely thinking you would get it the fourth time."

When I asked Carl Whitaker why he didn't do long-term psychotherapy or never got trained to do psychoanalysis, he said, "I would rather be a carpenter or a plumber." I suppose given Whitaker's view of things he trained me a relatively long time—52 weeks, 26 of which he did three-generational family therapy with my own family as one would have in a training analysis, while also supervising my work with one family for 26 weeks and one for 52 weeks. However, when I asked him over his career what the average number of sessions was for seeing patients or families he said "three."

When discussing psychotherapy with Jim Simkin, now deceased but second to Fritz Perls in the gestalt movement, the topic of unconditional positive regard and Carl Rogers was posed. Jim said he thought one of the worst things a therapist could do was provide "unconditional positive disregard." In other words, if you don't have the courage as a therapist to make impact, to go for the bottom line, you are disrespectful of peoples' life force, and that is the worst thing a therapist can do. Jim also had the capacity to move peoples' lives in one session. In one of his workshops in Big Sur there was a man threatening suicide. I do not know what was going through Simkin's mind, if he thought the man was on the level or manipulating the group. With the ferocious intensity of a bulldog, he motioned with his finger for the man to leave the group and follow him to the outside backyard. There was a good one-hundred foot drop onto jagged rocks. Simkin looked at him, pointed down to the jagged rocks and said in a very challenging way, "If you are really intent on killing yourself I have a hundred and sixty-one ways to see that you succeed!" The man went back to the group and told the group that he thought Simkin was a madman and that he scared the hell out of him." There was never any mention of suicide again.

LET ME CAUTION PSYCHOTHERAPISTS INTERESTED IN DOING THIS KIND OF WORK!

1. Start to take risks slowly, until you get confidence that you have the capacity to take the next step if things appear to go off in a direction you did not expect as a result of your intervention.

2. Make certain you know yourself well enough to know that you are a person of sufficient depth to reach and contact the deepest levels of your patients so that even if their conscious minds are homicidal toward you, at the deepest unconscious level they know you have supported their life force, even if they are angry with you.

3. When using the metaphorical experiential symbolic primitive language of a Whitaker, which may make patients very angry because it confronts them with their own homicidal, suicidal, and incestual primitive ways of being, then you need to expect certain things. You can expect that such interventions will evoke chaos and anxiety in the patient or the family and that it may very well create rapid movement; however, beware: most of the psycholegal trouble may come from those who are so literal they will intentionally misinterpret what they do not understand as a justification to persecute the therapist.

4. As a good safeguard use a letter of acknowledgement right in the first session, something to the effect that the patient knows and understands that you will utilize therapeutic *interventions that sound irrational and crazy* as a means of therapeutic treatment, but are meant to deal with those parts of themselves they present to you that can most effectively be changed by these methods. They realize they may have little conscious and rational understanding of what you are doing, and that such understanding is not necessary to the success of the treatment and in fact is not even expected. Have them sign the agreement, giving the psychotherapist more freedom to operate and to function.

5. In a recent workshop I attended given by Carl Whitaker, after he read this paper, he worked with the group on the appropriate paranoia a therapist should have on the first phone call when talking with a patient. He made it pretty clear it would not be that easy to get in to see him, that there were a number of patients he had lost, that he did not want any more spilled blood, and that they better give him the minimum conditions he required in order to work with them. He made it clear to them and the group he really did not want or need another patient, and that those who put that first put themselves in grave danger of taking the litigator on as a patient, thereby running the risk of professional ruination for a few bucks.

Erickson is often quoted as saying, "Into every person's life should come a little confusion and a little enlightenment."

12301 Wilshire Blvd.
Suite 300
Los Angeles, CA 90025

REFERENCES

Haley, J. (1973). *Uncommon therapy: The psychiatric techniques of Milton H. Erickson, M.D.* New York: W. W. Norton.
Kempler, W. (1973). *Principles of gestalt family therapy: A gestalt-experiential handbook.* Oslo, Norway: A.s Joh. Nordahls Trykkeri.

The Board of Psychology (State of California)'s Decision to do Away with The Oral Part of the Exam for Psychology Licensure: A Dissenting Opinion

— Leo Bergantino

Psychology has moved from a profession of personal growth on the part of the clinician, which could be put into one's private practice on Monday morning, to one of legal deadness. It is now a care and caution that make the fullness of being of the clinician in enhancing the patient's ability to become, a legal impossibility. The nonclinicians who run Boards of Psychology and state Psychological Associations and psychologists themselves have capitulated in their own castration. Now there isn't even a penis left to envy in the practice of psychology. I have seen the death of a profession I once loved and now have nothing in common with.

I think the State of California Board of Psychology's decision to do away with the oral examination is wrong on several counts:

1) It shows extreme cowardice on their parts when they have put each and every psychologist (admittedly with their own complicity in the project) at risk since the mid-1980s.

2) Having an oral examination is the only way to get a fair look at an examinee's clinical abilities.

3) Even if the Board of Psychology is sued by a disgruntled person who flunks the oral examination, the Board would probably win. (Dr. Steven Frankel in his course on law and ethics describes Board of Psychology bulldozing tactics as not having to adhere to law at all.)

4) The written examination has no validity for evaluating actual clinical practice. It primarily measures the ability to pass that kind of test and knowledge of some academic content of psychology.

The Board of Psychology's actions, along with lawyers looking for a new field in which to make money, and with the complicity of psychologists whose clinical acumen and lack of courage are suspect, have decimated the private practice of clinical psychology. Because practitioners can no longer be on the cutting edge of clinical practices nor have an interest in developing that ability, the profession has become one in which those kinds of services can no longer be rendered to patients and therefore clinicians with courage can no longer function nor make a good living doing so.

Psychologists continue to publish articles about new areas which they will not be able to practice, nor make a dime on. They go to continuing education classes (36 units a year) like good students and take courses of no use to private practice or to making a living. Many psychologists are making $75 an hour, which I made in 1975 and they are happy to get it. I write this because there has been a great deal about hard times and psychologists not being able to make money. But if you can offer quality of service and a quality of response, you can make money. For all intents and purposes, the Board of Psychology and the psycholegal system have made quality verboten!

...en that the California Board ...s participated in the death of psychology and asked psychologists to bear the brunt of fear by which they continue to castrate themselves, it is now a "totally bad faith decision" to do away with an oral examination. It is the only way one can determine if someone has any clinical abilities whatever. The decision deals a final blow to a profession that will attempt to sell the words *clinical psychologist* to the public when all they have are people who are able to pass academic examinations.

Wilfred Bion, the great British psychoanalyst, once said: "The entire psychoanalytic library is good for about the first hour and one half of an analysis. After that you have to know what to say to the patient." The Board's decision to do away with the oral examination will ensure that psychologists are no longer able to determine firsthand who knows what to say to a patient.

Their fear is unfounded in the following respects:

1) They actually do hold clout over the way administrative law is set up.

2) If three independent clinicians meet with an examinee and two flunk him, even if there are countertransference difficulties that preclude a purely objective examination, there is still the rule-of-thumb presumption that if someone doesn't pass the smell test of two out of three, then they ought to get some help, try again, or perhaps go into administration.

3) Written tests measure the ability to take tests and to go to school. (Dr. William B. Michael, USC Professor of Statistics, and writer of SAT and GRE exams, has stated emphatically that the tests don't even measure academic ability but only the ability to take those exams.)

4) There is the "halo effect" regarding graduate school clinical supervisors' recommendations, which says: "You are my supervisee. I have chosen you. Therefore you are worthy."

5) Tuition paid by students may make the university or professional school reluctant to judge a student as not having clinical skills when they may have good grades. But they have decided anyway to try to save themselves a few lawsuits by basing licensure upon an examination that does not look at the ability to do clinical work.

CLINICAL INTERVIEW EXAMPLE

Twenty-eight years ago, I worked as a clinical psychologist in a community mental health center in South Central Los Angeles, which was predominantly African American. An African American psychiatrist and an African American social worker had already interviewed a prospective Caucasian psychologist for a position and wanted to hire him.

He had a resume about twelve pages long, which stated that he had a law degree from the University of Michigan, a degree in clinical psychology, a great number of publications, etc.

My primary interest was how he would survive with the street population he would serve. Did he know what to say? Would he know what to do clinically? He came in and said to me, "Do you want to ask me about my resume?" I said, "I can read." He said, "Well, what do you want to ask me?" I said, "Nothing." His anxiety continued to rise. Then he said, "You have to ask me about my resume." I said, "No, I don't." He said, "Well, what are you going to ask me about then?" I said, "Nothing, all I'm interested in is what you have to say to patients, and what you do with them, and so far you haven't showed me shit!"

While this was confrontive, and may even seem harsh, it gives the fellow a chance to show me anything if he has anything to show, and believe me the patients attempted to rough me up a lot worse than that. He said, "I am going to get Dr. _______ (the psychiatrist)." I said, "If you need help with the interview, I strongly urge you to get him!" The man ran out of the office. And he did not come back with the psychiatrist. That told me he would not know what to say to clients in this neighborhood, nor what to do with them. If I was asked, he was clinically a "no-hire." I could not have known this from reading anything he submitted. It took a clinical interview.

After lunch, the psychiatrist said, "What did you do to Dr. _______, you really freaked him out?" I told him exactly what I said, and he said to me, "If you said and did that to me, I would have hit you in the head with a two by four." And I said, "If you had hit me in the head with a two by four, I would have hired you!"

He hired the man, and I soon after went into private practice. One day I read in the *Los Angeles Times* that that Community Mental Health Clinic was on probation and being fined by the State of California for hiring and having in their employment a fraudulent man who had never had any schooling or training in clinical psychology, law, or anything else for that matter.

Now that happened when the clinical exam was still in!

*LEN BERGANTINO, ED.D., ABPP, retired from the private practice of clinical psychology after 30 years. He has authored 75 publications and the book **Psychotherapy, Insight and Style: The Existential Moment** (Boston: Allyn & Bacon, 1983). He gave workshops at the international level, the focus being "Keeping the Space Open While Doing Therapy So That Experience Is Not Destroyed By Education." Three major influences were the training he received from Milton Erickson, M.D., Carl Whitaker, M.D., and his exposure to Wilfred Bion, M.R.C.S. and his analysands who trained him in Bion's methods.*

> The entire psychoanalytic library is good for about the first hour and one half of an analysis. After that you have to know what to say to the patient.
>
> — Wilfred Bion (1897–1979)

Len Bergantino

Invading the Unconscious With the Patient's Own Craziness to Create "Existential Shifts"

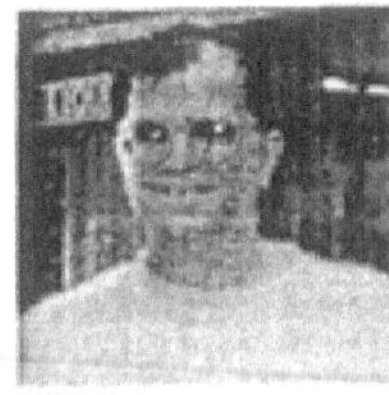

Len Bergantino, Ed.D., ABPP is in the private practice of Clinical Psychology in West Los Angeles. His book, *Psychotherapy Insight and Style: The Existential Moment* has been chosen among hundreds to be re-published in the Master Classic Series by Jason Aronson Publishers of Northvale, New Jersey, under a new title, *Making An Impact in Therapy: How Master Clinicians Intervene*. He has trained psychotherapists and family therapists internationally. At this time in his professional life, he enjoys doing family therapy and psychotherapy by invading the unconscious with the patient's own craziness to create existential shifts. Further, he is engaged in forensic consultation and expert testimony in the diagnosis and recommendations for cessation of "parental alienation syndrome", the virtual extermination by one parent and an unwitting court system of the other parent from the children's lives. He was trained by Carl Whitaker, M.D. and Milton Erickson, M.D.

Three master clinicians have trained me in terms of making an impact in psychotherapy and family therapy by "doing it to patients" much as a zen master would do. There is no value given to patient awareness, patient insight, or understanding of the process by the patient. In this way the results of the therapy cannot be destroyed by education. These master clinicians who trained me were Milton Erickson, now deceased; Carl Whitaker, who has recently suffered a serious stroke; and Walter Kempler, who retired recently. Thus, in the spirit of Bruno Bettelheim, when asked in 1983 why he wrote *Freud and Man's Soul* said, "Because I am the only one left who could do it!" I have written this article to illustrate working at a level Milton Erickson referred to as Occam's Razor—"Multiplicity ought not be posited without necessity."

When Erickson, Whitaker and Kempler trained me they didn't explain much of anything. Everything was an experience so I actually had the chance to learn to do what I was being shown because it was done to me. Of all that I learned, what I enjoy most is "invading the unconscious with the patient's or family's own craziness to create *existential shifts*."

However, if I were to explain what I did and why I did it, the flavor of giving you the kind of experience I had in learning would significantly be diminished by what Wilfred Bion, the great British psychoanalyst, might refer to as the destruction of experience and learning through knowledge by a saturation of the space. And of course one should realize when having had a week's workshop with Jim Simkin, who was like a bulldog at your pant leg with his tenacity, that one could never again make the mistake of working with "unconditional positive disregard!"

When discussing the kinds of interventions therapists made, Simkin was telling me of Rogerian kinds of responses where the therapist's own reaction to the client, if it were negative, would not be shared. Simkin referred to what was known as "unconditional positive regard" as really being "unconditional positive disregard" in that the therapist's self was missing from the response. Thus, I have attempted to write a psychotherapy article much as Mickey Spillane might have written about Mike Hammer.

THE PATIENT CALLED

I hadn't seen Joey in ten years. He called very disturbed and said he had an urgent situation; his sister had been alcoholic for twenty years and when her husband recently left her, she tried to kill herself. I said, "Come in at 3 p.m." He said, "that will be fine."

We were glad to see each other with a feeling of affection after all these years. He began by sounding guilty. I let it pass for the moment. He said, "My sister tried to kill herself three times." I said, "How come she is so incompetent!" He said, "she was smarter than anyone back on the East Coast. They put her in a hospital with 24 hour security and she walked out. She was pissed because they didn't have a mirror where she could put her makeup on." I said, "I guess she wanted to look good in the coffin." There was a long pause. I said, "what the hell are you guilty about?" He said, "I left her and I left my family twenty years ago." I said, "you said that the last time I saw you, and you're still guilty?" I paused, then asked, "are you still a lawyer?" He said, "I am in another kind of business." I said, "no wonder she is pissed at you. She had all the brains and you went to law school!" He said, "you haven't gotten any nicer." I said, "Thank you. Coming from you that's a compliment!"

He gave me a reasonable sounding diagnosis a psychologist who was a self respecting lawyer with a criminal's mind might have given. He then went on to expound and even pontificate about what he should tell her about taking responsibility for herself. It was all too pat.

I told him a story about Sal Maglie, the ex-Giant-Dodger great, and Jim Bouton, the ex-Yankee pitcher when Bouton was all washed up and pitching for Seattle in the minor league. I said, "Bouton had the bases loaded and nobody out. Sal Maglie came to the mound." Sal said, "Jim, I want you to throw him two high hard ones on the inside corner and then hook him low and away on the outside corner." Jim looked at Sal and said, "Sal, if I could do that, what the hell would I need you for?" (A question all therapists ought to ask themselves.)

The patient told me, "Her two sons moved out here and my wife hates my sister." Remembering his wife, I knew full well what hatred was and thought for an instant, against my better judgement, that making an offer to have her in family therapy was the coefficient of adversity beyond which I dare not tread. I thought, "maybe he'll leave now." He went on by saying in reference to his sister, "Her husband had left her but was too much a gentleman to just walk away." I thought, but didn't say, "Maybe he has the same wish for me." He said, "my sister described her husband as a nice man who was always helpful and thought the world of her without ever raising his voice. He just got his own apartment but was too much a gentleman to just walk away from her." (The second time he said the same thing.) I said, "what she meant was that his pastime was letting her cut off his penis and he was useless to her." (If someone is in a relationship he or she can either bring value to the other person's life or he or she cannot!)

He then talked about his mother coming out here from New York to visit, staying two months and now deciding to move out here. I said, (thinking of the mirror and the makeup story,) ")Mirror mirror on the wall, who is the fairest child of all?"

I said, "look, I don't know what is going on with them and your sister but I am pretty confident in my own responses. If you want to have coast-to-coast sessions with them I am willing to do that." He thought it was a good idea (working by conference call. Carl Whitaker, M.D., trained me to do that kind of work three generational.) I said, "let me see, who are the players?" He said, "I don't know about her husband." I said, "I don't trust you. I want him in just because you don't. I'll teach him to put his penis back on! No wonder your ex-wife wants to kill your sister (he is still married but emotionally I sensed he was married to his sister); you're married to your sister!" I said, "get your sister, her daughter and her husband who moved out back there; bring your mother, yourself, your wife, and her (his sister's) two sons out here.

I looked at my watch. A fifty minute session had been scheduled. 35 minutes had gone by since he walked in. I said, "we're done." In full acknowledgement that the existential facts had been dealt with, he said, "we're done." I said, "you must trust me a lot." He said, "you did it last time!" He hugged me with a sigh of relief. He said, "how much do I owe you? What's your current fare?" I said, "it's $200 for 50 minutes."

I heard from him about a week and a half later. He called to tell me the check had been returned in that he must have written the wrong address. He mailed it back to me and somehow he had written the correct address and it had been returned to him with a "return to sender" stamped on it. It then hit me that he made the check out for $200. I called him back and said, "I am returning the check. Scale it down to 35 minutes and make it $140." He said, "My sister's in an alcohol rehab unit back there. The whole family is doing better as a result of what you did with me. I feel much better. I thought it was worth $200! Keep it!" I said, "I thought so, too! You got my best shot!"

CONCLUSION

To do this kind of work you must do what Bion recommended: abandon memory and desire. If you have any agenda for the patient or family and do not trust your unconscious, your countertransference will interfere with the work.

1215 Brockton Ave., Ste. 104
Los Angeles, CA 90025

Ad in Natural Psychologist
2013

12

The Therapist Is Alive and Well: The Existential-Experiential Therapy Style of Carl Whitaker, M.D.

DR. WHITAKER TEACHES and practices an existential-experiential brand of family therapy. He has written several major books and numerous articles on the family, and is editor of *Psychotherapy of Chronic Schizophrenia* as well as co-author of *The Family Crucible*, with Dr. Augustus Napier, and *The Roots of Psychotherapy*, with Dr. Thomas Malone. Dr. Whitaker is professor of Psychiatry at the University of Wisconsin Medical School.

The basis of this chapter was derived from my participation in "Family Therapy–Process and Techniques," a program sponsored by Professional Seminars in Los Angeles in December, 1979. Dr. Whitaker presented the program for two days. While I had no personal therapeutic experience or training with Dr. Whitaker, I so enjoyed his unique style of doing therapy that I felt it was a must for a book dealing with therapeutic style. While Dr. Whitaker specializes in family therapy it is not the purpose of this chapter to focus on his way of doing family therapy (as that would be much too ambitious a task). The purpose is to present Dr. Whitaker's style and discuss some of its components.

In his therapy, Dr. Whitaker's unusual viewpoints were very effective, as well as humorous. He would nearly always maintain a straight face despite the fact that his primary process responses were often so unexpected to patients that when observing, Whitaker's responses often seemed hilarious. Patients felt they just didn't know what to do with him. He didn't quite fit into their customary view of the world. It is the absurdity of his nonconformity that is the impetus to help the family change.

Dr. Whitaker continually talked of how important it is for the therapist to win the battle, and to keep winning the battles; that is, for control of the process. This is not to be mistaken as meaning control over the people in the family process.

In maintaining control over the battle, the integrity of the therapist is the critical issue. Dr. Whitaker maintains this integrity by acknowledging his own wants and needs in terms of structuring a situation so that he does not get trapped into the pathology of the family. If they don't accept his demands, "You hold them responsible for the imminent failure."

The maintenance of this integrity gives him the opportunity to be the "coach." While coaching he tells the family that he needs all members present because he can't coach a team without a first baseman, or a pitcher, or a short-stop. He has a "just-folks" way of talking to people, and feels that it is particularly important to relate the situation to your own life. "If you want to work with a Wisconsin dairy farmer, get yourself some cows."

He describes his method as being an endless series of doubts that he presents to the family. It then becomes their task to prove otherwise, if they want to change the family for the better. As coach, however, Dr. Whitaker does make it clear what he thinks would be useful and structures the situation so that it will work.

Dr. Whitaker feels that his primary motivation for doing therapy is that he gets to enjoy the "fun of being crazy–going wild–way out."

The following are short segments of dialogue between Dr. Whitaker and his clients.

Scene 1: Dr. Whitaker has just brought another psychiatrist–a resident–into the session with him. He says he often does this if he has any sense of being trapped or confused during the first interview.

Patient	What do you need this other guy for?
Whitaker	(In a very dry tone with the impression of a chuckle behind the straight face all throughout the work) He's going to help me out.
Patient	I came here to see you!
Whitaker	Yes. Yes.
Patient	I didn't want to see him.
Whitaker	Sorry about that.
Patient	We don't think he ought to be here.
Whitaker	Well, I'm sorry about that, too.
Patient	I think we should take him away.
Whitaker	I appreciate your opinion.
Patient	Well, you aren't going to send him away?
Whitaker	No.
Patient	I don't want him here.
Whitaker	Sorry about that. What do you want to do?
Patient	What do you mean?
Whitaker	Well, you're free to leave. As a matter of fact, if you want to leave I won't charge you. But if you come back again I will charge you for this one, too.

Whitaker sets the structure and even intimidates patients a bit with his comment about fees. By the way he made the last statement, the total burden of responsibility moves to the patients for staying or leaving. He feels winning the *first battle* is critically important, as this sets the tone; "We go round and round, but I always win the political struggle."

Scene 2: A child responds with "I don't know" to questions about the family.

Whitaker	What does your family look like?
Child	I don't know.
Whitaker	If I asked you to describe the Green Bay Packers you would tell me what they look like. Why can't you tell me what your family looks like?

Such a response points out the absurdity of the child's response in a playful way. Whitaker feels that patients may not get answers to the questions, but they do get the questions. Those questions themselves are effective enough.

Scene 3: Dr. Whitaker talks to an eight-year old in the family.

Whitaker	Your parents don't know anything about it. Your big brother doesn't know anything about it. Your big sister doesn't know anything about it, but she thinks they are friendly. What's going on?
8-Year Old	Dad and mother always fight.
Whitaker	When they fight, do they enjoy themselves?

Whitaker implants a new idea into the family–that mom and dad can fight and enjoy themselves, or that such an occurrence might even be a healthy part of family life.

8-Year Old	No, no.

Whitaker   Do they cry?

8-Year Old   Yes, yes.

Whitaker   Who cries?

8-Year Old   Well, mostly Mom.

Whitaker   Do you think Dad cries, but he doesn't let the tears fall?

Here Whitaker acknowledges the father's pain, even though the father may have been denying the pain to himself. Again, there is a tremendous advantage to confronting members of the family indirectly by talking with a child, who reacts honestly. In this way, the family's problems are confronted and are more difficult to resist. After all, Whitaker isn't talking to them. He is talking to the eight-year old.

8-Year Old   Yes. Yes.

Whitaker   What do you do?

8-Year Old   I go up to my room.

Whitaker   Oh, that's terrible.

8-Year Old   Why?

Whitaker   Well, you ought to stay down and cheer for the winner or at least encourage the loser. But you shouldn't back out of there twice because they are your parents. They need you.

Here Whitaker is telling the eight-year old that he ought not to back out, but should play and kid with his parents. He is structuring a situation so the boy will have other options than going up to his room and learning to be terrified of conflict–a problem he might then project onto his own family when he becomes an adult.

8-Year Old   I'm afraid they will both get mad at me.

Whitaker   If they do, tell them I told you to do it. They
                    shouldn't get mad at you. They need you to be the
                    referee and be the audience.

Whitaker backs out and moves into the family and is teaching the eight-year old to do the same thing.

Scene 4: Whitaker asks a man to bring both his parents and his in-laws to a session. There is a political battle for control in structuring a situation.

Patient   You want my in-laws here and my parents too?

Whitaker   Yes.

Patient   They haven't spoken to each other in ten years!

Whitaker   Yes. Just bring them in together and they can turn
                    the chairs around so they don't have to look at each
                    other.

This is a delightful way to structure the absurdity of the in-laws' relationship to the patients. Here Whitaker emphasizes that he structured the situation in a way he felt would make it work, but if his suggestion wasn't taken, he would hold the patients responsible for the imminent failure.

Whitaker   If you don't have your parents and in-laws here, I'm
                    sure I am not going to be as much help to you as
                    if they were here. If you are not desperate enough,
                    maybe it's a waste of your time and mine. And not
                    only that, but I don't want to get stuck with saying
                    grace over one more failure. You know, I've bled
                    so much with other people that I'm very sensitive
                    about getting myself in a corner.

His perpetual doubting and concern over the eventual failure of the treatment if his suggestions are not taken puts all the burden on the family–and keeps Whitaker from being sucked under.

Scene 5: The patient isn't really involved in taking responsibility for the therapy.

Whitaker	I'm worried.
Patient	About what?
Whitaker	Well, I don't know if I should stay in academia, or if I should retire. Perhaps I should do private practice, but then again academia is pretty interesting . . .
Patient	Hey, wait a minute! This is my time!

Whitaker's comment forces the patient to assume responsibility. Movement begins to take place in the therapy.

Whitaker's objectives are to force people out of their standard way of looking at life. He helps them be intuitive. He says, "Sometimes it's remarkable what you can do if you don't find yourself restricted by the professional thing or the social thing you have been brought up in." He describes the therapist's task as *How to be free to go where you happen to be*, which is basically what my book is all about, and is the basis for creating an environment in which existential moments will occur.

Scene 6: A patient questions Whitaker about his motivations for doing therapy with him. Patients often test to see if they can trust a therapist.

Whitaker	I do therapy in the hopes that we can make it. Then I get some more for me.
Patient	What do you mean, more for you? (The implication–during my therapy time!!)
Whitaker	I mean, get to be more of who I am and I am going to use you in that process. If we make it, I'll get

some more of me and you'll get some more of you. If we don't make it, we'll both lose.

Whitaker says his style starts out sounding cruel, but ends up being honest and very caring. This is the paradoxical nature of caring. Genuine caring isn't always what it appears to be. Whitaker talked about the difference between making believe and making believe that you're going to play straight. "Patients can see through us more than we can see through them. It's ridiculous to pretend you can handle families technically. You are stuck with the fact that you will be up to your ears in your own guts." He then suggested therapists better find a way to protect themselves and recommended a professional cuddle group composed of colleagues.

Scene 7: Whitaker describes a session in which he was sure the patient wanted to kill him halfway through the session. He got up and hurried across the hall to get the help of his colleague at that time, Dr. John Warkentin.

Whitaker then took John and sat him down with the patient Whitaker feared and began to talk in front of both his patient and Dr. Warkentin.

Whitaker	I had a terrible experience. I was halfway through the session and I was sure the son of a bitch was going to kill me! That's why I came over to get you.
Warkentin	(Pausing for a moment, then talking to the patient) You know, sometimes I feel like killing the son of a bitch (referring to Whitaker) myself.

Warkentin's comment cleared the air. Whitaker said that he was later able to put together this fear of being killed with his own unconscious fear of suicide that he had not acknowledged. Whitaker feels that each of us has both suicidal and homicidal impulses that we usually keep under wraps, but that pop up in the most unexpected places.

Scene 8: Whitaker is approached by a patient who has had individual therapy, marital therapy, and family therapy, but still feels there is something missing.

Whitaker	I don't think I have super stuff like that. I don't think you are going to find more of you in me. You're going to have to find more of you all by yourself.
Patient	You mean you won't work with me.
Whitaker	No. I think you should rent a cabin up in the wilderness and stay there all by yourself for a month and find more of you.

Whitaker feels it is useful for family members to switch their roles. The young son can pretend he is the father, while the father, in a whining complaining voice may say, "You know I don't like peas and you gave me the middle of the beef and you know I don't like beef. And it isn't fair to give me potatoes like this. You know I can't eat potatoes." In this way parents and children realize they can step out of the roles that confine them.

Mock Family Interview

At this point several professionals in the seminar got together to form a mock family that Whitaker would do family therapy with. He stressed his telephone interviewing technique, saying he often spends ten minutes on the telephone before he sees a family.

In the simulated telephone conversation, the mother called and said she needed to take her son in for treatment. Whitaker asked her questions about her husband, and commented that she didn't treat him as if he counted. As the telephone conversation ended, Whitaker asked her to have her husband call him so he could get to understand her a little better.

The husband was an over-intellectualized type who was interested in impressing Whitaker.

Whitaker	What time is good for you?
Husband	Well, I'm terribly busy, but I can get away from three to seven on Mondays. It will have to be after my research work.

Whitaker

I could have time between 3 and 4 or 4 and 5 p.m. on January 4.

Husband

But our son might even get into more difficulty before that.

Whitaker

Maybe you could find someone who has time earlier.

Husband

OK, we'll take it.

Whitaker

I'll see you at 3 p.m., three weeks from now.

Actual Interview

Daughter

(About the son) He's always picking on me.

Whitaker

That's nice.

Daughter

(inaudible)

Whitaker

(Taking her by surprise while she is complaining about her brother) You sound like you are having a great time.

Daughter

You should live in our house.

Whitaker

You should live in your own house and I'll live in mine.

Father

(About son) I want him to make something of himself.

Whitaker

It feels like you're a brain who has never learned how to be a people and he is a people who has never learned how to be a brain. The two of you could make a people. Your son is trying to help you find some of the energy he has.

Here Whitaker points out the value of the identified patient within the family system–that the son is more of a healing agent than a problem to be cured.

Daughter   (Sing-song quality of her voice) I'm talking.

Whitaker   I thought you were singing a song. It sounded like a cover-up to make believe there is nothing going on in the family.

Whitaker dealt with their primal sexual feelings by commenting that perhaps the way to deal with this would be to have mommy and the son to live together in one apartment while daddy and daughter live together in another apartment. Once, when the son got very involved with the mother and the daughter tried to interfere, Whitaker asked her why she wanted to break up their orgasm, their fun. I thought this to be a shocking remark, but I tried it out when working with a couple in reference to the man's relationship with his daughter and the mother's interference. It hit home and they both acknowledged orgasm to be the issue.

Now that I have presented Whitaker's stylistic approach, I am going to briefly mention some of the principles and attitudes about families he feels are important.

1. Use your intuition, guts, and feeling responses.
2. The investment you put into other people is irrevocable. You can never get it back. (This implies, with intimates, that there is a lot invested that motivates marital partners and families to work at it.)
3. Two families who send out a scapegoat to reproduce themselves is a marriage. (This is an interesting way to think about how new marriages play out some old parental scripts.)
4. The difference between a schizophrenic and others is not craziness. It's stupidity. Accuse a schizophrenic of being different from Picasso because he is stupid.

Whitaker and Keith say, "Our verbal interview is designed to symbolically invade the family relationships using metaphor, teasing, humor, free association and fantasy, and confrontation to increase the confusion around the compromise character of the family's resolution of stress."[1] A metaphor, "You act like you are your mother's mother and that would make you your own grandmother,"[2] while being playful, is also intended to be challenging. Such an approach is intended to increase toleration of anxiety. There is also an increase in interpersonal stress. THE QUALITY OF WHITAKER'S RESPONSES IS "NOT BASED UPON INTELLECTUAL UNDERSTANDING BUT RATHER AN INTERACTIVE PROCESS, METAPHORICAL LANGUAGE AND PERSONAL INTERACTION."[3] When speaking of the effort to respond in ways that significantly increase anxiety in patients, Whitaker and Keith say, "The power to change anything in the family, whether schizophrenia, divorce or internecine fighting, requires a voltage amplification in the suprasystem."[4] This is quite different from a great deal of therapy that attempts to minimize anxiety. On the one hand it is important to reduce stress anxiety that accrues from self-torture, but on the other it is important to increase patients' tolerances for existential anxiety as a movement toward a fuller, more engaged way of living.

Metaphor is used to expand meaning and impact, and in a way that produces open or incomplete gestalts. Whether verbal or nonverbal, the use of metaphor makes it difficult for a patient to memorize a response and then dismiss it. The use of metaphors as incomplete gestalts makes for learning in addition to recognition. Also, it is felt that interpersonal experiences, preferably with significant others, make for the kind of learning experiences that are built into a patient's living as opposed to intellectual insights.

"Like humor, personal disclosure is used to increase the interpersonal focus, to shatter a gestalt which is becoming too set, never to diminish anxiety."[5]

Whitaker and Keith increase non-rational, free-associative, fantasy organized confronting or paradoxical responses as patients become more secure in handling such input.

> For example, "Dad, I don't think you have to worry about the family getting along so much better. It's not going to last anyway. They'll go back to isolating you and beating on mother by next week or at least the week after." Or, on another occasion, "Mother, I'm certainly

glad I'm not married to you the way you take off after your husband. I think I would run for the hills if you were my wife." Or, to one of the kids, "Hey, you know the way your father looks at you when he tells you to either clean up your room or he's going to paddle your behind, I would be tempted to head for San Francisco and probably get on drugs just to get back at them." Noting physical responses to interactions can be extremely powerful. "The way he glared at me just then gave me a prickly feeling in the back of my neck."[6]

Symptoms are viewed as efforts for growth. For example, a woman complained that her husband didn't love her, and that on one occasion he even threatened her with a gun. The response questioned her opinion based on the assumption that the husband would not want to kill her if he didn't love her.

Whitaker and Keith both feel that mid- or late-phase therapeutic responses should arise out of aliveness on the therapist's part, rather than out of a pre-planned agenda or some set decision-making at an intellectual level. It is such responses that result in existential moments.

As for the danger of using affect and intuitive response, Whitaker and Keith feel that it is important for therapists to learn how to become effective, not just safe. They use the analogy that while surgery is also a dangerous business it would be foolish to say that it should not be practiced. *Affect may be positive or negative, but emotional investment enables the kind of authenticity that makes an impact.*

Whitaker and Keith view the paradoxical nature of therapists as being paramount to the success of the therapy. These include such factors as the ability to combine being loving with being tough, craziness and structure, a willingness to not hang onto a patient and a willingness to be inconsistent. *Craziness is viewed as that creativity which is not locked into anything symbiotically, but is available to therapists as another part of their personalities.*

Whitaker switches from sane to crazy and back when working. He does this particularly when he feels defeated. In treating schizophrenia Whitaker states that if the therapist is sane, the patient will be crazy. But when the therapist is emotionally hooked in, or connected to the patient, the therapist can be crazy and allow the patient to be sane.

In this way the patient learns to be both sane and crazy, moment by moment. Instead of getting the family over its craziness, Whitaker works with the paradoxical belief that the therapist has to make it more crazy. It is this turning the tables on the patient that helps patients to expand their ways to relate.

Whitaker views psychopathic behavior as an avoidance of schizophrenia. He feels they look for more love than mother was able to give them at one and one-half years old. Psychotherapy is almost impossible, but what is needed is a father who holds them against the breast. Psychopaths have no touch of intimacy. They talk primary process babble trying to find mother's love out in the world. Bad poison milk is a decision. They manipulate the world into loving them as opposed to being in the here and now.

Whitaker is truly existential in that he tries never to take initiative for accomplishing something. He has no advice for how people ought to be. He offers options, but he doesn't make them orders. He suggests that therapists make all the demands they can think of before they take the job. That is where they win the battle.

In summary, I experienced Dr. Whitaker as having fire in him, being very clear with his own unconscious, generous with sharing his knowledge with other therapists, having a lot of heart in his relationships with his patients, working effectively on sex issues with patients, and, relating authentically, in a manner where there was no doubt that he was connected between his head and his guts–making him particularly effective when working at the primal level. From a critical point of view I would be hard pressed to find a weakness.

Above all, I found his moment-to-moment style to focus on the patient's responsible involvement. Even more, Whitaker shows people how to enjoy themselves while they are doing effective therapy. His therapy flows along, without any particular need on his part to wrap things up in a neat little package for the patient. He has a basic trust that the patient will be able to do that for him or herself.

Professional Exchange

A Little Bit of Outrageousness Goes a Long Way

By Len Bergantino, Ed. D. ABPP   American Board of Professional Psychology • Diplomate in Family Psychology

Upon physician referral, father telephoned. He said the entire family was upset because his youngest son would not report to his new job because he insisted his hair was too thin and too kinky. I told father that mother and older brother would have to come. He agreed.

Mother, father, and older brother sat down and younger brother plopped his chair right in the middle of the floor while emanating an emotional response of taking up all the space in the office.

"Move your chair out of the center" I said to him in an offhanded authoritarian manner. The tone of command, ordering him around, and not treating him with kid gloves, established my authority, and reframed him as someone who wasn't fragile. He moved and there was a feeling of relief in the family.

The older brother said he had been to a psychotherapist and he thought people of my profession were for the birds. I said, "I've often had the same thought myself. Obviously you are an intelligent man." He was off balance in that I had joined him and identified him as being an intelligent man because we had the same thought.

When patients are thrown off balance, there exists opportunities for life shifts to relieve the chaos of not knowing.

After speaking with all family members I told them that baby brother was trying to keep his older brother from withdrawing from the family and bring some heat to the family because there wasn't much there between the parents and they needed him to keep their marriage together. I told the younger brother that he was doing an ingenius thing to save the family and that every family needed a sacrificial lamb. It was obvious, I said, that he remain the problem to focus upon but that it was a shame he was practicing family therapy without a license and not being paid for it.

He looked all knowing. Even though he didn't say a word, his look was that of a paranoid sort who would never speak his thoughts or feelings. I told him he had a great deal of wisdom. He was taken off balance when I treated him as if he were all-knowing in that he did not know how I knew that, given he said nothing. When patients are thrown off balance, there exists opportunities for life shifts to relieve the chaos of not knowing.

When the family tried to persuade him that his hair was normal, and it was, he became more entrenched in his position.

Having established myself as an authority with an unusual but credible perspective, I then used this position. I told him, in an insulting way that had to be believed because of its impoliteness, that he had a lot more to worry about than his hair —namely,

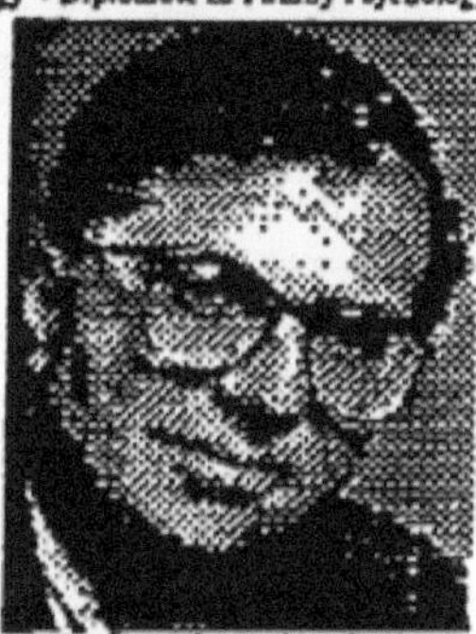

all that "baby fat" and the fact he shakes hands like a "wimp". I forcefully suggested he should join a gym, get rid of his baby fat, and he should develop a firm handshake and that these changes would solve his problem.

I shifted the ground or reframed the situation whereby the boy could utilize his own power in such a way that would get him out of the family enmeshment as much as all parties could tolerate, but with a solution he could work upon as opposed to one he could not—his kinky hair.

Two days later the family came back for a second session. They reported that the boy had joined a gym, begun to work out, and that he did report for work. The boy said he felt much more confident. When the family left, he looked me square in the eye and gave me a very firm handshake. All members of the family were pleased with the life shift.♥♥♥♥

♥♥♥♥♥♥♥♥♥

LEN BERGANTINO, Ed.D., ABPP
Doctorate-University of Southern California -1971
Diplomate in Family Psychology-American Board of Professional Psychology

Private Practice of Clinical Psychology
Specialty: Family Therapy

memo

California Association of Marriage and Family Therapists

To: Dr. Len Bergantino

From: Eileen Schuster

Date: April 29, 2019

Re: Permission to reprint

CAMFT hereby grants permission to Dr. Len Bergantino to reprint the article "A Little Bit of Outrageousness Goes a Long Way." Any reprint or reference of the article should cite its original publication in *The California Therapist,* a magazine of the California Association of Marriage and Family Therapist.

The article may be reprinted in the following works:

- The Art of Psychotherapy and the Liberation of the Therapist
- The Essence of Music
- A Handbook for Political Psychology

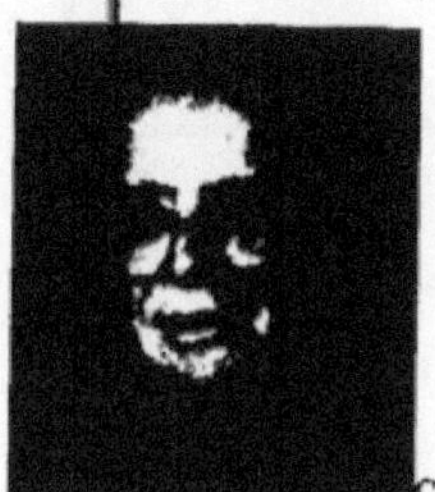

Carl A. Whitaker, M.D., was a pioneer in psychotherapy as well as family therapy. He co-authored the master classic, The Roots of Psychotherapy, with Thomas P. Malone, M.D., Ph.D. Whitaker's major contribution was freeing up the use of self to shoot from the hip concerning such unconscious materials as suicide, homicide, incest etc. that therapists and patients customarily do not deal with.

I first met him when he came to the Bonaventure Hotel in Los Angeles and presented to 700 licensed psychiatrists, psychologists and social workers. He began by telling a story about a farmer and his son:

Son: "Dad, I'm going over the hill and get me a wife!"

Father: "Good, son. How long will you be gone?"

Son: "A couple of days."

Father: "All right, son. I will see you when you get back."

Two days later the son came back.

Father: "Well, son, where is she?"

Son: "Well, dad, I found her but she was a virgin."

Father: "Son, you did the right thing. If she wasn't good enough for her own family, she isn't good enough for us!"

The 700 clinicians in the room were in disbelief.

Later, I went up to him and said, "Dr. Whitaker, I spent a week at the Atlanta Psychiatric Clinic getting to know Tom Malone but I never got a sense of his style of work. You were very good at demonstrating your style. I wonder if you could give me an example of how Tom Malone actually worked?"

Whitaker pensively looked up in the air for a moment and then said, "Tom Malone was catatonic, but you ought to look him up. I think he has something to offer you." He subsequently wrote the foreword to my book, Psychotherapy, Insight and Style: The Existential Moment. (Allen and Bacon Inc., Boston.

I next saw Whitaker at The Evolution of Psychotherapy Conference after Milton Erickson's death on March 8, 1980. He said he and Erickson met only once. Erickson picked him up at the airport when he was invited to be a guest speaker at Wayne State Hospital.

Erickson said, "How many kids you got?" Whitaker said, "I've got six." Erickson said, "I've got eight."

Whitaker said they never spoke another word to each other.

I asked Whitaker to supervise me and he agreed to do so by speakerphone, as he was at the University of Wisconsin Medical School and I was in Los Angeles. He kept throwing down the gauntlet, realizing I was dedicated. He kept saying, "How can I take you seriously that you want to learn family therapy when you don't have your own family in family therapy?"

So I mobilized my parents in Connecticut, my wife and her parents and her brother and his girlfriend with a speaker-phone in Los Angeles and Whitaker worked 26 weeks with all of us once a week by speakerphone coast to coast.

My parents had been considering moving to Los Angeles near me for years and brought it up in one session. Whitaker raised every fear they had not voiced:

"You have to be crazy to uproot at your ages and move close to that one-way son-of-a-bitch son of yours who is so involved in his practice that he will never make time to see you. You will be giving up all your life-time friends and family." And then, in the last seconds of the session, he said, "Take a chance," and hung up.

I did not think much about it, but I got a phone call from my father two days later, saying, "Len, your mother and I are moving to California. We will be there in two months."

So, Whitaker gave me something of value: my parents for the last few years of their lives.

The other thing I learned from him is that in doing family therapy it is imperative to have the battle for control right in the beginning and win it in terms of getting all the family members present, such as mother, father, children and grandparents on both sides and, where applicable, the lover of one or both spouses. A paranoid situation will be set up if you only bring one spouse in later.

Whitaker worked with me only long enough for me to set the dynamite necessary to get all family members involved. He refused to work with a family if only some were present. "I have enough blood spilled," he said. "I don't need another failure. I have already failed enough times. Are you sure you want to do this? I am not a good as you heard."

> Len Bergantino, Ed.D., Ph.D., is a licensed psychologist in California, Arizona and Hawaii with an ABPP diplomate in fam-ily psychology. He is the author of Psychotherapy, Insight and Style: The Existential Movement. He may be reached at Dr.LenBergantino@gmail.com or 310-207-9397.

ENDNOTES

[1] Carl A. Whitaker and Daniel Keith, "Symbolic-Experimental Family Therapy." in Handbook of Family Therapy Alan S. Gurman and David P. Kniskern, ed. (New York: Brunner/Mazel, 1980.

[2] Ibid., p. 28.

[3] Ibid., p. 35.

[4] Ibid., p. 40.

[5] Ibid., p. 49.

[6] Ibid., p. 50.

REFERENCES

Whitaker, Carl A., and Keith, Daniel. "Symbolic-Experimental Family Therapy." In *Handbook of Family Therapy*, Edited by Alan S. Gurman and David P. Kniskern, New York: Brunner/Mazel, 1980.

Whitaker, Carl A. *Family Therapy–Process and Techniques*. A seminar sponsored by Professional Seminars in Los Angeles, December, 1979.

Whitaker, Carl, ed. *Psychotherapy of Chronic Schizophrenia*. Boston: Little, Brown, 1958.

Whitaker, Carl, and Malone, Thomas. *The Roots of Psychotherapy*. New York: The Blakistone Company, 1953. Available through University Microfilms International, 300 North Zeeb Road, Ann Arbor, Michigan 48106.

Whitaker, Carl, and Napier, Augustus. *The Family Crucible*. New York: Harper & Row Publishers, 1978. (This book is a delight and brings the reader right into the family session with Whitaker and Napier.)

EPILOGUE

Infinite Possibilities of Therapeutic Response

WHAT HAVE I learned in my search for the development of impact and style in therapy? Why do I believe what I have learned makes a difference in developing effective methods of psychotherapy that are unique to each individual practitioner?

From William Ofman I learned that trust of self was on target most of the time and would get to the basic issues in patients lives much quicker than beating around the bush. Bill also provided me with a basic humanistic existential philosophical framework that left my mind open to view existentialism as encompassing all of the possibilities and choices of human existence, and therefore, all of the possibilities of therapeutic response. I learned that affirmation of how I chose to live, in many respects, gave me a sureness and inner strength that I had not previously experienced. And I learned that through the progression and development of a sharing relationship, I too, was a person that had inner power. I learned that having a flair for the dramatic and being outrageous would often help to get the therapeutic message across in indelible ways.

My experience with Wilfred Bion was at least five years too short due to his advanced age, return to London, and subsequent death. Bion embodied humility and great sense of presence. I learned that if I talked to people at my inner pace, which is much slower than I usually move or talk at when I'm unconsciously attempting to "hurry up" or "please" people, my body will continue to fill up with me–with my presence. I, and others, will continue to experience both me and themselves as fuller human beings while I am doing this. I learned that Bion continually put his wealth of knowledge to use. That is, he hardly ever wavered from being all that he could–from manifesting a full sense of presence at an unusual and extraordinary percentage of the time. He was not trapped by a need for conscious understanding. He would say thoughts without thinking, and such a process left him open to unlimited creativity.

I learned to maintain a sense of presence at a slow and centered pace. When patients experience any pressure in their bodies at all, I am able to pick up such degrees of self torture on a physical level. Bion's work in particular helped me work with patients until the sides of my head would feel absolutely no pressure in reaction to the psychological self-torture my patient was experiencing. I learned that if I paid attention to that sensation on the sides of my head and worked with as full a sense of presence as I could manifest, people could become freed from pressure and their own sense of presence would expand. The release of the pressure on the sides of the head is particularly important when treating the obsessive qualities in people. As the pressure diminishes, so do the patient's manifestations of obsessive qualities. As the body continues to fill up with the patient's sense of presence, the body feels almost as if someone were pumping air in the patient's body with a bicycle pump. Such expansion of presence is tantamount to patients learning to produce both physical and mental states of well-being in themselves through psychological means. I learned from Bion that when I give myself the freedom to say thoughts without thinking based upon my intuitive knowledge, that I may often know all I need to know, without consciously knowing what I know, that I am free of my own obsessive prison and am then best able to facilitate such freedom in my patients.

I learned that the giving up of memory and desire were helpful in not having any secret agendas that the patient would unconsciously feel a requirement to fulfill. In other words, I learned that if I have a desire, even at the unconscious level, for a patient to change in a particular way, I not only impede that patient's growth process by becoming invested in the patient's change, but may help to fix on that patient's mind an image of change that is not congruent with the patient's natural flow of being and development and help to create the resistance which I work to help the patient overcome.

Bion said that he often didn't even remember whether a patient was married, or had children. The memory of such content may in fact get in the way of the full sense of being and responsiveness that can only come by giving oneself permission to respond without conscious understanding.

Last but not least, I learned from Bion that I could be impactful and even quietly outrageous, while being tactful, courteous and humble—and that the full sense of my presence would help facilitate growth in people—if I dared to give myself that freedom to be.

From Martin Grotjahn, I learned to be more stylish in the old European tradition. I learned that while Grotjahn's training and background were psychoanalytic, it was his use of his unconscious in the "I-Thou" encounter in a stylish manner that both fascinated and reached a most difficult patient population—narcissistic people who had failed in most other therapies because they insisted on being treated as special. Grotjahn had enough of these characteristics to play with them in himself. This made the use of his narcissism charming to narcissists. In this way Grotjahn could seduce patients to be attracted to him as a special person, until he began to build an authentic relationship with each. He manifests the qualities of genuineness and generosity, which is particularly good for other narcissists to see. Grotjahn would use his own narcissism to teach his narcissistic patients to become more human. He is a thoroughly enjoyable fellow who enjoys the people with whom he works very much. I learned the value of pursuit. Grotjahn wouldn't let me hide in the corners. He had a good sense of what was going on with me and he often chased me right onto the hot seat when my own lack of courage would not have let me take the journey. I was able to make many more breakthroughs and also increase my level of trust in people.

From Bob and Mary Goulding I learned how two people could be so in touch with the games in themselves that they could pick up on and be direct as well as tricky in helping people become straight with themselves. I learned that things didn't have to be heavy to make an impact, that the work could have fun in it. As I learned to nurture myself, my nurturance of others increased. As my ability to nurture others increased, so did their level of trust that I would provide a safe environment and not let myself get hooked into patient games. I learned how to provide an environment in which patients felt free at the child level to make redecisions about how they were going to live their lives, and where patients would experience and reown their power to decide how they were going to live–despite that they may have felt no control over their lives in certain areas as far back as they could remember. From Bob and Mary, I truly experienced and learned that the power is indeed in the patient.

From Miriam Polster I learned compassion and how to help patients who are stuck find the tiniest little key that will unlock the door. I learned how to be gracious. I was provided with many keys that have been of great personal value to me. I learned how to include patients instead of imposing my fixed frame of reality upon them. I understand the give-and-take between two people. I learned about subtle sensitivity combined with a sharp eye, and learned to suggest experiment in a much gentler way. Oftentimes it would seem like a mundane sort of session, and all of a sudden the patient had unlocked the door. In this way I learned to be more generous about the change being credited to the *patient*. Most of all, I learned how it felt to experience a genuinely kind human being as my therapist, and in turn, provide such kindness when working with others.

From Erv Polster I learned much about making contact in a variety of unusual, outrageous and strange ways. I remember Erv beginning a workshop by jumping around like an ape while he made contact with me. The entire group was tickled. I learned how to appreciate my uniqueness. I learned the difference between my stereotypes of what interested me in people, and the development of genuine interest in people. I learned how to stay with my curiosity and interest until I found something that was interesting about a patient–and then learned how to facilitate that patient becoming interesting to him or herself. This was no small task for an obsessive like me. I had the pleasure to experience one of the most extraordinary therapeutic techniques I have yet to encounter, for Erv has the ability to follow the patient one step at a time, without losing himself in the process, while I as a patient felt Erv, at times, understood me so well that he had to be right in my shoes. At such times his work was very healing to the narcissistic part of me that felt misunderstood by most people.

I learned to experience the quality of being absorbed in what I was saying and doing. When thinking of gestalt therapy in comparison to current psychoanalytic thinking, Erv's technology in doing gestalt therapy may be compared to the kind of empathic technique that Heinz Kohut speaks and writes about. In getting inside the patient's skin, the narcissistic wounds begin to heal.

Jim Simkin is an unusual man. He has the courage to work in such a manner and live with the consequences. And that is precisely what he does. Jim has an extraordinary technical skill to focus on moment-to-moment process of the patient, while being particularly fine tuned to his organism in picking up sensitivities that lead to therapeutic direction, while working with a focus on the "I"-"Thou" style. Jim stands his ground, confronts, and lets you know where he stands and how he experiences you. He has great courage in his willingness to say things that are not particularly pleasant to people, but may be of great help in breaking through an impasse. He has great courage in not feeling obligated to rescue people from their stuck point. He forces the facades to come down.

Jim is a man of principle and his work teaches people how to take others into account as opposed to letting discounts of the therapist slide by. I learned to keep it simple. I learned to be courageous, and I learned to balance out my work with an emphasis on "I" as well as on "You." I learned that to care enough about the relationship may mean I will have to be tough as well as tender. And I began to get a feel for a balance within myself of the authoritarian side as opposed to the more *laissez faire* style of working.

From Walt Kempler I learned how to deliver a message with power. I learned how to use arousal, and how to differentiate that aroused concern for the welfare of my patients from using the same degree of power with more overtones of anger. Walt taught me to give up my fear of powerful authoritarian figures. I remember calling him one evening, telling him I was interested in getting to know him but that

I felt intimidated by him. I told him I felt if I had one inauthentic bone in my body he would know where it was. I said I played mandolin and I understood he played banjo and perhaps we could play some music together. I didn't quite know what his response would be, and I was anxious. Walt said, "When you hear me play the banjo you won't be quite so intimidated." Walt had the fastest interactional eye I had ever experienced. He would pick up the little unusual twist that no one had ever seen with "hopeless" couples and he would deliver his hopeful message with such potency that the couple–if they genuinely wanted to make things work, now had the tools. I learned that despite helping people to make things work, I must also appreciate that perhaps the work might take a direction of helping the people separate, if they genuinely did not want each other. I learned how to find the stuck point where people feel they can't break clean with each other. I learned how to teach people to become more generous with each other, thereby enhancing an upward spiraling relationship instead of being stuck in hopelessness. And more important, I turned the corner in helping to make my own marriage work out–as did my wife. I learned what it means to make a commitment to make a relationship work out, and what is meant by *responsible action* on the part of both partners.

From Bob Martin I learned to break through rigid concepts of myself and enhance my capacity to be outrageous and joyful. I learned to increase my sensitivity by paying attention on a physiological as well as a thinking level. I learned how to make my responses include my entire organism, as opposed to just parts of it. I learned some keys to the enhancement of my creativity and how to continue to expand by talking about whatever goes through me, by dancing in session, or singing, or whatever combination of unusual ways of making contact happen to go through me. I learned how to go with the aliveness at a continuing pitch of intensity until my level of vitality and that of the patient simultaneously felt as if we were just given a shot of B-12 vitamins.

From Stanley Keleman I learned how to take the step-by-step process, such as that used in gestalt therapy by Erv, Miriam, and Jim, and to integrate it into working with the bodily processes in coordination with the psychological processes. For example, step by step, I learned how I made my shoulder tight, and how to unlearn the process. I learned to get an inner sense of pacing by paying attention to my body. I learned how to distinguish between images of my body experience and the actual experience. I saw Stanley stand his ground with a rageful patient who looked like he was going to explode and rip Stanley's head off if he said or did the wrong thing. Stanley told him he had nothing invested in the man changing. There was a gentle toughness about Stanley, in the way he held his ground without being intimidated that left me curious. When I asked him about it he said that after he graduated high school his parents told him how proud they were of him. He experienced it as a very painful separation, because while he appreciated their love and concern for him, he knew he did not need them to be proud of him to get on in the world. He said from that moment on he was a free man. Since working with Stanley I have had a much greater sense of my body plus my depth or shallowness of breathing, and the corresponding feeling of well-being.

From George Bach I learned how to use aggressive identification and coaching with my patients. I learned how to become an actor instead of a reactor, and how to become more aggressive and have fun doing it. I kept a journal so I would not use therapy as a life experience in place of living. I got a fuller appreciation of therapy being a reinforcement for living. I got to appreciate the charming rogue in myself as this was a part of George's personality. I learned how to solve problems and help people solve problems, in a practical more than a gestalt-process sense. I had more opportunity to experiment with being outrageous in a fun way. George would say things to people that very few therapists could get away with and still have the patient smiling while they got a pretty impactful insight.

Albert Ellis taught me how to handle lack of self-acceptance very quickly. He taught me that it is all right to be opinionated, and that one can use the flagrant expression of those opinions to break through the images of how therapists ought to be in the world. Most important in my life, I learned to live without an angry philosophy of life. I learned to challenge my beliefs that people must be fair, that things must be better or more desirable. There is no reason why things must be better. It would be more desirable, but there is no reason the world must be fair and lead to good results. Both George Bach and Al taught me how to be entertaining when I work before large groups. When using Al's method of disputing the irrational belief and giving new information that leads to self-acceptance, I find that when I tune in on a sensory perception level, all the pressure on the sides of my head disappears as that self-torture process disappears in that patient. Further, Al taught me to challenge two beliefs–"I must succeed" and "It's too hard"–that freed me for the more experiential therapies. I realize that self-worth is not necessarily based on *doing*, am more productive, without having to be to feel acceptable.

What can one say about Milton Erickson? I learned that a trust in my unconscious mind has been freeing to me, and has basically helped me turn many difficult corners in my life. I learned the value of utilizing an authoritarian approach in doing hypnosis, and the value of hypnosis in helping people to let go of control and to paradoxically begin to take charge of their lives. Each day new things keep coming to my unconscious and the unlimited possibilities of my life continue to come forth. I am able to live my life more freely as a result of a trust in my unconscious because before I was too anxiety-bound to move. What appears to be the safest road does not always turn out that way. I learned how to play tricks on patients that would help them untangle themselves. I learned how to tell stories that come through my unconscious in response to patients hour after hour. I learned that Milton's ability to keep people off balance, to surprise them with the unexpected, was a large part of how he bypasses resistance. I learned that with all his mastery, he was still very human in touching people. He was so intuitively in tune with his unconscious, that there was a continual flow of unexpected responsiveness coming from him.

I learned how to change people's belief systems from negative to positive, and even reach many of those patients formerly believed to be hopeless. Erickson brought out the trickster and the storyteller in me. Also, I never forgot the sound and pace of his voice, and use it to hypnotize myself and others quite readily.

Bill Kroger is a gracious man and a gentleman. He invited me to sit in on several of his sessions to get a feel for the way he uses imagery in hypnosis. I learned how to hypnotize people who are so controlled, and so unwilling to let go, that they may not be ready or able to benefit from the unconscious method of doing hypnosis that I learned from Dr. Erickson. I remember the first time I called Bill and told him I was having trouble working with patients who wanted me to prove it to them that they were hypnotized. He said, "Tell them to prove there is a God." I learned that patients can still remain in control and use hypnosis as a tool.

From Jack Rosberg I learned a way to enter the patient's delusional system and to cut away character disorders. I was particularly taken with Jack's spontaneity and range of responsiveness. His words and tone would go anywhere from loving to violent. He was quite impactful in getting the job done in short periods of time with schizophrenic patients and schizophrenic patients who had character disorders. I feel Jack's methods are particularly potent when working with people who refuse to take others into account. Jack described a situation where a patient was blasting the radio after he had been requested several times to turn it down because it was very disturbing to a number of inpatients. Jack in a loud voice said, "If you don't turn that radio down I'm going to step on your gonads." The patient turned the radio down. While I was discussing the writing of the chapter with Jack, a patient began to scream, J A A A A CC CC KKK in a loud, whiny voice. Jack's immediate response was to the patient's tone. He replied in exactly the same tone of voice, Y Y E E E S S S S. Both responses had a sing-song quality to them. The patient got the message that she would do better to approach people in a more palatable manner. I felt there was much that could become part of a therapist's style when working with patients other than schizophrenics, particularly character disorders.

In a sense Carl Whitaker was a return back to square one for me in that he dealt with the integrity of the therapist, and how the implementation of that integrity can manifest itself in a style of doing therapy. He focuses on the "semantics of responsible involvement" in a truly existential way. Most important for Whitaker was his enjoyment in what he was doing while being extremely effective with patients. If therapists can find this part of themselves they may feel about therapy the way Mickey Mantle did about baseball when he said, "And they pay me for this too!"

In summarizing, I have intended to present a book that is open-ended. It is existential in that it is open to all the possibilities and choices of therapeutic response. It is existential, in that the quality of being exemplified in the person of the therapist has been paramount throughout all the different methodologies and modes of psychotherapy; that is, each of the therapists was very full in terms of being themselves and in forming a style of therapy based upon the uniqueness of their personalities. They gave it their all!

The unconscious mind needs to become free. When it moves along in this direction a variety of unlimited therapeutic possibilities may unfold. The key is in the gradual and gentle letting go of the conscious control, which people often falsely deem as being necessary to their survival.

Now for the second question I asked in beginning the epilog–Why do I believe what I have learned makes a difference in developing effective methods of psychotherapy that are unique to each individual practitioner?

I am speaking of potency in a therapist. I have presented you with a wide variety of therapists, the kind of responses they make, and how those responses are an extension of their unique personalities. While there is clearly a method of therapy that accompanies each of the schools of thought of therapy, there are also potent methods that embellish the technology of psychotherapy as it is known, that come from the artistry of the therapist. That artistry comes from the personal development of the therapist in being as uniquely him or herself as is possible. The potency is in the being of the therapist, and to the extent the therapist is able to flow with him or herself, the therapist is more likely to create the kind of contact, the kind of connection, the kind of experience that will help patients turn the corner in their lives.

Therapeutic styles of practice develop from the individuality of the therapist. While what I have presented you may be initially used as models to emulate, the task then becomes one of superseding the model and developing a personal style.

In addition to knowing the art and craft of psychotherapy, one must know oneself and have the courage to be all that one can be when responding to patients, whether it be through therapy that is indirect, or direct, or gestalt or transactional analysis. Each of the people with whom I have worked have given it their all, with caring, dedication, and commitment. With this combination of ingredients the therapist can provide an environment in which healing, existential moments between patient and therapist will occur.

These existential moments must first come from within the therapist. However each therapist's personality manifests itself, it is important that the therapist risk sharing those thoughts, ideas, feelings, and attitudes with patients. Even if the therapist's style is not one of sharing directly, the existential moments can occur from within the therapist and be communicated to the patient through indirect methods and through therapeutic action. Sensitive therapists will listen to their inner voices to offer patients the response that will be most effective. The only issue at that point is the therapist's willingness to risk!